EYE MOVEMENTS AND HUMAN INFORMATION PROCESSING

Proceedings of the XXIII International Congress of Psychology of the International Union of Psychological Science (IUPsyS) Acapulco, Mexico, September 2-7, 1984

Selected/Revised Papers

Volume 9
(For further volumes see back of the cover)

Published for the
International Union of Psychological Science (IUPsyS)

Eye Movements and Human Information Processing

Edited by

Rudolf GRONER

Psychology Department
University of Bern
Switzerland

George McCONKIE

Center for the Study of Reading
University of Illinois, Urbana-Champaign
U.S.A.

Christine MENZ

Psychology Department
University of Bern
Switzerland

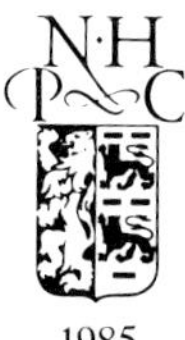

1985

NORTH-HOLLAND
AMSTERDAM · NEW YORK · OXFORD

ISBN: 0 444 87789 4
ISBN set: 0 444 87790 8

Publishers:
ELSEVIER SCIENCE PUBLISHERS B.V.
P.O. Box 1991
1000 BZ Amsterdam
The Netherlands

Sole distributors for the U.S.A. and Canada:
ELSEVIER SCIENCE PUBLISHING COMPANY, INC.
52 Vanderbilt Avenue
New York, N.Y. 10017
U.S.A.

Library of Congress Cataloging-in-Publication Data
Main entry under title:

Eye movements and human information processing.

(Proceedings of the XXIII International Congress of Psychology of the International Union of Psychological Science (IUPsyS) Acapulco, Mexico, September 2-7, 1984 ; v. 9)
"Published for the International Union of Psycological Science (IUPsyS)."
Includes index.
1. Human information processing--Addresses, essays, lectures. 2. Eye--Movements--Psychological aspects--Addresses, essays, lectures. I. Groner, Rudolf. II. McConkie, George W. III. Menz, Christine. IV. International Union of Psychological Science. V. Title. VI. Series: International Congress of Psychology (23rd : 1984 : Acapulco, Mexico). Proceedings of the XXIII International Congress of Psychology of September 2-7, 1984 ; v. 9.
BF455.E98 1985 150 s [153.7] 85-13079
ISBN 0-444-87789-4 (U.S.)

PRINTED IN THE NETHERLANDS

PREFACE

This volume represents the selected and edited Proceedings of a symposium 'Eye Movements and Psychological Processes' held at the 23rd International Congress of Psychology in Acapulco, Mexico, September 2-7, 1984. It was a continuation of an earlier symposium held at the 22nd International Congress of Psychology in Leipzig, German Democratic Republic, 1980, and subsequently published jointly by North-Holland Publishing Company and Deutscher Verlag der Wissenschaften under the title "Cognition and Eye Movements" (edited by Rudolf Groner and Paul Fraisse).

The organisation of the symposium and the production of this book could not have succeeded without the help of several persons to whom we would like to express our gratitude. First it was the president of the International Union of Psychological Science, Professor Friedhart Klix, and his successor in the presidency, Professor Wayne H. Holtzman, who both accepted the idea of such a symposium and gave it their strong personal encouragement. We also would like to thank the Swiss Academy for Humanities for their indirect support by sending the first editor of this book as a delegate to the International Congress.

It is impossible to thank all persons who provided some help during the symposium, such as e.g. the chairman of the symposium at the next door for reducing the amplifiers, or the person who managed to put down the airconditioning before all speakers were hoarse up to the point of inaudibility. However, we would like to thank Dr. Geoffrey Underwood who, in addition to the editors of this volume, kindly agreed to be chairperson of one session.

Setting up a symposium and editing a volume of Proceedings are two different matters, and both of them consume a lot of time and energy. We would like to thank both, the International Union of Psychological Science and the Swiss Society for Psychology and its Applications, for giving us strong moral and also some financial support for the second part of the enterprise. We gratefully acknowledge the help of Mario Truffer who assisted in various editorial matters and put together the author and subject indices. We would like to thank Professor Alex Wearing for providing helpful linguistic and substantial advice. We would also like to thank Charlotte Apostolou for her secretarial help. Titia Kraaij and Dr. Kees Michielsen of Elsevier Science Publishers (North-Holland) supported our work from the part of the publishing company.

Finally we would like to thank all those authors who were most cooperative in following the editorial suggestions and sometimes producing several forms of a manuscript which had to be in a ready-to-print form. The substantial number of contributions and their excellent quality made it possible to produce a separate volume around one common methodological approach, viz. eye movement research, demonstrating the current activity in this field as well as the potentials of this method for Psychology.

CONTENTS

I.

STUDIES OF OCULOMOTOR CONTROL AND DEVELOPMENT

Eye Movements and Human Information Processing
R. Groner, G.W. McConkie and C. Menz (eds.)

STUDIES OF OCULOMOTOR CONTROL AND DEVELOPMENT

Introduction

Investigations involving eye movement registration can roughly be grouped into two categories, each with quite distinct research aims. The object of studies in the first category is to explain the mechanisms of the oculomotor system, how different subsystems interact and how performance is achieved by means of neuronal pathways. In the second category oculomotor measures are used as an indicator of something else, i.e. perceptual and/or cognitive processes. The majority of articles in this book falls into this latter group, only a few studies in the first section dealing with the first issue.

The paper which approaches the interaction of different subsystems most directly is the first in the book, by Schmid, Buizza and Zambarbieri. It is necessary for the visual system to maintain stabilization of gaze despite of head rotations and eye movements. The authors report a variety of findings and propose a superordinate model which combines the information of optokinetic and vestibular afferences in the vestibular nuclei, thus transforming the information acquired in retinotopic coordinates into environment-related coordinates.

The next paper, by Logothetis, Fries and Pöppel, is concerned with the experimental separation of the two main systems, i.e. the saccadic and the smooth pursuit system. Following Rashbass, they use the negative step-ramp paradigm, in which a target is rapidly displaced from the foveal zone followed immediately by a continuous movement. The phenomenon of a small presaccadic pursuit movement (PPM) prior to the correcting saccade has been taken as evidence that the saccadic and pursuit system are independent, the latter having a shorter latency but being overridden by the saccadic response. Logothetis et al. show that the PPMs only occur independently of the step amplitude in about one third of all trials. They conclude that in the horizontal plane the retinal region in which PPMs are elicited extends up to 7 degrees, that is close to the macular region in the human eye. However, due to their specific experimental conditions (all trials involving negative step-ramp movements) they still leave open the possibility of PPMs as dependent on the expectation of the subject.

This conception of PPMs as the expression of an internal predictor rather than a stimulus response presents an interesting parallel to the next paper in this section by L.E. Ross & S.M. Ross, although their paper is exclusively focussed on the saccadic system. It is concerned with the latency of saccades to peripheral targets when the occurence of the target is either preceded or followed by other stimulus events. Warning signals preceding a peripheral target reduce the latency of the saccade to that target, the offset of the warning stimulus resulting in a shorter latency than the onset. However, if the "warning" (interfering) stimulus onset occurs 100 msec after the target the saccadic response to the target becomes slower while the offset of the same stimulus has no effect. Other important variables which affect saccade latency are the type of directional information, the modality (visual or acoustic) of the warning stimulus and its retinal position (foveal or peripheral).

Although the fourth paper by H. Intraub is not directly concerned with eye movements, the psychological phenomena investigated and the models proposed are closely connected to the rest of the book: it deals with the information processed in a single fixation and with the early stages of picture processing. The experimental paradigm involves the use of tachistoscopic exposure and rapid sequential presentation of a series of pictures. By means of careful experimentation Intraub makes plausible the assertion that the bottleneck of pictorial processing is the short-term conceptual store. She argues that during normal visual activity one rapidly assesses the contents of each "scene" and adjusts the extent of encoding. These overlapping processes of identification and storage may also play a role in the integration of successive fixations.

The developmental perspective of oculomotor control is introduced by L. Hainline who summarizes several studies from her laboratory showing that despite an immature visual system most oculomotor systems are already highly functional in early infancy. Here it is necessary to apply somewhat different research tactics from those needed with adults by making the experimental setting as interesting as possible in order to avoid confounding level of arousal and motivational factors with oculomotor functioning. An additional requirement, which should also be applied to adult studies, is to replicate the findings over a set of different stimuli and experimental conditions to establish the generality of an observed behavior. Under these conditions it is surprising how mature many infant behaviors are when tested under optimal conditions, including smooth pursuit, optokinetic nystagmus and saccades.

The issue of optokinetic nystagmus (OKN) in a developmental and comparative perspective is taken up by T.L. Lewis, D. Maurer and H.P. Brent. They start from neurophysiological observations, where it has been shown that cats which were binocularly deprived shortly after birth show normal OKN for patterns moving from the temporal to the nasal visual field, but little OKN for patterns moving in the opposite direction. The hypothesis of an asymmetrical OKN which can be related to neural pathways has been investigated by Lewis et al. with children who had been visually deprived during early infancy because of dense bilateral cataracts. In two experiments, this hypothesis could be confirmed with the visually deprived children while the control group of normals showed an almost symmetrical OKN. (A somewhat analogous developmental/comparative study on scanning behavior with deaf children by L. Hall, which further elaborates such a research strategy, has been placed latter in the book in section 3 dealing with scanning.)

Together with the last part of the book (which is devoted to applied issues), this first section contains a wide variety of phenomena all of which reflect different aspects of oculomotor behavior that have one goal in common: to adapt the visual system to changing types of stimulation so that processing secures the invariance of objects in the outside world. It is surprising how much of the flexibility of the system is already present (either built in or achieved) at an early stage of development.

Eye Movements and Human Information Processing
R. Groner, G.W. McConkie and C. Menz (eds.)

THE ROLE OF THE VESTIBULAR NUCLEI IN VISUAL STABILIZATION: EXPERIMENTAL RESULTS AND MODELLING (°)

R. Schmid, A. Buizza and D. Zambarbieri
Dipartimento di Informatica e Sistemistica
Università di Pavia, Italy

The stability of visual localization of stationary objects in the presence of head and eye movements requires an internal reconstruction of current gaze direction, which, in turn, requires an estimate of head absolute velocity. In natural conditions of visual-vestibular interaction a neural signal representing absolute head velocity is made available in the vestibular nuclei (VN) in the full range of frequencies through combination of visual (optokinetic) and vestibular afferences. There is experimental evidence that the output of VN is used not only in a reflex arc aimed to make the eyes a stable platform for vision during passive head rotations, but also to produce self motion sensation and to stabilize visual perception.

(°) Work supported by CNR (Rome, Italy), Nucleo di Studio per le Applicazioni Biomediche dei Calcolatori

INTRODUCTION

In order to obtain a stabilization of gaze during passive rotations of the head and an absolute perception of the visual surround during voluntary rotations of the gaze, a central estimate of head angular velocity should be made available within the central nervous system (CNS). Gaze stabilization can be reached by commanding an eye movement that compensates head movement. Absolute visual perception requires the information acquired in retinotopic coordinates to be transformed into absolutes coordinates. Such a transformation can be obtained through a processing of retinal information in which both head and eye velocities are considered.

GAZE STABILIZATION

The vestibular nuclei (VN), which receive vestibular and visual afferences, are the place within CNS where an estimate of head angular velocity is made possible over the full range of frequencies. What are the respective contributions of the vestibular and the visual inputs to VN in such a reconstruction of head angular velocity?

Single unit recording from primary vestibular neurons (Fernandez and Goldberg, 1971; Goldberg and Fernandez, 1971a,b) and theoretical considerations on the dynamics of the semicircular canals (Van Egmond et al., 1949; Steer, 1972) have proved that the peripheral vestibular system behaves like a high-pass filter with a time constant which represents the mechanical properties of the cupula-endolymph system (about 3 sec in the cat, 6 sec in the monkey and, presumably, about 6 sec also in man). Then, information on head angular velocity during rotations at constant velocity or during sinusoidal oscillations at frequencies below 0.02 Hz cannot reach VN through their vestibular afferences. An indirect proof of this fact is given by the vestibulo-ocular responses (the only objective output of the vestibular system that can be measured in man) evoked by head oscillations in darkness at different frequencies.

The nystagmic eye movement recorded in man during oscillations at 0.07 Hz in the dark is shown in the upper part of Fig. 1. If the fast components of nystagmus are removed and the slow components are fitted together as shown in the lower part of the same figure, the diagram of the slow cumulative eye position (SCEP) is obtained (Meiry, 1965). This diagram represents the compensatory eye movement induced by the vestibular stimulation. The gain and the phase shift between SCEP and head position define the performance of the vestibulo-ocular reflex (VOR) at the examined frequency. Alternatively, the same parameters can be computed from nystagmus slow phase velocity and head velocity.

The experimental results reported in Fig. 2 (Benson, 1970; Baloh et al., 1981) by filled squares and circles give the gain and the phase shift between eye and head velocity versus frequency. Head oscillations at frequencies below 0.02 Hz are not compensated. At higher frequencies eye velocity is proportional to head velocity and almost phase opposite, although the

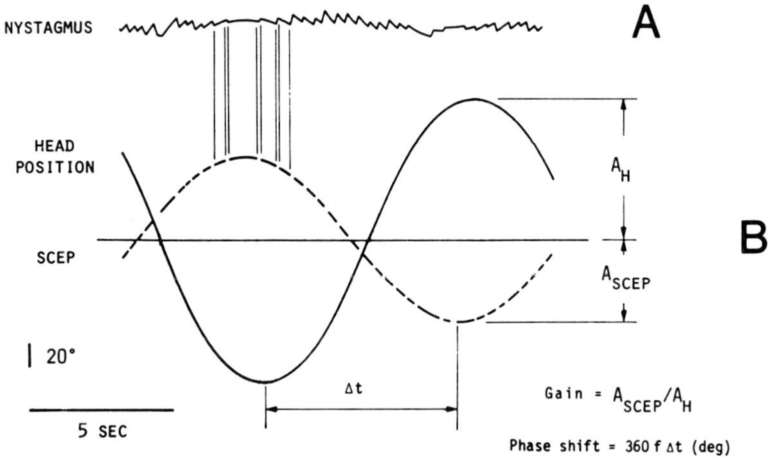

Figure 1

A: nystagmic eye movement evoked by a sinusoidal head rotation in the dark about the vertical axis. B: slow cumulative eye position (SCEP) obtained from the nystagmic response A by removing the fast components and fitting together the slow components. The gain and the phase shift between SCEP and head position, computed as indicated in the figure, define the performance of the vestibulo-ocular reflex at the examined frequency.

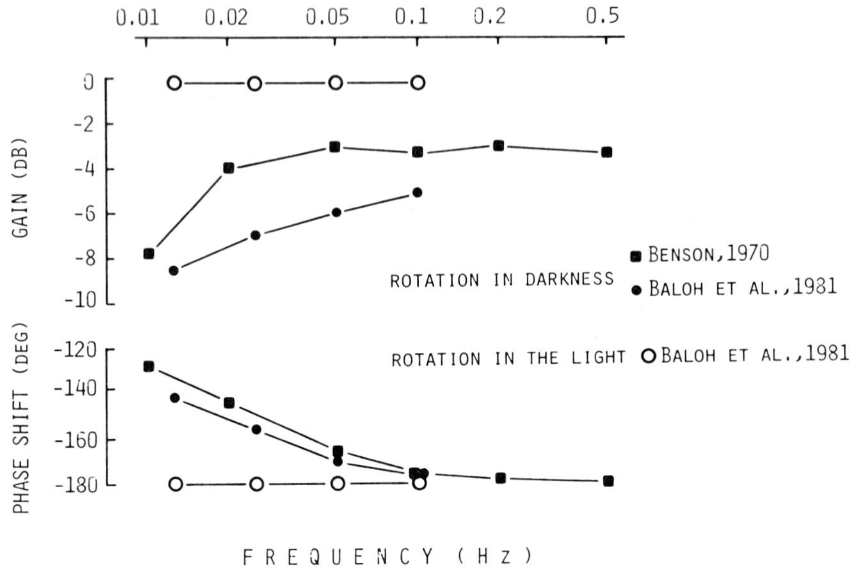

Figure 2

Gain and phase shift of the compensatory eye movement during sinusoidal head rotations at different frequencies in the dark (filled dots and squares) and in the light (open circles).

gain is less than unity indicating that, also in this range of frequencies, VOR compensation is not complete. There is so direct and indirect evidence that information on head angular velocity at low frequencies cannot reach VN through their vestibular afferences.

The role of the visual afferences to VN has been examined by recording VN neuron activity during the presentation of a rotating visual surround to a hearth stationary animal (Allum et al., 1976; Keller and Precht, 1979; Waespe and Henn, 1979a). It was found that the same neurons which are activated by head rotation in one direction are also activated by rotation of the visual surround in the opposite direction. Moreover, the dynamics of the visual pathway to VN in open loop conditions (paralyzed eyes) was found to be that of a low-pass filter with a time constant close to that of the semicircular canals (Raphan et al., 1977; Robinson, 1977). The visual pathway to VN is therefore perfectly designed to work in the range of frequencies in which the vestibular information about head velocity is lacking.

Fig. 3 shows, on the left side, single unit activity recorded in monkey's VN during rotation in darkness (heavy lines), during rotation of the visual surround in front of the stationary animal (dashed lines), and during rotation of the animal within a stationary visual surround (thin lines). The stimuli consisted of a constant acceleration period followed by a period of constant velocity. It can be noted that, during constant velocity rotation in darkness, VN activity returns to the resting level. On the contra-

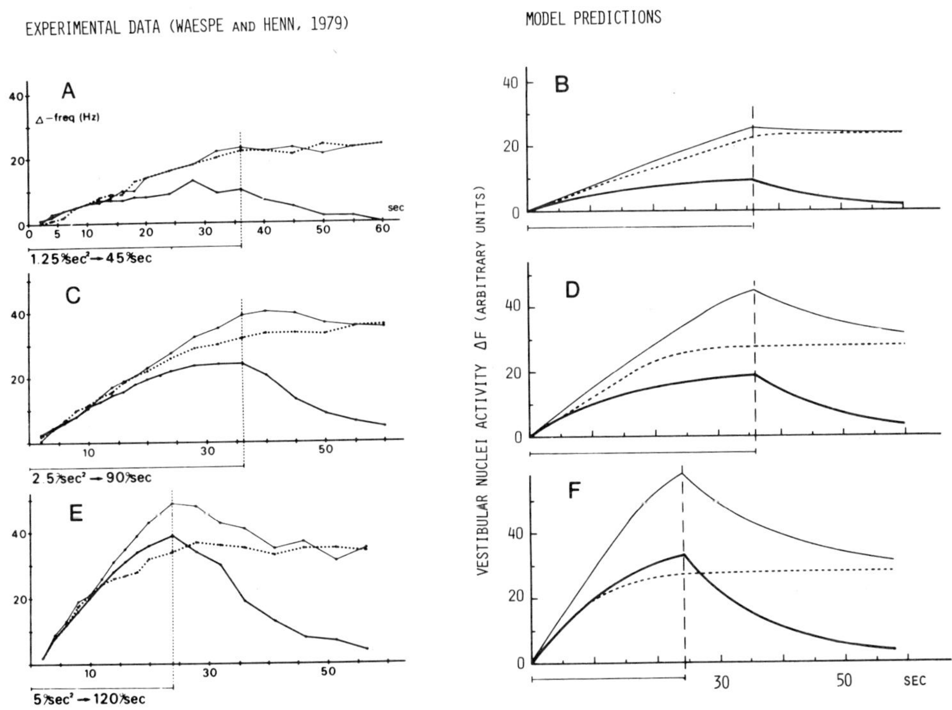

Figure 3

A-F: single unit activity in monkey's vestibular nuclei during vestibular (heavy lines), optokinetic (dashed lines) and combined (rotation within a stationary visual surround, thin lines) stimulations. Stimuli consisted of a constant acceleration period (36 s in A-D and 24 s in E-F) followed by a period of constant velocity rotation. Left side: experimental data from Waespe and Henn (1979b); right side: model prediction.

ry, during rotation in the light, VN activity reproduces the profile of head velocity also during constant velocity rotation (°). The right side of Fig. 3 shows the predictions obtained by a mathematical model of visual-vestibular interaction developed by our group (Buizza and Schmid, 1982).

In normal conditions of visual-vestibular interaction a copy of head angular velocity is so made available at the VN level in the full range of frequencies through addition of the vestibular and the visual inputs to these nuclei. An indirect proof is given again by the vestibulo-ocular responses evoked by head rotation in a stationary visual surround. As shown in Fig. 2 by open circles, the velocity of the compensatory eye movement evoked in this condition is equal in amplitude (unitary gain) and opposite in phase with respect to head velocity also at frequencies below 0.02 Hz.

SELF MOTION PERCEPTION AND VISUAL STABILIZATION

A next question is whether the output of VN is also used by CNS to produce self motion sensation. As a matter of fact, the visual input to VN gives information about the relative movement between subject and visual environment without distinction on which one is actually moving. On the other hand, in every day life, a retinal slip of the image of the entire visual surround is produced, with very few exceptions, by a motion of the subject with respect to a stationary environment. The stationarity of the external world is likely to be an "a priori" assumption, based on experience, in the interpretation of retinal information by CNS. Then, independently of its vestibular or visual origin, the output of VN would always be interpreted by CNS as a measure of subject's head rotation. If this is the case and if VN output is actually the signal used to produce self motion sensation, a self motion illusion should be expected when the environment is made to rotate with respect to a stationary subject. A sensation of circular vection is currently produced in the laboratory by rotating a striped cylinder

(°) For stimulus velocities greater than 90°/sec, the activity reached at the end of the acceleration period cannot be maintained at the same level as the vestibular contribution is vanishing. This is due to a saturation of the visual pathway to VN (Keller and Precht, 1979; Waespe and Henn, 1979b)

around a stationary subject (Mach; 1875; Helmholtz, 1896; Fisher and Kornmüller, 1930; Dichgans and Brandt, 1978).

In order to discuss the relationship between the output of VN and motion sensation in a more quantitative way we can make reference to the results reported in Fig. 4. Four experimental conditions are considered: A) rotation in darkness; B) rotation in the light (natural condition of visual-vestibular interaction); C) optokinetic stimulation, and D) rotation in a stabilized visual surround. SRV indicates the continuous tracking of perceived self rotation velocity (experimental results from Dichgans and Brandt, (1978)). VNO is the output of VN predicted by our model in the examined

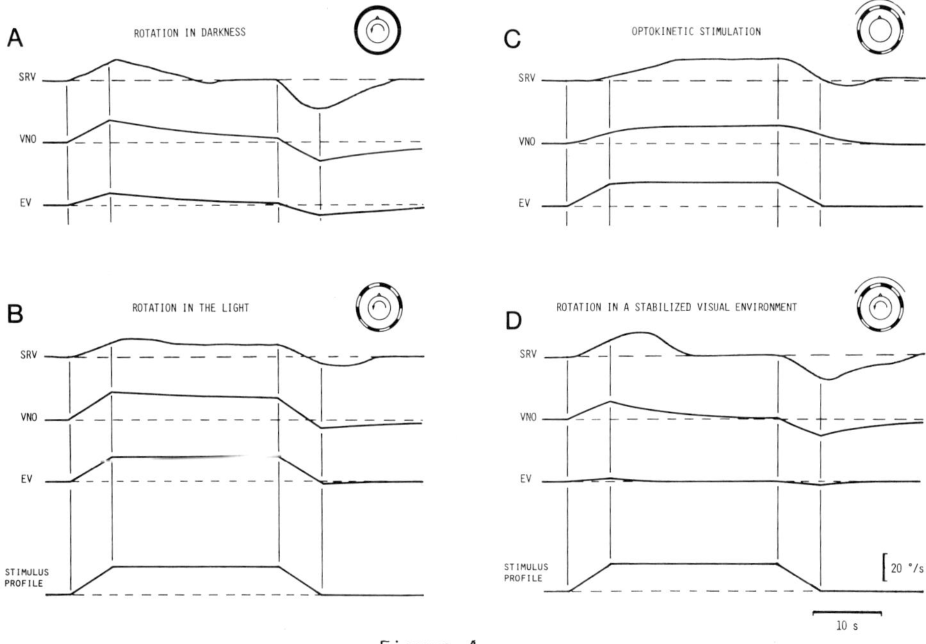

Figure 4

Perceived self rotation velocity (SRV) under different combinations of vestibular and optokinetic rotatory stimulations is compared with the predicted output (VNO) of the vestibular nuclei and the predicted slow phase velocity (EV) of nystagmus. A: rotation in darkness; B: rotation in an earth stationary visual surround; C: pure optokinetic stimulation; D: rotation in a visual surround stationary with respect to the subject. The trapezoid profile of stimulus velocity is shown in the lower part of the figure.

experimental situations, and EV is the predicted eye velocity. The trapezoid profile of stimulus velocity is shown in the lower part of the figure.

During rotation in darkness the time course of self motion velocity roughly follows the mechanical characteristic of the cupula-endolymph system resulting in a lack of constant velocity discrimination and consequent misinterpretation of deceleration. When the subject is rotated in the light, motion sensation is quite correct also during constant velocity rotation and during deceleration. When a pure optokinetic stimulation is applied, an apparent self rotation opposite to that of the visual surround is elicited with a clear latency. When the subject and the visual surround are rotated in the same direction with the same velocity, motion perception is again erroneous since, as in darkness, it relies exclusively on the vestibular input.

If perceived self motion velocity (SRV) is compared to the output of VN (VNO) and to eye velocity (EV) predicted in the same experimental situation, it results that SRV is much more related to VNO than to EV. Nevertheless some differences between the time course of self motion sensation and that of VN activity can be noted. The lack of a complete matching suggests that some further processing of VN output takes place before motion sensation is produced. The central processing is likely to be rather complex in the case of sensory conflict situations.

As suggested by Reason's "neural mismatch model" (1978) shown in Fig. 5, a conflict situation can be recognized by CNS through a comparison of current sensory afferences with those retrieved from a "Neural Store" which contains pairs of efferent-reafferent traces consolidated by the experience. In natural conditions of visual-vestibular interaction, any perceived acceleration or deceleration is accompanied by a vestibular afference. If a vestibular afference is actually lacking, as in the acceleration and deceleration phases of a pure optokinetic stimulation (condition C), a mismatch signal is likely to be generated and a conflict situation signalled. Then, the sensory afference represented by VN output ought to be interpreted in a different way than in natural conditions. The interpretation

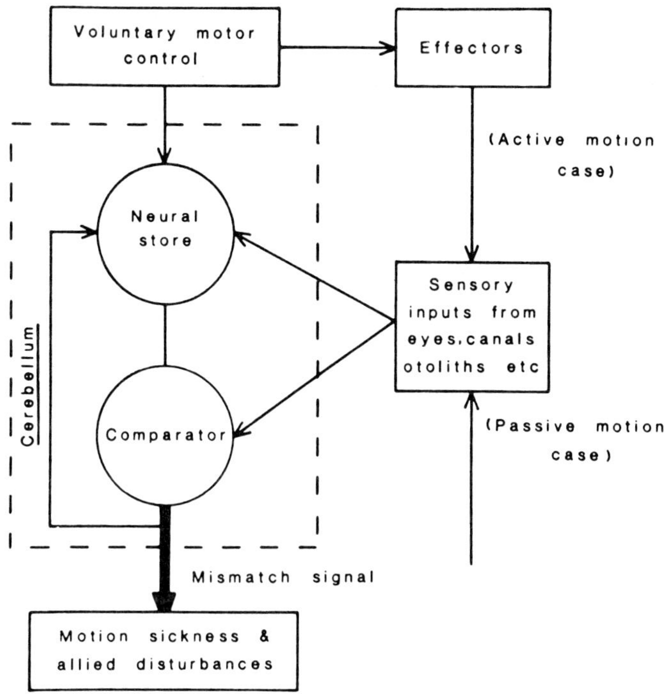

Figure 5

Reason's (1978) "Neural Mismatch Model"

might be based on which one between the conflicting sources of sensory information (visual or vestibular) has to be considered as the more believable one. Motion sensation (true or illusory) preceding the conflict could be a relevant factor for tacking a decision.

At the beginning of the acceleration phase of the pure optokinetic stimulation, when a conflicting situation is first created, the subject's sensation previous to the conflict was that of stationarity. Thus, the output of VN is likely to be correctly interpreted as to represent a motion of the visual surround and no self motion sensation takes place. As acceleration goes on, the reliability of this assumption decreases, since the experience proves that the visual surround never rotates indefinitely in the same direction. A circular vection grows up and reaches a steady state during constant velocity stimulation, when CNS "knows" that no vestibular input should be expected (no conflict situation). In this condition, VN output is interpreted as a measure of head velocity as in natural conditions.

Finally, when the optokinetic stimulation starts decelerating, a new conflict is created. Since subject's sensation previous to this new conflict was that of a constant velocity rotation, the more natural interpretation of the sensory afference represented by VN output is now that of a self deceleration.

A tight coupling between self rotation illusion and perceived stationarity of visual scenes actually moving around a stationary subject was also reported in the literature (Dichgans and Brandt, 1978). There is so evidence that VN are the nuclei deputated to provide a central estimate of head absolute velocity to be used by CNS to produce gaze stabilization during passive head movements, self motion sensation and visual perception stability.

REFERENCES

1 - ALLUM J.H.J., GRAF W., DICHGANS J. and SCHMIDT C.L. (1976): Visual-vestibular interactions in the vestibular nuclei of the goldfish, Exp. Brain Res. 26, 463-485.

2 - BALOH R.W., YEE R.D., KIMM J. and HONRUBIA V. (1981): Vestibular-ocular reflex in patients with lesions involving the vestibulo cerebellum, Exp. Neurol. 72, 141-152.

3 - BENSON A.J. (1970): Interaction between semicircular canals and gravireceptors, in "Recent Advances in Aerospace Medicine", D. E. Busby Ed., Dordrecht, Reidel, pp. 249-261.

4 - BUIZZA A. and SCHMID R. (1982): Visual-vestibular interaction in the control of eye movement: mathematical modelling and computer simulation, Biol. Cybern. 43, 209-223.

5 - DICHGANS J. and BRANDT T. (1978): Visual-vestibular interaction. Effects on self-motion perception and postural control, in "Handbook of Sensory Physiology", R. Held, H. Leibowitz and H. L. Tauber Eds.,

Vol. VIII, Springer, New York, pp. 755-804.

6 - FERNANDEZ C. and GOLDBERG J.M. (1971): Physiology of peripheral neurons innervating semi-circular canals of squirrel monkey. II. Response to sinusoidal stimulation and dynamics of peripheral vestibular system, J. Neurophysiol. 34, 661-675.

7 - FISHER M.H. and KORNMUELLER A.E.(1930): Optokinetisch ausgelöste Bewegungswahrnehmung und optokinetischer Nystagmus, J. Psychol. Neurol. (Lpz.) 41, 273-308.

8 - GOLDBERG J.M. and FERNANDEZ C. (1971a): Physiology of peripheral neurons innervating semi-circular canals of the squirrel monkey. I. Resting discharge and response to constant angular acceleration, J. Neurophysiol. 34, 635-660.

8 - GOLDBERG J.M. and FERNANDEZ C. (1971b): Physiology of peripheral neurons innervating semi-circular canals of the squirrel monkey. III. Variations among units and their discharge properties, J. Neurophysiol. 34, 676-684.

10 - HELMHOLTZ H. Von (1896): Handbuch der physiologischen Optik, Hamburg-Leipzig.

11 - KELLER E.L. and PRECHT W. (1979): Visual-vestibular responses in vestibular neurons in intact and cerebellectomized alert cat, Neurosci. 4, 1599-1613.

12 - MACH E. (1875): Grundlinien der Lehre von den Bewegungsempfindungen, Leipzig: Engelmann.

13 - MEIRY J.L. (1965): The vestibular system and human dynamic space orientation, Sc. D. Thesis, M. I. T., Cambridge, Mass.

14 - RAPHAN T., COHEN B. and MATSUO A. (1977): A velocity storage mechanism responsible for optokinetic nystagmus (OKN), optokinetic after-nystagmus (OKAN) and vestibular nystagmus, in "Control of Gaze by Brain Stem Neurons", R. Baker and A. Berthoz Eds., Elsevier/North Holland, Amsterdam, pp. 37-47.

15 - REASON J.T. (1978): Motion sickness adaptation: a neural mismatch model, J. Royal Soc. Med. 71, 819-829.

16 - ROBINSON D.A. (1977): Vestibular and optokinetic symbiosis: an example of explaining by modelling, in "Control of Gaze by Brain Stem Neurons", R. Baker and A. Berthoz Eds., Elsevier/North Holland, Amsterdam, pp. 19-28.

17 - STEER R.W. (1972): The influence of angular and linear acceleration and thermal stimulation on the human semicircular canal, Sc. D. Thesis, M. I. T., Cambridge, Mass.

18 - VAN EGMOND A.A.T., GREEN T.T. and JONKEES L.B.W. (1949): The mechanics of the semicircular canal, J. Physiol. (London) 110, 1-17.

19 - WAESPE W. and HENN V. (1979a): The velocity response of vestibular nucleus neurons during vestibular, visual and combined angular acceleration, Exp. Brain Res. 37, 337-347.

20 - WAESPE W. and HENN V. (1979b): Motion information in the vestibular nuclei of the alert monkey: visual and vestibular input vs optomotor output, in "Reflex Control of Posture and Movement", R. Granit and O. Pompeiano Eds., Elsevier/North Holland Biomedical Press, pp. 683-693.

Eye Movements and Human Information Processing
R. Groner, G.W. McConkie and C. Menz (eds.)

Perceptual Control of Predictive Smooth Pursuit Eye Movements[1]

H. A. Sedgwick
Institute for Vision Research
S.U.N.Y. College of Optometry
New York, New York 10010

Jeffrey D. Holtzman
Department of Neurology, Division of Cognitive Neuroscience
Cornell University Medical College
New York, New York 10021

Theresa Rugiero Corliss
S.U.N.Y. College of Optometry
New York, New York 10010

Purely predictive smooth pursuit was examined by having observers saccade to a sinusoidally moving target spot and begin to track it. Because the display was generated by a computer that also continously recorded eye position, it was possible to have the computer artifically stabilize the target spot on the fovea as soon as the eye began tracking. Results show that the smooth pursuit system can generate purely predictive sinusoidal movements on the basis of perceptual information alone. Detailed analyses of horizontal and vertical components of velocity during purely predictive smooth pursuit and comparisons with normal tracking are offered.

Introduction

It frequently has been observed that the eye shows little or no lag while smoothly tracking a moving target that follows a simple repetitive path, such as back and forth sinusoidal oscillation. This observation suggests that the control system for smooth pursuit eye movements has a predictive component that allows the eye to anticipate the movement of the target. In normal tracking, this predictive component would combine in some way with retinal information about velocity and positional errors in tracking to determine the overall tracking performance of the eye.

A variety of models of smooth pursuit have been suggested that incorporate a predictive component (Dallos & Jones, 1963; Michael & Jones, 1966; Robinson, 1968; Stark, Vossius, & Young, 1961; Yasui & Young, 1976), but experimentally isolating the characteristics of this predictive component has normally been complicated by the presence during tracking of retinal error information that acts as a co-determinant of tracking performance. One goal of the research to be reported here was to create a situation in which we could observe the predictive component of smooth pursuit in the absence of competing retinal error information. We accomplished this by artifically stabilizing the target on the fovea of the eye so that, regardless of how the eye moved, there was no retinal error.

A second goal of this research was to investigate the origins of the predictive component. Two alternatives may be considered. On the one hand, the predictive component may reside within the motor system, being built up as a record of on-going motor activity that eventually becomes self-perpetuating. On the other hand, the predictive component may reside outside of the motor system, in the perceptual system. According to this account, the observer perceives the repetitive motion of the target and then uses this perceptual information about the path of the target to control the smooth pursuit movements of the eye. We have attempted to isolate the perceptual contribution of the predictive component from any contribution due to on-going motor activity. We did this by creating a situation in which the observer's predictive tracking was based on observations of target motion made while the observer's eye was itself stationary.

Apparatus

Our target was a small, moving spot of light. Both it and a fixation spot were presented on the face of a large, high-resolution cathode ray tube (CRT) controlled by a PDP 11/40 mini-computer. Observers watched these spots monocularly in otherwise total darkness with their heads held fixed by a bite-bar. Eye position was monitored by an SRI, double-Purkinje-image eye-tracker (Cornsweet and Crane,1973), having an accuracy of a few minutes of arc. and was digitized and recorded every 2 msec by the computer. Because the computer both recorded the observers' eye movements and controlled the position of the spot that the observer was watching, it was possible to stabilize the target spot on the fovea of the observer's eye by simply moving the target spot on the CRT screen so that whereever the observer looked, the spot was there. (For more detail on the apparatus and calibration procedures, see Holtzman, Sedgwick, & Festinger, 1978.)

Procedure

Our data for each observer were gathered from a series of trials, each lasting less than a minute. We shall be concerned here with two types of trials, one of which we shall refer to as "stabilized" trials, and the other of which we shall refer to as "nonstabilized" trials . We shall describe the stabilized trials first.

Each stabilized trial had 2 phases, a "fixation" phase followed by a "tracking" phase. During the fixation phase, the observer fixated a stationary spot of light while attending to the motion of a second, target spot of light that moved back and forth with sinusoidally varying velocity along a straight path at some fixed angle to the horizontal. This angle varied from trial to trial. The center of the target spot's motion path was either 4 degrees directly above or 4 degrees directly below the fixation spot. The target spot moved back and forth at the rate of one complete cycle every 2 1/2 seconds (0.4 Hz), and the fixation phase lasted for 5 or 6 cycles, that is, about 15 seconds. During this time the observers had the opportunity, although their eyes were stationary, to build up a perceptual impression of the repetitive movement of the target spot.

The second phase of each stabilized trial was initiated by sounding a tone. Observers were instructed, before the start of the experiment, that when they heard the tone, they were to saccade to the moving target spot and to begin following it with their eyes. The tone was timed so that this saccade occurred when the target spot was almost directly above or below the fixation spot and was moving away from, rather than toward, the fixation spot. When the saccade began, the fixation spot disappeared. As soon as the saccade to the target spot ended, the target spot was artificially stabilized on the fovea of the eye and remained there for 1 1/4 seconds before disappearing, a time equivalent to half a cycle of target motion. During this stabilization period any smooth tracking movement that occurred must necessarily have been purely predictive because all retinal error information was eliminated by stabilization. Furthermore, any predictive movement occurring during this period must have originated with the perceptual system rather than with on-going activity of the motor system because the eye was entirely stationary prior to the beginning of the predictive tracking.

The nonstabilized trials were essentially the same as the stabilized trials except that the target spot was not stabilized when the eye reached it and began tracking. Instead, the eye was allowed to carry out half a cycle or more of normal tracking before the target spot disappeared. The nonstabilized trials served two purposes. First, they served to maintain the expectation that the target spot would continue moving when the eye reached it. For this reason nonstabilized and stabilized trials were randomly interspersed, and there were approximately 3 times as many nonstabilized as stabilized trials. Second, the nonstabilized trials gave us a baseline of normal tracking that we could compare with the predictive tracking that occurred on the stabilized trials.

Observers

In the study reported here, we used 3 paid observers, all of whom were naive as to the purposes of the experiment and were unaware that we were ever making the target movement contingent on their eye movements.

Design

We obtained responses to both stabilized and nonstabilized trials using 3 different angles to the horizontal for the motion path of the target spot--34, 63, and -63 degrees, with positive angles being measured counter-clockwise from the horizontal. The Y-component of target motion was always 6 degrees of visual angle; the X-component was varied to obtain these 3 angles. The 34 degree target was always presented above the fixation spot, while the 63 and -63 degree targets were presented either above or below fixation, thus yielding a total of 5 distinct conditions. We attempted to obtain 2 stabilized trials for each condition for each observer; some trials, however, had to be rejected from the analysis for a variety of reasons such as calibration errors leading to imperfect stabilization. Overall, we obtained 25 analyzable stabilized trials and 93 comparable nonstabilized trials.

Results

Our results show clearly that perceptual information alone is sufficient to produce over 1 second of purely predictive tracking that closely resembles the previously perceived path of target motion. During the tracking phase of almost every stabilized trial, the eye moves up along a path whose angle to the horizontal closely resembles that of the target spot, slows and stops aprroximately where the target spot would have stopped, and then returns along a path whose angle to the horizontal is again close to that of the target spot (an example of such a path is shown in Holtzman, Sedgwick, and Festinger, 1978, Figure 2). We used best fitting straight lines to estimate the angle of the eye's path before and after it turned for each of our stabilized trials; the period during which the eye was turning was omitted from this analysis by not including data

N	Above/Below Fixation	Target Angle	Avg. Angle Before Turn	Avg. Angle After Turn
5	above	34	37.2	39.4
4	above	63	61.6	57.5
6	above	-63	-59.8	-56.6
6	below	63	45.7	58.0
4	below	-63	-43.2	-52.0

Table 1. Average angle to the horizontal of the motion path of purely predictive tracking for 5 different previously seen target path angles and locations. Positive angles are measured counter-clockwise to the horizontal. (Cf. Holtzman, Sedgwick, and Festinger, 1978, Table 1)

obtained while the speed of the eye was less than 2 degrees of visual angle per second. These results are shown in Table 1. As can be seen there, the match between the predictive tracking and the previously perceived target path is quite good overall. The largest deviations occur when the target is below the fixation point. Here, the path of the eye during the first half of its predictive movement (i.e., before it turns) is consistently more shallow, by almost 20 degrees, than the previously seen path of the target.

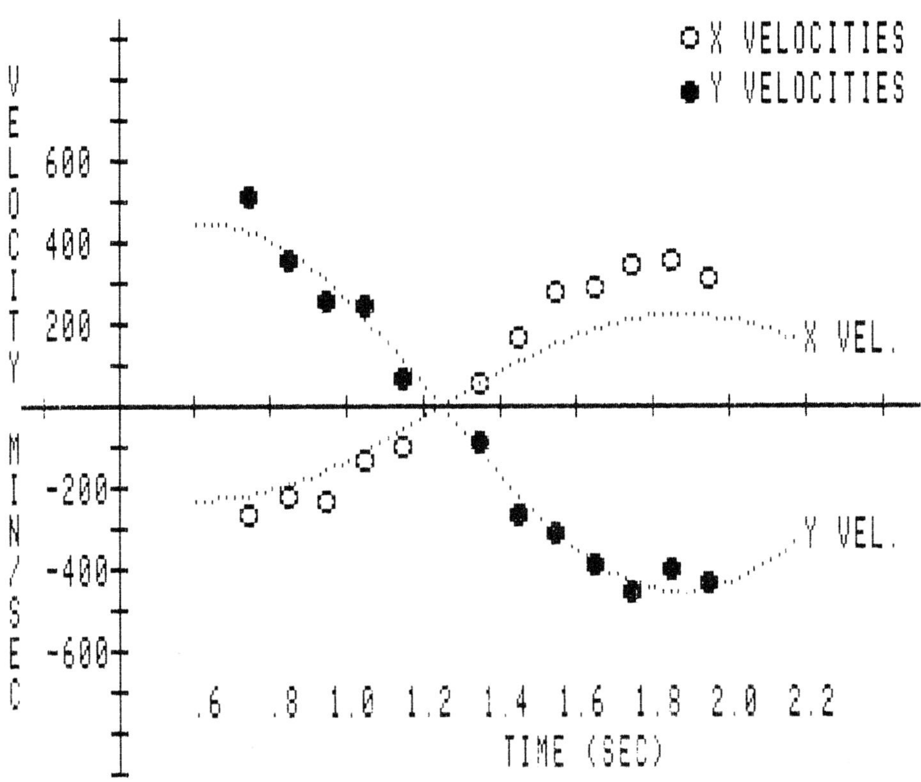

Figure 1. Velocity components of a single trial of purely predictive eye movements with a foveally stabilized target spot. The dotted lines indicate the velocity components of the path of the target spot before tracking and stabilization began; it was located above the fixation point and moving at an angle of -63 degrees to the horizontal.

To obtain a more detailed look at the eye's performance during predictive tracking, we analyzed the eye's movement into its horizontal (X) and vertical (Y) components and plotted the velocity, at 100 msec intervals, of each of these components during the tracking phase; intervals in which the eye's overall velocity is less than 1 1/2 degrees per second are omitted from the plot. An example of such a plot is given in Figure 1. Velocity is on the vertical axis and time is on the horizontal axis. The dotted lines show the sinusoidally varying velocity of the target spot over slightly more than one half cycle of its motion. Because the target spot is moving at an angle of -63 degrees to the horizontal in this example, the y-component of its velocity is twice that of the x-component. As can be seen in the figure, the velocity profile of the eye closely mimicks that of the previously seen target spot.

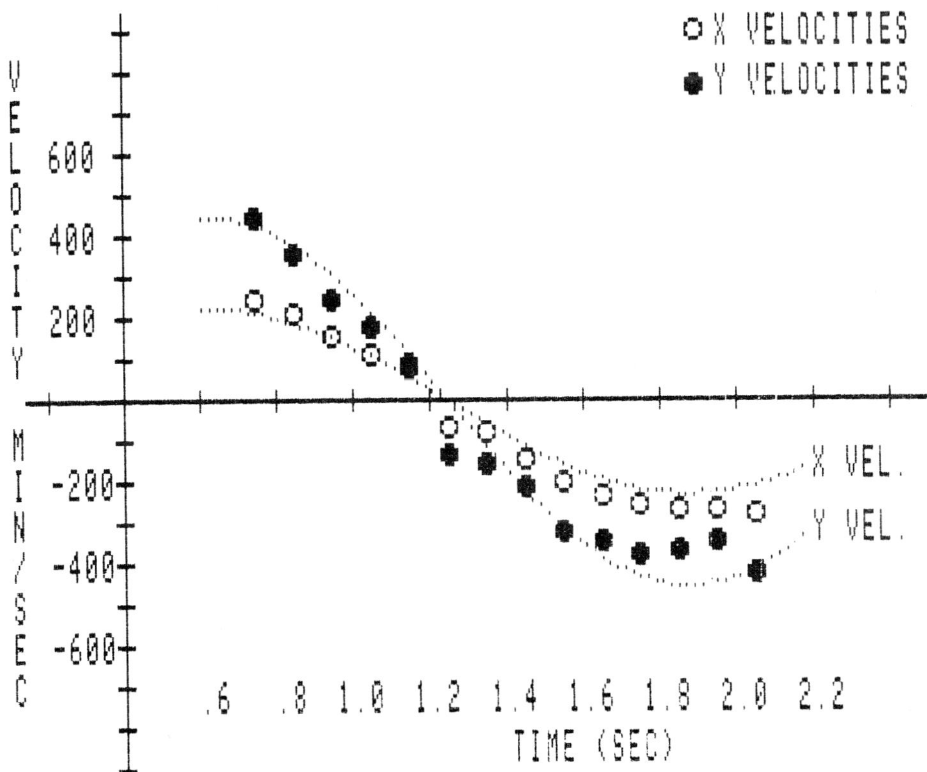

Figure 2. Averaged velocity components, stabilized trials, 63 and -63 degree target path angles, above fixation spot (N = 10).

We made such plots for all of the trials and then averaged these plots together within each condition. Furthermore, because the 63 degree and -63 degree conditions appeared quite similar, we averaged the results of those conditions together, changing the sign of the -63 degree condition.

Figure 2 shows the averaged X- and Y- velocity profiles of the 63 and -63 degree conditions for target spots located above the fixation spot. It can be seen that the deviations of the eye's predictive movement from the target spot's previous motion are quite small. A tendency for the eye to slightly anticipate the target's motion can be seen in both the X- and Y- velocity components of eye movement, which both cross the zero-velocity

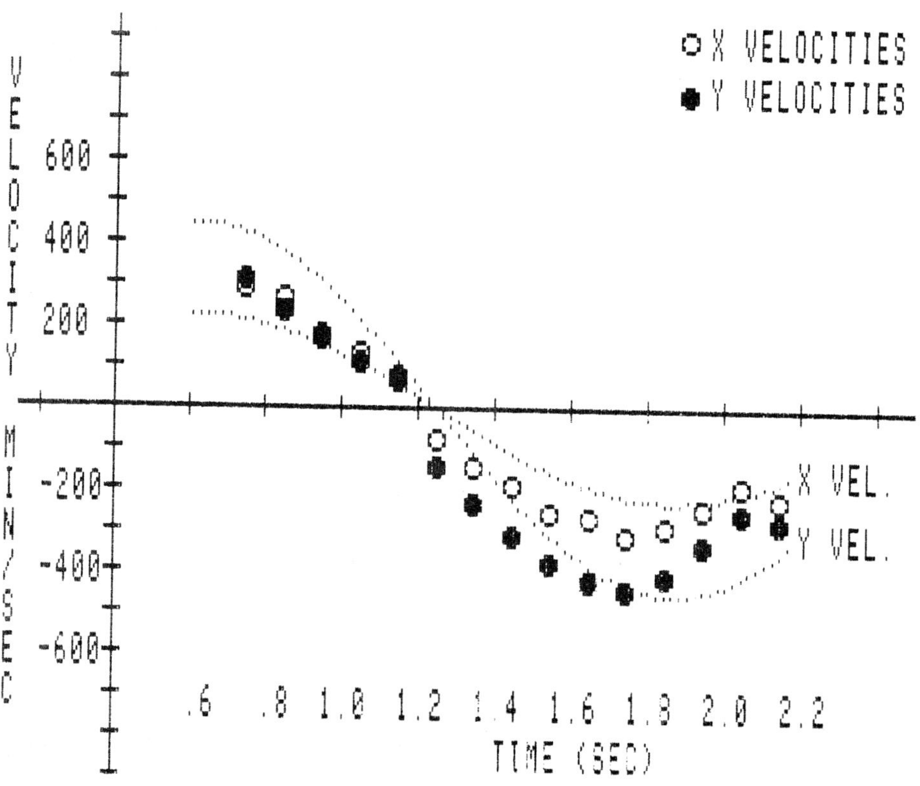

Figure 3. Averaged velocity components, stabilized trials, 63 and -63 degree target path angles, below fixation spot (N = 10).

axis (i.e., change direction) about 50 msec before the target does. This anticipation appears to reflect a phase-shift of the entire sinusoidal velocity profile of the eye's movement. There is also a tendency for the amplitude of the X-component to be slightly too large and for the amplitude of the Y-component to be slightly too small, thus resulting in the eye having a somewhat more shallow angle to the horizontal than the target, as indicated in Table 1.

Figure 3 shows the averaged X- and Y- velocity profiles of the 63 and -63 degree conditions for target spots located below the fixation spot. The velocity profiles are quite similar to those in Figure 2 except that during the first portion of stabilization, before the eye turns, the

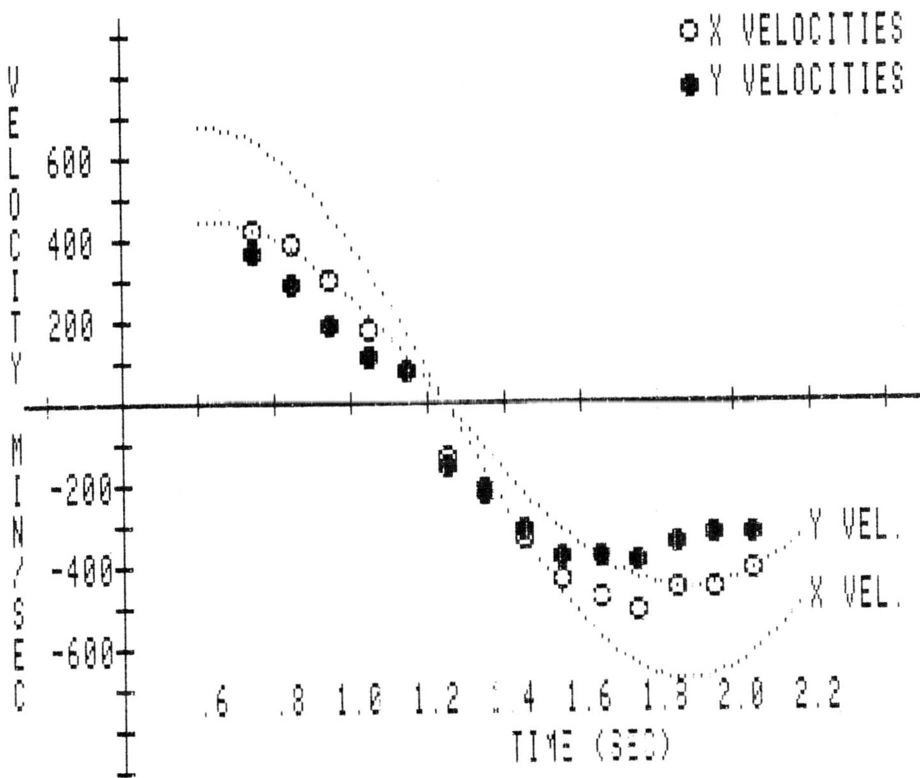

Figure 4. Averaged velocity components, stabilized trials, 34 degree target path angle, above fixation spot (N = 5).

amplitudes of the X- and Y- components are more similar to each other, the first being greater and the second less than the corresponding target components, so that the resulting path of the eye is close to 45 degrees, as shown in Table 1.

Figure 4 shows the averaged X and Y velocity profiles of predictive eye movement for target motion along a 34 degree path. Again there is a tendency toward phase anticipation, in both the eye's X- and Y-components of velocity, of between 50 and 100 msec, and again the amplitude of the eye's Y-component of velocity is somewhat too low. As the dotted lines show, the target spot's X-component of velocity is 50% greater than the target spot's Y-component of velocity in this condition. The eye's X-

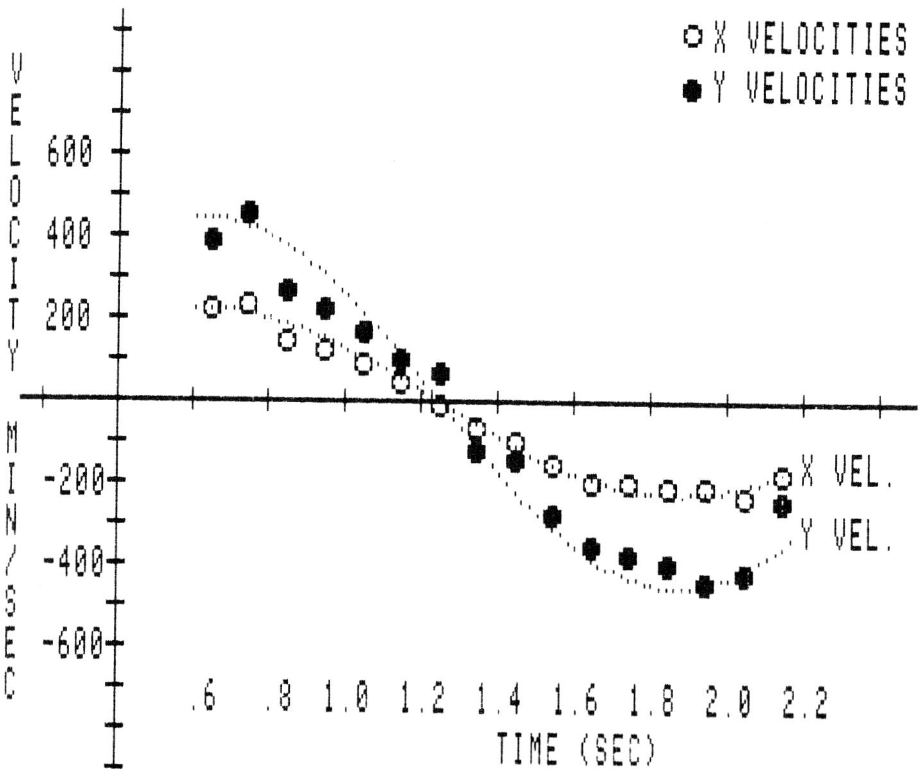

Figure 5. Averaged velocity components, nonstabilized trials, 63 and -63 degree target path angles, above and below fixation spot (N = 75).

component of velocity does not show a correspondingly large increase in velocity, so that the amplitude of the X- component is substantially too low. The amplitudes of the eye's X- and Y-components of velocity, although both too low, are close to being in the correct proportions to each other, however, so that the angle to the horizontal made by the path of the eye is only a few degrees greater than the angle made by the target spot. One qualitative way of seeing that the eye's purely predictive movements are in fact responsive to changes in the angle of the target spot's path is to note that in the 63 and -63 degree conditions the Y-component of velocity is greater than the X-component, both for the target spot and for the eye, while in the 34 degree condition these relative magnitudes are reversed for both the target spot and the eye.

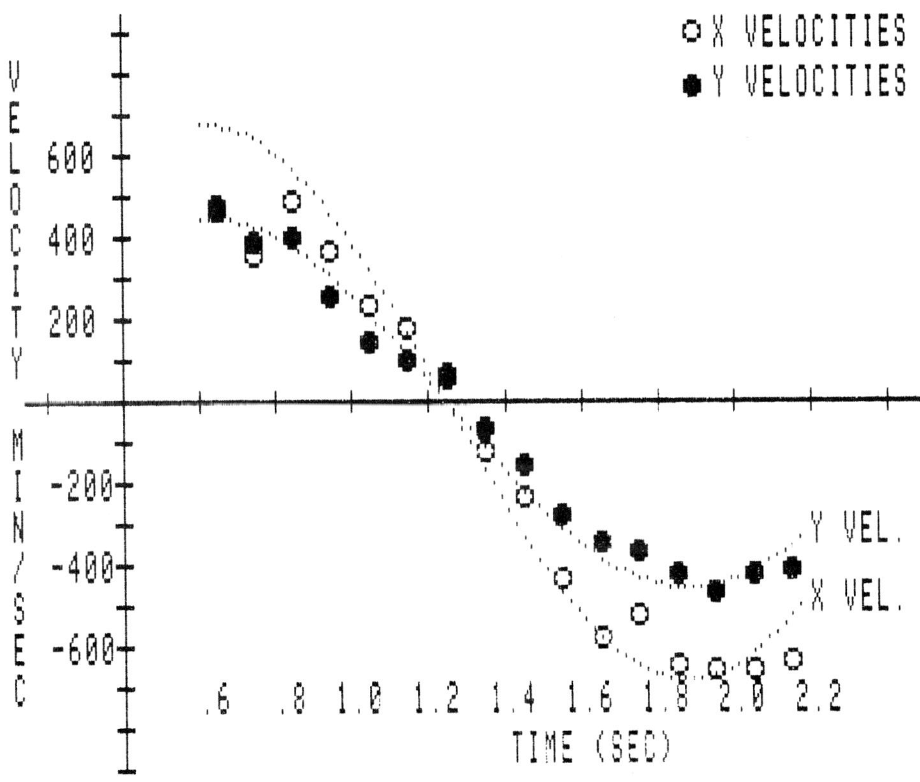

Figure 6. Averaged velocity components, nonstabilized trials, 34 degree target path angle, above fixation spot (N = 18).

To compare the eye's performance during purely predictive tracking with its performance during normal tracking, we prepared similar plots of the eye's X- and Y-components of velocity during nonstabilized trials. The results for the 63 and -63 degree paths above fixation and for the 63 and -63 degree paths below fixation do not appear do be systematically different and so these were all averaged together; they are shown in Figure 5. The averaged results for the 34 degree path are shown in Figures 6.

Inspection of these figures shows that the phase anticipation that characterized the purely predictive tracking is absent from the averaged normal tracking trials. Here, the eye's X- and Y-components of velocity both cross the zero-velocity axis very close to the zero-velocity crossing of the target spot itself. Also, the systematic errors in amplitude that characterized the purely predictive tracking are largely absent from the averaged normal tracking trials.

It may be noted, however, that the averaged velocity component plots for normal tracking are slightly more irregular in appearance, despite the substantially larger number of trials used to obtain them, than are those for purely predictive tracking. These irregularities are more marked when individual trials are examined. Such irregularities are not due to saccades, which are few in these records, and whose effects, when they do occur, have been removed from the records by substituting linear interpolations of the smooth pursuit immediately preceeding and following them. Rather, it may be that these irregularities are due to velocity corrections that are made in response to the retinally registered velocity and position errors that occur during normal tracking.

Discussion

Our results show clearly that the smooth pursuit system can generate sustained periods of smooth pursuit on a purely predictive basis; that this predictive pursuit can be based entirely on the previously perceived path of the target to be pursued; and that this pursuit can have sinusoidally varying components of velocity whose phase and amplitude characteristics are quite similar to those of the target. A close analysis, however, of the X- and Y-components of velocity of purely predictive pursuit shows them to differ from the corresponding components of comparable normal pursuit in several ways. First, the purely predictive pursuit typically shows a small phase anticipation. Second, the peak amplitudes of the components of purely predictive pursuit show small but systematic deviations from the peak amplitudes of target motion, generally being somewhat larger when target velocity amplitudes are small and somewhat smaller when target velocity amplitudes are large. Neither of these effects were observed systematically in normal pursuit; presumably there is a tendency to eliminate them by using the retinal velocity information that is present in normal pursuit. Third, the velocity components of purely predictive pursuit appear to be somewhat more smoothly sinusoidal in form than those of normal pursuit. The greater irregularity observed in normal pursuit may be a sign of the smooth pursuit system's attempt to correct the small errors introduced by the predictive tracking mechanism.

Several questions are raised and left unanswered by our results. The generality and the broader functional characteristics of the deviations from target motion that we found in our purely predictive eye movements require further investigation. Also, we do not know for how much longer than 1 1/4 seconds pure predictive tracking can be maintained, although our exploratory pilot studies suggested that at times longer than this the predictive tracking becomes more variable and begins to deteriorate.

Our results can be compared with those obtained in some recent attempts to measure or model predictive smooth pursuit. Becker and Fuchs (1982) obtained intervals of purely predictive smooth pursuit by briefly blanking out a target light while it was being pursued. The target was moving with constant velocity and disappeared for intervals of up to 1.5 sec (up to 3 sec for one observer). Tracking continued while the target was blanked but rapidly declined in a few hundred msec to a velocity about 60% that of the target and, on the average, continued to decline more slowly for the remainder of the blanking interval. When the blanking interval occurred at the very start of target motion, which was repeated over many trials, the eye executed a purely predictive accelerating smooth pursuit movement that for a period of 250 to 500 msec was the same as its velocity profile during normal tracking. After that initial period, the eye continued to track predictively, but its velocity profile increasingly deviated from that obtained in normal tracking. Our results, in which one velocity component of predictive tracking sometimes actually exceeds the corresponding velocity component of normal tracking for a period of 1 1/4 sec, suggest that some of the limitations on predictive tracking found by Becker and Fuchs may be more a function of the absence of a visible target than of inherent limitations in the predictive tracking mechanism.

Bahill and McDonald (1981) suggest an adaptive control model for smooth pursuit eye movements. Their model is capable of internally synthesizing a sinusoidal signal that matches the motion of a sinusoidally moving target and is then capable of using that internal model to drive the smooth pursuit system. This approach appears to be consistent with our results. Bahill and McDonald, however, suggest that signal synthesis would be limited to a fixed set of a few basic waveforms contained within their controller (presumably, although they are not explicit about this, within the motor system). On the other hand, our results, by placing the burden of "signal synthesis" on the perceptual system, put the massive information processing capacities of that system at the service of the smooth pursuit system, implying that the limits of predictive tracking may be less clear-cut and less restrictive than Bahill and McDonald suggest.

Note

1. The data to be reported here were gathered as part of a larger study of the interrelation between the perception of motion and the control of smooth pursuit eye movements. This work was carried on in collaboration with L. Festinger and was supported by Grant Number MH-16327 from the National Institute of Mental Health to him. Accounts of this larger study and preliminary analyses of the present data have been published elsewhere (Holtzman, Sedgwick, and Festinger, 1978; Holtzman and Sedgwick, 1984).

References

Bahill, A. T. & McDonald, J. D. (1981) Adaptive control model for saccadic and smooth pursuit eye movements. In A. F. Fuchs & W. Becker (Eds.)

Progress in Oculomotor Research, Elsevier North Holland, Inc.

Becker, W. & Fuchs, A. F. (1982) Predictive mechanisms in human smooth pursuit movement. In A. Roucoux and M. Crommelinck (Eds.), Physiological and Pathological Aspects of Eye Movements. Dr. W. Junk Publishers, The Hague.

Dallos, P. J. & Jones, R. W. (1963) Learning behavior of the eye fixation control system. I.E.E.E. Transactions on Automatic Control, AC -8, 268-277.

Holtzman, J. D. & Sedgwick, H. A. (1984) The integration of motor control and visual perception. In M. S. Gazzaniga (Ed.) Handbook of Cognitive Neuroscience, Plenum Publishing Corporation, New York.

Holtzman, J. D., Sedgwick, H. A., & Festinger, L. (1978) Interaction of perceptually monitored and unmonitored efferent commands for smooth pursuit eye movements. Vision Research, 18, 1545-1555.

Michael, J. A., & Jones. G. M. (1966) Dependence of visual tracking capability upon stimulus predictability. Vision Research, 6, 707-716.

Robinson, D. A. (1968) The oculomotor system: A review. Proc. I.E.E.E., 56, 1032-1049.

Stark, L., Vossius, G., & Young, L. R. (1961) Predictive control of eye movements. MIT Research Laboratory of Electronics, Cambridge, Mass. Quarterly Progress Report No. 62, 271-284.

Yasui, S. & Young, L R. (1976) Eye movements during afterimage tracking under sinusoidal and random vestibular stimulation. In R. A. Monty & J. W. Senders (Eds.) Eye Movements and Psychological Processes. Lawrence Erlbaum, Hillsdale.

Eye Movements and Human Information Processing
R. Groner, G.W. McConkie and C. Menz (eds.)

EXTRAFOVEAL PURSUIT AS STUDIED WITH THE RASHBASS PARADIGM

Nikos Logothetis, Wolfgang Fries, Ernst Pöppel
Institut für Medizinische Psychologie
Ludwig-Maximilians-Universität München
8000 München 2, Goethestraße 31/I
Federal Republic of Germany

SUMMARY

The size of the foveal pursuit zone was investigated by using the RASHBASS step-ramp paradigm. Presaccadic pursuit movements were found up to a step amplitude of seven degrees. Thus, the pursuit zone might correspond to the macular region of the retina.

INTRODUCTION

The goal of smooth pursuit eye movements is to keep a moving visual object fixated on the fovea, i.e. on the retinal region of best vision. A visual target outside the fovea has first to be "caught" by a saccadic eye movement, before it can be followed by the eyes in the smooth pursuit mode. The retinal region from which a smooth pursuit response of the eyes can be elicited, is restricted to a small foveal zone. Detailed studies have revealed that a stationary displacement of a light stimulus of 0.4 deg is enough to elicit a saccadic movement. Further, a stimulus position of more than 1.5 deg away from the fixation point ("position error") during the pursuit movement will be answered by a corrective saccade (Eckmiller und Mackeben, 1978) while position errors smaller than 1.5 deg can be compensated for by varying the gain of the pursuit movement. These findings led to the notion of a "pursuit zone" in the fovea from which alone pursuit movements are elicited and controlled.

Rashbass, however, who introduced the negative step-ramp paradigm into oculomotor research (Rashbass, 1961), noted that, in the response to a step-ramp stimulus of a step amplitude of 3 deg, the saccadic movement compensating for the position error is preceded by a small but distinct pursuit movement. This finding was taken as evidence that, neurologically, the saccadic and the pursuit system are independent, the latter having a shorter latency but being overridden by a powerful saccadic response to the position error signal (Rashbass, 1961; Robinson, 1965). Consequently, a pursuit movement might be evoked from regions outside the "pursuit zone". We have explored this question systematically, using Rashbass' step-ramp paradigm. By varying the step amplitude between 0 and 10 deg, and the ramp velocity between 0 and 10 ^{o}/sec we wanted to know up to which eccentricity such a presaccadic pursuit movement occurs.

METHODS

Three healthy volunteers served as subjects in the experiments. Subjects were seated in a dark chamber, their head fixed with a bite plate, and faced a target screen onto which the light stimuli (High contrast light spots of 0.25 deg diameter) were presented. Stimuli were generated by a slide projector. The stimulus light was shown on a small mirror mounted on the axis of a servo-controlled pen motor by which stimulus movement was achieved. This system was linear for frequencies up to 100 Hz at 5 deg amplitude; thus, true step movements of the stimulus could be produced. Eye movements were monitored by an infrared sensitive corneal reflexion system (eye track 2000^{R}, modified for our purposes). For horizontal eye movements, amplitude resolution was better than 10 min of arc. Temporal resolution was 1 msec. Both stimulus generation and data recordings were controlled by a PDP-11 computer.

In the experiments, subjects were presented first with a square wave calibration stimulus that was repeated after every four stimulus presentations. The stimuli consisted of step-ramp movements of which the step amplitude was varied between 0 and 10 deg in 1 deg intervals, and the ramp velocity between 0 - 10 deg/sec in 1 ^{o}/sec intervals. Step-ramps of different step amplitude and ramp velocity were presented in random order. Within one session that lasted about 20 minutes, 48 stimuli were given. Each subject performed at least 10 sessions. For analysis, the occurence of presaccadic eye movements was first assessed qualitatively, and their latencies, velocities and gains measured quantitatively. Altogether, about 4000 responses to step-ramp stimuli were evaluated.

RESULTS

The classical response to a step ramp stimulus concists of a small pursuit movement preceding the saccade that brings the stimulus into the fovea (Rashbass, 1961). An example is shown in figure 1. The presaccadic pursuit movement (PPM) is indicated by an arrow.

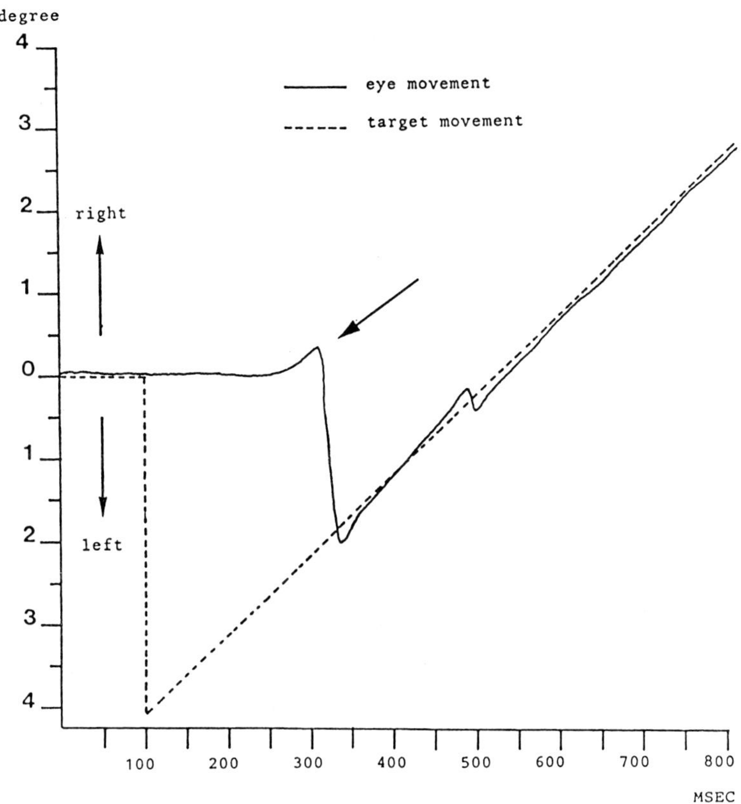

Figure 1
Eye movement response (solid line) to a step-ramp stimulus (dashed line). Convention is that movement to the right are up and those to the left are down. Abscissa marks time in milliseconds, ordinate marks eye and stimulus position in degree of visual angle.

Such PPM's were found for step amplitude up to seven degrees but never beyond. Figure 2 shows such representative oculomotor response to step-ramp stimuli.

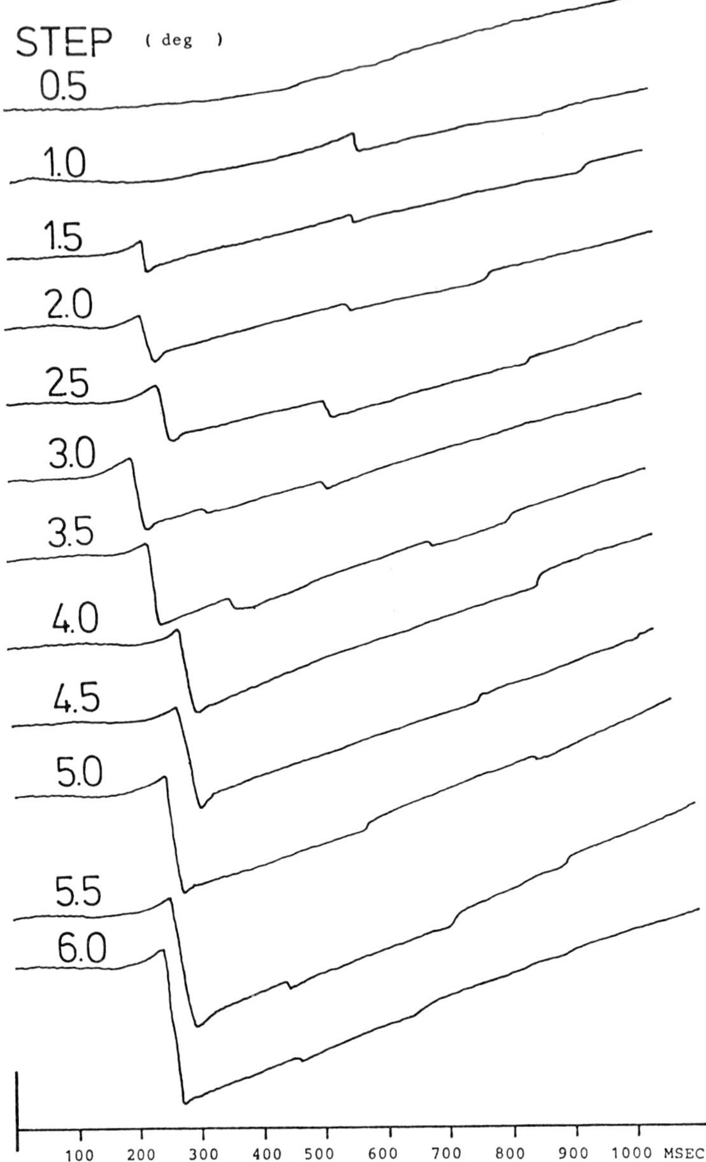

Figure 2
Representative eye movement responses to step-ramp stimuli whose step amplitude increase systematically from 0 to 6 deg. Only examples containing a presaccadic pursuit movement are shown.

This finding means that a ramp movement of a stimulus that begins at 7 deg eccentricity is still responded first by a pursuit movement. Hence, the retinal zone from which pursuit movements can be evoked is, at least in the horizontal plane, 14 deg in diameter.

However, it should be noted that PPM's did not occur invariably in response to every step-ramp stimulus. Rather, we found PPM's to be relatively rare events, occuring on average only every third trial. In no subject there was any clear correlation with step amplitude, i.e. the frequency of PPM's did neither increase nor decrease with increasing eccentricity at which the ramp movement began. Interestingly, however, there was a clear difference between subjects in the frequency at which they made PPM's. Two subjects made consistently PPM's in about 10 % of all trials (Fig. 3) whereas the three other subjects made PPM's uniformely in about 40 % of all trials (Fig. 4). However, the maximal step amplitude of the step-ramp stimulus at which subjects made a PPM (i.e. about 7 deg) appeared to be independent both of the individual frequency of PPM's in different subjects and of the ramp velocity.

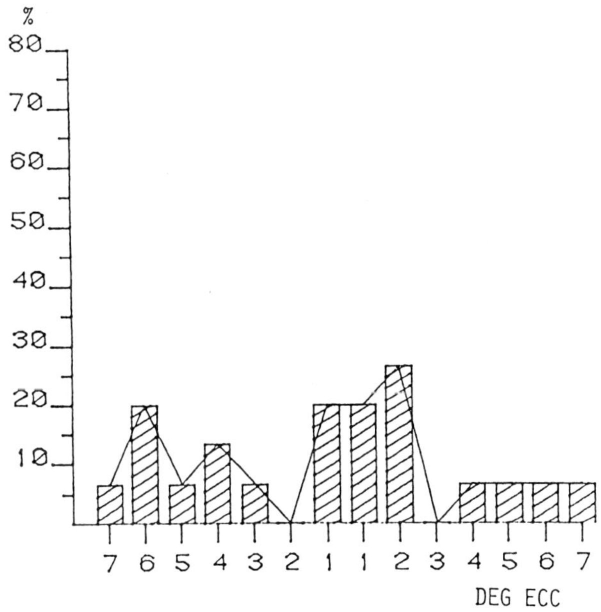

Figure 3
Frequency distribution histograms of PPM's for one observer. On the abscissa, the amplitude of steps is indicated; the left half gives eccentricities in the nasal, the right half in the temporal field. The ordinate gives the frequency in percent.

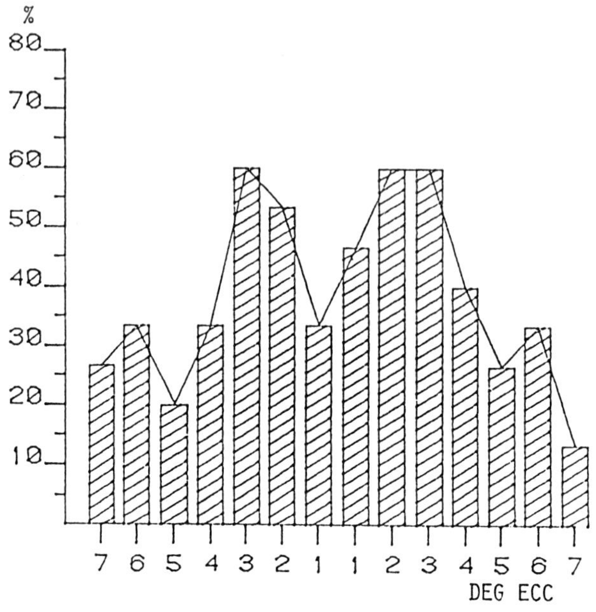

Figure 4
Frequency distribution histogram of PPM's for another observer. Conventions as in Figure 3.

DISCUSSION

The present findings show very consistently that, in the horizontal plane, the retinal region in which PPM's can be evoked has a radius of 7 deg. This area appears to be significantly larger than those eccentricities of ± 0.4 deg at which saccades can be elicited using stationary stimuli and of ± 1.5 deg at which a position error of the stimulus on the retina is compensated during pursuit movements without making a saccade (Eckmiller and Mackeben, 1978). It should be noted that those values are obtained under very different stimulation conditions. The threshold for correcting saccade is elevated, for example, during pursuit movements (Kommerell and Klein, 1971). Eckmiller (1981) briefly mentions that the "Pursuit zone" can be as large as the entire macula. Since the macular region in the human eye has a radius of about 8 to 9 deg (see, for example, Mountcastle (1980)), our findings might thus confirm nicely that the macular region is a spezialized region with respect to the pursuit mode, a view that is supported also by other psychophysiological experiments (Kommerell and Klein, 1971; Puckett and Steinman , 1969). Clearly, within this region, a moving stimulus can be responded to with a small pursuit movement before the correcting saccade.

This interpretation, however, is based on the view that such PPM's are indeed responses to the external stimulus as implied by Rashbass (1961). The low incidence of PPM's, particularly in two subjects, led us to the question why in the majority of instances, subjects make no PPM's to step-ramp stimulus. Preliminary studies of the velocity and the gain of PPM's (Logothetis, Fries, Pöppel, in preparation) indicate that there is little correlation between PPM velocity and ramp velocity. This seems to be true for all step amplitudes tested so far. Taken together with the fact that PPM's are by no means invariable responses to the step ramp stimulus we suspect that PPM's might not represent a response of the oculomotor system to the external stimulus. Tentatively, we would like to propose that PPM's might be the effect of a more or less powerful predictor, hence the variation between subjects. As all subjects were experienced in the experiments knowing that a ramp movement would occur automatically after the stimulus displacement, their predictor could be activated, depending on their attentional state. We are currently conducting experiments to test this hypothesis. The existence of a predictor in the oculomotor system has been first shown by Westheimer (1954). It plays a powerful role also in pursuit movements (see, for example, Stark et al., 1962, Eckmiller and Mackeben, 1978, Yasui and Young, 1984) and has been thoroughly discussed in respect to its importance in theoretical models of the pursuit system. Even though still speculation, the explanation of PPM's as an expression of an internal predictor, rather than a stimulus response might have some consequences on the presumed independece of pursuit and saccadic eye movements that was postulated on the basis of PPM's to step-ramp stimuli (Rashbass, 1961).

REFERENCES

Eckmiller, R.: A model of the neural network controlling foveal pursuit eye movements. In: Progress in Oculomotor Research, Fuchs, A.; Becker, W.; Elsevier, 1981

Eckmiller, R., Mackeben, M.: Pursuit eye movements and their neural control in the monkey. Pflügers Archiv 227, 15-23 (1978)

Kommerell, G. and Klein, U.: Über die visuelle Regelung der Okulomotorik: Die optomotorische Wirkung exzentrischer Nachbilder. Vision Res. 11, 905-920 (1971)

Mountcastle, V.B. (ed.): Medical Physiology, Mosby Co., Toronto - London (1980)

Logothetis, N., Fries, W., Pöppel, E.: The oculomotor response to step-ramp stimuli (in preparation)

Puckett, J., Steinman , R.M.: Tracking eye movements with and without saccadic correction. Vision Res. 9, 695-703 (1960)

Rashbass, C.: The relationship between saccadic and smooth tracking eye movements. J. Physiol. 159, 326-338 (1961)

Robinson, D.A.: The mechanics of human smooth pursuit eye movement. J. Physiol. 180, 569-591 (1965)

Stark, L., Vossius, G., Young, L.R.: Predictive control of eye movements. Institute of Radio Engeneers, Transactions on Human Factors in Electronics, HFE-3, 52-57 (1962)

Yasui, S., Young, L.R.: On the predictive control of foveal eye tracking and slow phases of optokinetic and vestibular nystagmus. J. Physiol. 347, 17-33 (1984)

Westheimer, G.: Eye movement response to a horizontally moving visual stimulus. A.M.A. Archs. Ophthal. 52, 932-941 (1954)

Eye Movements and Human Information Processing
R. Groner, G.W. McConkie and C. Menz (eds.)

TARGET INFORMATION AND EYE MOVEMENT LATENCY

Leonard E. Ross & Susan M. Ross
University of Wisconsin-Madison

While visual or auditory warning stimuli presented prior to a peripheral target reduce saccade latency to the target, visual stimulus onset or change following the target increases saccade latency. This interference effect was found to be related to the presence or absence and type of directional information provided by the non-target stimulus, but only when the stimulus was presented foveally. These results are discussed in terms of oculomotor and stimulus encoding and identification factors.

The research reported in this paper is concerned with the latency of saccades to peripheral targets when the occurrence of the target is either preceded or followed by another stimulus event. In these studies we have been interested in the facilitating and interfering effects of such pre and post-stimulus changes on the programming and execution of saccades, as indicated by changes in saccadic latency. Our most recent studies have examined the effect of adding directional information to the pre- and post-target stimulus events in order to determine the degree to which the resulting increase in stimulus encoding and interpretation would affect the facilitation or interference found to result from such stimulus changes.

PREVIOUS STUDIES

Research by others had generally used the offset of the fixation stimulus as a warning event in studying the effect of warning on saccade latency, and our first studies (Ross & Ross, 1980) were intended to determine if a similar facilitation would occur when the warning event was the onset of a stimulus or a change in the form of an already present stimulus. We found in our first experiment that stimulus offset and stimulus change could function as warning stimuli to reduce saccade latency to a target, but that the effect was smaller, except perhaps at long (600 msec) warning intervals, than that obtained with stimulus offset. It was also determined that simultaneous warning signal offset and target onset significantly reduced saccade latency but, surprisingly, that a stimulus onset or change that occurred simultaneously with the target onset produced a consistent increase in the latency of the saccade to the target of 30-40 msec.

To investigate this interference phenomenon further, a second experiment was carried out with onset and offset warning stimuli and warning intervals of 50, 0, -50, -100, -200, -250, and -300 msec. (Negative intervals represent conditions where the stimulus followed the target onset by the indicated value. Although the term 'warning' is something of a misnomer when applied to a stimulus that follows a target, the term will be used here to refer to stimuli presented both before and after target onset.) The results of this experiment, as seen in Figure 1, showed clearly that there was little if any interfering effect of stimulus offset as a warning event, but that stimulus onset resulted in an increase in saccade latency that was at a maximum when the onset occurred 50-100 msec after the target.

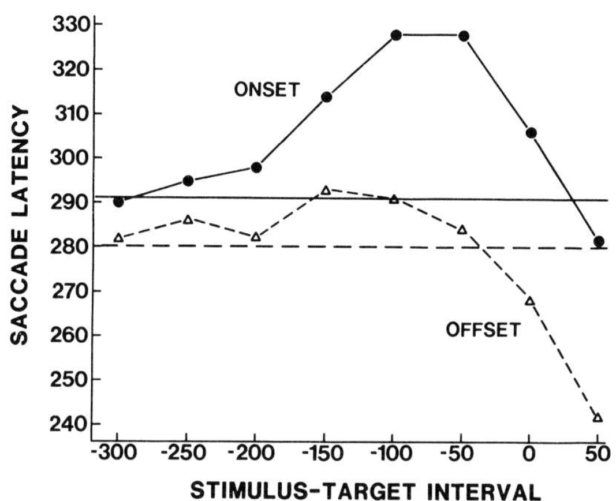

Figure 1. Saccade latencies as a function of the interval between foveal stimulus onset or offset and target onset. The horizontal lines indicate average no-warning latencies.

It was obvious from these results that when new information in the form of a stimulus onset or change occurred soon after the target there was a disruption in either the programming or execution of the target saccade. From an adaptive point of view it is not too surprising that new information, as contrasted to the disappearance of old, should result in the delay of a saccade. Both Potter (1976) and Senders (1976) have suggested that the eye tends to remain relatively fixed at the place where information is rapidly being presented in order to process the new information, and presumably some time interval would be necessary to buffer the new stimulus from the suppression effects of subsequent fixations. Alternatively, or in addition, there could simply be incompatibility or delay between the automatic programming or other processes elicited by the new stimulus on the one hand, and the ongoing programming or execution of the saccade to the target on the other. The subsequent experiments in this series of studies were designed to investigate further this interfering effect of post-target stimulus onset.

At this point it would be useful to describe briefly the experimental methods common to the studies discussed. All subjects were undergraduate students, balanced in number of males and females. Group size was eight, with warning interval a within-subjects factor. The stimuli were produced and timed by a laboratory computer and displayed on a Hewlett-Packard Model 1321A oscilloscope with a fast (P15) phosphor that was at a 60 cm viewing distance. Eye movements were detected using a Narco Biometric Eye-Trac Model 200 eye movement monitor, with horizontal eye movements recorded from the right eye and vertical eye movements recorded from the left eye. Permanent records of the unfiltered analog output of the Eye Trac were made using a Beckman R511A dynograph with a paper speed of 50 mm/sec. During each trial, the unfiltered Eye Trac output for the right eye was digitized by the laboratory computer, which identified the onset of the first saccade and determined its latency. At the conclusion of the trial, the trial conditions and saccade latency were printed, and the saccade, with computer-determined saccade onset identified, displayed on a monitor scope for the experimenter's inspection. Stimuli consisted of target letter X's, subtending visual angles of .5 degree vertically and .35 degree horizontally, appearing 15 degrees to the left or right of the center of the screen in an unpredictable sequence for a duration of 1 second. In most cases a fixation pattern consisting of four diagonal lines, each subtending .43 degree of visual angle was present at all times. The lines defining the fixation area radiated outward at angles of 45 degrees to the horizontal from the four corners of an imaginary square. The resulting pattern resembled an X with the center blanked out. Warning signals, e.g. an O, appeared, changed, or disappeared within the fixation area. All stimuli had an intensity of one nit.

The next question to be addressed in our studies was whether the saccadic interference phenomenon was related to visual-oculomotor processes or was a more general effect. Accordingly, a study was designed (Ross & Ross, 1981) to compare the effects of visual and auditory onset and offset warning stimuli on saccade latency. If the onset interference effect were found for auditory as well as visual stimuli, interpretation of the effect in terms of visual information intake or saccadic programming interference would be inappropriate. Similarly, if visual onset stimuli produced interference effects with other motor response systems, e.g. manual responses, interpretations involving programming mechanisms specific to the oculomotor system might be less convincing.

In the first two studies visual and auditory onset and offset warning events were compared at warning intervals of -300, -100, 0, +100, and +300 msec, with the auditory warning consisting of an electronic switch controlled onset or offset of a 1000 Hz tone superimposed on a 45 db white noise background. One visual and one auditory warning group received no-warning (baseline) trials while the second visual and second auditory warning groups did not. The results showed no interference effect for either auditory onset group, but delayed saccadic responding at the -100 warning interval for both visual onset groups, as shown in Figure 2.

The next study employed the same visual onset and offset warning conditions as those for the two visual warning groups, but the subjects were given the task of moving a 13 cm vertical response lever, fixed to the end of the armrest of the subject's chair on the subject's preferred side, to the right or left upon the occurrence of the visual target to the right or left. In this case the onset and offset effects were found to be virtually identical, as shown in Figure 3, with a facilitating warning effect when the warning stimulus preceded the target, but no interference effect when the warning stimulus lagged the target onset.

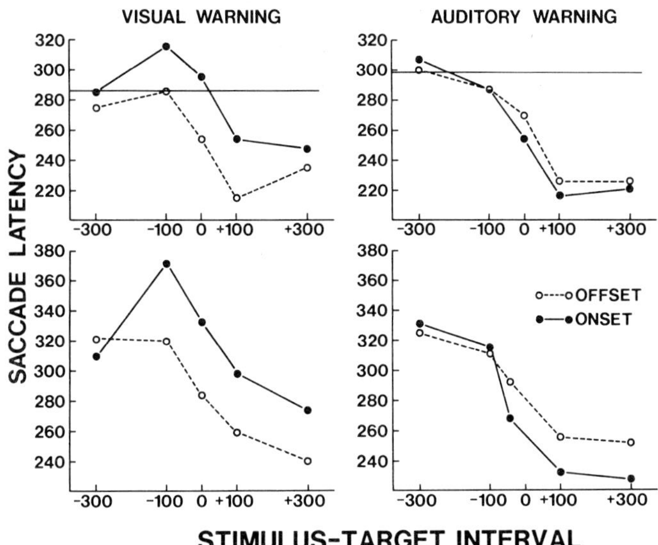

Figure 2. Saccade latencies as a function of warning interval for visual and auditory onset and offset conditions. The horizontal lines represent average no-warning latencies.

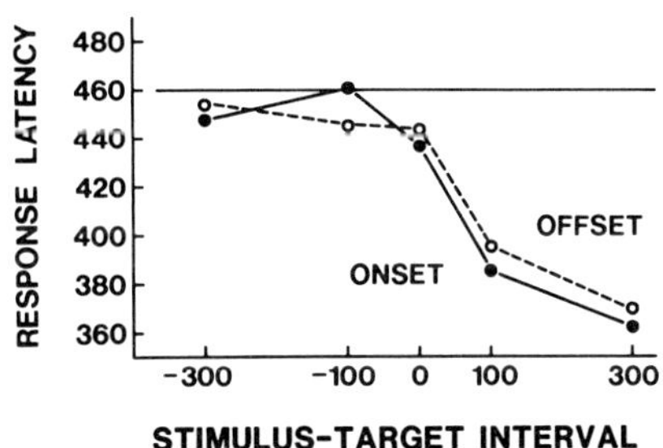

Figure 3. Manual response latencies as a function of the interval between foveal stimulus onset or offset and target onset. The horizontal line represents average no-warning latency.

In the final study of this group, onset and offset warning stimuli were presented not at the fixation point, but in pairs 5.5 degrees to the right and left, or above and below, the fixation pcint in order to determine if the post-target stimulus interference effect was specific to the warning stimulus appearing at the fixation point. It was found that the onset-offset warning effect difference still occurred when the warning stimuli were presented peripherally, in either the horizontal or vertical meridian, and in fact the functions were remarkably similar to those obtained with foveal presentation of the warning signal except that there was little if any onset-offset facilitation difference at 100 and 300 msec warning intervals. The fact that foveal and peripheral warning stimuli were found to have the same facilitating and interfering effects does not, however, necessarily indicate that the processes are the same. Foveal warning interference effects could reflect information intake processes while peripheral warning could be due to the initiation of oculomotor programming that interferes with the programming or execution of the saccade to the target.

At this point it should be noted that the interfering and facilitating effects discussed above are also found with children. Children as well as adults show a reduction in the latency of saccades when a stimulus offset precedes the target's appearance (e.g., Cohen & Ross, 1977, 1978; Groll & Ross, 1982), and a recent study by Ross and Ross (1983) has demonstrated that children (mean age of 10.0 years) show the same warning stimulus onset-offset differences that were found with adults as discussed above. The interference effects were much larger for children, however, being of the order of a 100 msec delay when the warning stimulus followed the target by 100 msec. Adult-children comparisons were also made when the warning signal was presented peripherally, in this case vertically above and below the fixation area. Both children and adults showed the delayed saccadic latency to the target, as in the case of foveal presentation of the warning stimulus, although the size of the effect in children was similar to that found for adults in this case. It could be speculated that the relatively greater foveal warning delay for children reflects the longer interval needed to extract information from that stimulus, while peripheral warning involves roughly comparable programming interference effects for both children and adults.

STUDIES WITH INFORMATIVE WARNING SIGNALS

Our most recent research has been concerned with post-target stimulus interference when directional information has been added to the warning stimulus. The three studies reported here were undertaken to determine if the processing of such directional information would affect the interference phenomenon; e.g., it is possible that the oculomotor delay might be constant if its only function is to permit time for stimulus registration and initial encoding while, alternately, the delay could vary depending upon the relative complexity of the encoding and interpretative processes elicited by the warning stimulus.

In the first experiment in this series four groups differed in the type of visual onset stimuli that preceded or followed the target. Two of the groups received stimuli that provided directional information about the target. For the Informative Digits Group a digit identified where the target would appear, while for the Arrows Group an arrow pointed in the direction of the target. The other two groups received stimuli that were unrelated to target location, and therefore served as non-informational controls. For the Onset O Groups the noninformative stimulus was the symbol O, and for the Random Digits Group the stimulus was a digit that was not associated with a particular target position.

Pre-experimental calibration procedures served to establish a relationship between the digits and arrows and target location, as well as to provide general instructions. Upon arriving at the laboratory, subjects received a vision test and were then seated in front of the display screen on which a five element calibration array was present. This array contained five digits for subjects in the Informative Digits, Arrows, and Onset O Groups, and five letters for the Random Digits Group. Subjects were told that from time to time the letter X would appear on the screen, and the experimenter indicated, by pointing to two positions in the calibration array, where the X could appear. The subject was instructed to look at the X as quickly as possible each time that it appeared. In addition, the fixation pattern was described and subjects were informed that sometimes a symbol would appear at the center of the fixation area. Subjects in the Informative Digits Group were then given an association between the informational warning stimuli and the digits location by being told that the warning symbol could be either a 2 or a 5 and that when it was a 2 the target would occur at position "2" as indicated on the calibration array, while when the warning stimulus was a 5 the target would occur at position "5" on the array. Subjects in the Arrows Group were told that the symbol would be an arrow pointing either to the left or to the right. When it pointed to the left the target would be at position "2" and when it pointed to the right the target would be at position "5". Subjects in these two groups were assured that the numbers and arrows would always give correct information when they appeared.

Subjects in the Onset O Group were informed that the X could appear at position "2" or "5" as indicated by the calibration array and that the symbol at the center of the fixation area would always be an O. Subjects in the Random Digits Group were told that the X could appear at positions "A" and "E" as indicated by the calibration array and that the symbol at the center of the fixation area would be either a 2 or a 5, with the sequence of 2s and 5s randomly determined.

All subjects received 108 trials including 18 no-stimulus control trials and 18 with each of the five intervals; -300, -100, 0, 100 and 300 msec. The interval values were randomly arranged within blocks of 36 trials with the restriction that within each block each interval was paired three times with a left target and three times with a right target, and that the same type of trial did not occur twice in succession.

Average saccadic latencies obtained for the four groups are shown in Figure 4, with the horizontal line representing the average latency on no-stimulus control trials for all subjects. If the stimulus onset interference effect is at least partly a consequence of processes related to information extraction, then significant differences in the amount of interference might be expected for groups differing in the amount of information conveyed by the stimulus and the ease with which it could be extracted. The results shown in Figure 4 appear to be consistent with this possibility in that when information is presented in a form requiring interpretation (the Informative Digits Group) greater interference is found as compared to the control conditions, while when information can be obtained with a minimum of encoding and interpretation (Arrows Group) very little if any interference occurs.

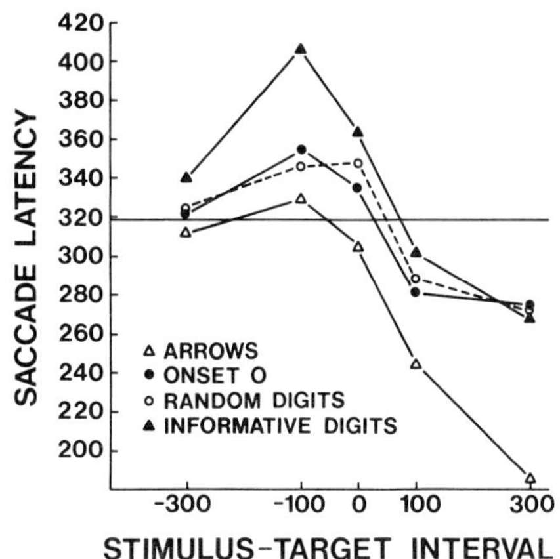

Figure 4. Saccade latencies as a function of the interval between foveal stimulus onset and target onset.

Statistical analysis support these conclusions in that significant ($p < .05$) effects were found for the interval and groups factors as well as their interaction. Subsequent analyses found that there was significant interference at the -100 msec interval for all but the Arrows Group, while significant facilitation was found at the 100 msec interval for the Arrows, Onset O, and Informative Digits Groups.

The greatest delay in the execution of the target saccade was associated with the informative digits, presumably because these stimuli elicited the greatest amount of cognitive activity on the part of the subject. It is of interest that this effect occurred in spite of the fact that by the time the foveal stimulus appeared the target had already been present for 100 msec, and the stimulus provided no new information regarding responding to the target. Thus it appears that whatever cognitive activity was involved occurred automatically in spite of the lack of usefulness of the information.

Also of interest is the fact that the Arrows Group did not show significant interference at any interval. This is quite surprising considering the interference shown by the other groups, especially in comparison with the large effect that resulted from the use of informative digits, the other condition in which there was information pertinent to target position. If stimulus onset per se was the critical factor in the interference effect then directional arrow onset should also have produced interference with the ongoing saccadic process. It is possible, however, that the interference effect is modified by the characteristics of the interpretative processes that result from the onset of a particular stimulus. In cases where the information is readily available and very easily visually interpretable, as is the case with the directional arrows used in this study, apparently no interference occurs.

The results for warning intervals of 100 and 300 msec, where the warning stimulus appeared 100 or 300 msec prior to the onset of the target, show subjects in the Arrows Group responding significantly faster than the subjects in the other three groups. This provides evidence that subjects in that group were able to utilize the directional information contained in the arrows. In contrast, subjects in the Informative Digits Group were apparently not able to make use of their stimulus' directional information to reduce saccade latency below the value of the control conditions, even when the digits appeared 300 msec prior to target onset. The reduced saccade latency shown by the Onset 0, Random Digits, and Informative Digits Groups presumably reflects nonspecific warning effects such as have been observed in other experiments.

In this study the informative and noninformative stimuli were always presented at the center of the fixation area, while for our next study stimuli were presented to the peripheral visual field. Our interest was in determining if the informative warning effects seen with foveal presentation would also occur with peripheral warning stimuli. With peripheral presentation competing or interfering programming might occur, but a delay to keep the stimulus in the fovea for processing would not be necessary.

To examine this question, groups were tested under procedures and conditions identical to those of the previous study except that instead of a single warning digit or arrow in the fixation area two identical warning symbols appeared 5.5 degrees above and below the center of the fixation area. The results of this study can be seen in Figure 5. There were very small and nonsignificant differences among the groups except at the 300 msec interval where the Arrows Group was significantly faster than other groups, and the Informative Digits Group was faster than the noninformative groups, which did not differ. These results support the view that the interference effects seen when the warning stimulus occurs at the fovea reflect informational aspects of the stimulus and the encoding and interpretative processes that then occur.

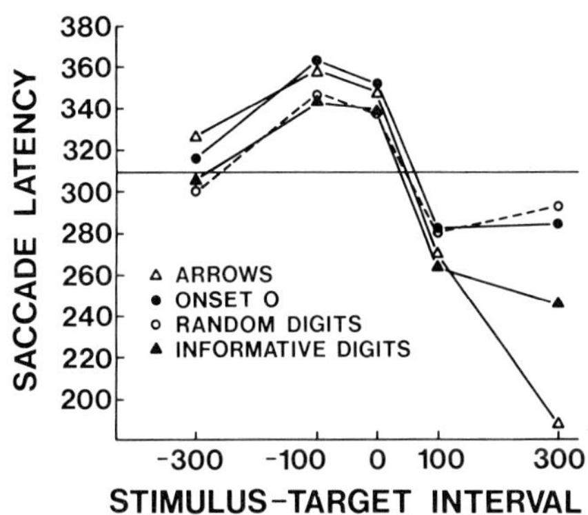

Figure 5. Saccade latencies as a function of the interval between the onset of the peripheral stimuli and the onset of the target. The horizontal line represents average no-warning latency.

Since interference effects were obtained with peripheral warning, a question is raised about the nature of the process involved. The interference could reflect initial programming, elicited by the stimulus, that interferes with the on-going programming or execution of the saccade to the target. At the same time, however, these peripheral warning stimuli were differentially effective in facilitating the target saccade when they preceded the target onset by 300 msec. This indicates, firstly, that when target directional information is given sufficiently in advance of the target's appearance the information can be utilized to reduce saccade latency to the target, presumably through preprogramming of the response. Secondly, these differences demonstrate that the lack of interference differences probably was not due to the subject's inability to discriminate and utilize the differences among the stimuli when presented in the periphery (the computer monitored eye position and did not present the trial if fixation deviated more than 1 degree from the center of the fixation area).

The final experiment in this series investigated another question concerning the effects of providing directional information prior or subsequent to target onset. In the previous studies each subject received only one type of warning information at the various positive and negative warning intervals. These data do not provide information with respect to whether the interference effects reflect identification and interpretation processes specific to the informative stimulus presentation on a specific trial, i.e., show trial by trial stimulus control, or involve more general processes that operate across trial types when warning stimuli of differing information value are mixed together within trial blocks. To investigate this question, a within subjects design was used in which each subject received more than one type of warning stimulus. Two combinations of foveally presented stimuli were employed. One group of subjects received informative digits on half of the trials and the noninformative 0 on the other half. The other group received the two types of informative stimuli in that half of the trials involved presentation of the informative digits, with the directional arrows presented on the remaining trials. Thus for one group the comparison was between the informative digits, which produced the greatest interference, and the noninformative and less interfering 0 stimulus; while the other group received a combination of informative digits and arrows, the latter a condition which was found not to result in interference. Other experimental conditions were identical to those of the previous two studies.

The results of these within subject combinations of informative warning signals are shown in Figure 6. The data clearly indicate that the interference produced by informative digits was not limited to trials on which those particular digits appeared, i.e. it was equally great on trials where the other stimuli followed target onset at the same interval. In addition, it should be noted that the magnitude of the interference effect found with a mixture of trials was approximately equal to that found for the Informative Digit Group in the previous experiment. Thus it is clearly the case that the interference effect is not a function of the specific stimulus that follows the target on a particular trial, but rather carries over to trials on which other stimuli occur as some kind of generalized factor, e.g. a memory representation of the stimulus situation. It is also noteworthy that for the Informative Digits-Arrows Group the interference was found on trials where the arrows were presented, although presumably little cognitive interpretation is required and where an interference effect was not found in the first of this series of three studies. As in the previous two studies, the arrow warning stimuli were more effective than the other stimuli when they preceded the target by 300 msec.

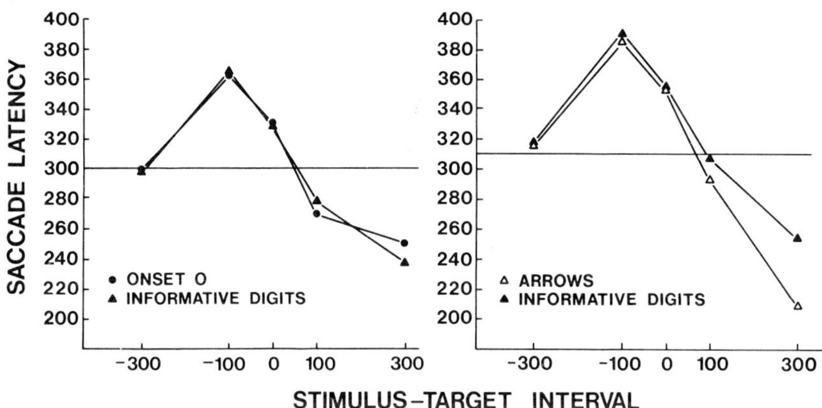

Figure 6. Saccade latencies as a function of the interval between foveal stimulus onset and target onset. The horizontal lines represents average no-warning latencies.

DISCUSSION

The results of the studies discussed above can be summarized briefly. As demonstrated by previous research, warning signals preceding an unpredictable peripheral target reduce the latency of the saccade to that target. In addition, our studies show that the offset of warning stimulus results in a shorter target saccade latency than does warning stimulus onset or a change in the configuration of the warning stimulus. Further, there is evidence that presenting easily interpreted directional information concerning the target results in even greater facilitation of the saccadic response to the target.

A more surprising finding, however, is that a warning stimulus onset or change occurring approximately 100 msec after the target can slow the saccadic response to the target, while the offset of the same stimulus has no such effect. Similar facilitation and interference effects are found when warning signals are presented in pairs in either the horizontal or vertical meridian. Further, it appears that these interference effects are specific to visual stimuli and the oculomotor system since post-target auditory warning onset does not interfere with saccadic responding, nor is an onset interference effect found with visual warning signals and manual responses.

When warning signals containing directional information are presented, results are obtained that indicate the interference effect is sensitive to the informational content of the stimulus and the nature of the encoding and interpretational load that results. The appearance of a stimulus that contains directional information and requires memory and interpretation results in a greater amount of interference than a non-informational stimulus, while directional information that is graphically explicit and easy to interpret does not result in any delay of the saccade to the target. Interference effects related to the informational load of the warning stimulus do not occur when the warning stimuli are presented in the periphery, and when different types of warning stimuli are mixed in blocks of trials the large interference effects found with the more difficult to decode informational stimuli generalize to trials on which either non-informative stimuli or informational stimuli that do not produce interference are presented.

There are several mechanisms or processes that could result in the facilitation and interference effects found in these studies. The facilitation of responding that occurs when a warning stimulus is presented prior to the target could reflect any of a number of processes including a general alerting process that facilitates motor responding, the occurrence of preliminary motor (in this case oculomotor) response programming or preprogramming that reduces the time necessary to initiate a saccade, and shifts in attention which could facilitate saccadic responding in the same way that they are thought to facilitate other motor responding (e.g., Posner, Synder & Davidson, 1980). When directional information is available, as in the last series of experiments reported above, the additional facilitation could reflect additional directional preprogramming of the saccade, a central attentional shift that speeds the processing of the visual event or a combination of these two factors.

There are also several processes or mechanisms that could delay the saccade when warning stimulus onset follows target onset. One possibility is that the onset of a new stimulus of some attentional value either interrupts ongoing programming or produces a hold on the execution of the response. This could occur with or without the initiation of new and competing programming since the delay could function to provide time for a decision as to whether an eye movement should be programmed to that stimulus. Alternatively, the presence of a new and possibly important stimulus could automatically elicit the preliminary stages of programming for a saccade that is not executed but nevertheless interferes with the saccade to the target. Although the interference effect is found with both foveal and peripheral warning stimulus presentations, it does not appear that the delay found with foveal warning stimuli is due to the initiation of programming for a new saccade since in that case no saccade is necessary to bring the stimulus to foveal regard. It could be the case, however, that an efficient system would start programming upon the occurrence of a new and possibly important stimulus anywhere in the visual field, given the relatively low possibility of such a stimulus occurring close enough to the point of fixation that no saccade is needed to improve its resolution. Another process that could delay the saccade to the target, at least when the warning stimulus is presented foveally, is the tendency of the eye to remain fixed at the point at which information is being presented rapidly (e.g., Potter, 1976), which could permit the buffering or analysis of the stimulus prior to the next eye movement.

The situation becomes more complex when the effects of adding directional information to the post-target warning stimulus are considered. As in the case with the nondirectional warning stimulus, the directional information is redundant with that already available to the subject in the form of the actual location of the target. The fact that differing degrees of directional information are reflected in the latency of the saccade implies some automatic interpretational process that is triggered by the appearance of the informational stimulus, just as is the case when interference occurs when a non-directional warning signalstimulus appears after target onset. Unlike the case with nondirectional warning stimuli, however, this presumably higher level processing involving directional information occurred only when the directional information was presented foveally, while the facilitative effects that reflect directional content were found with either foveal or peripheral presentation. Thus, interpretation per se seems to occur in both locations, but the interference and delay resulting from post-target presentation appears to be a foveal presentation phenomenon.

The fact that there was no interference when the post-target stimulus was an easily encoded directional stimulus demonstrates that when the stimulus interpretation processes are simple the results of that interpretation can override the interference process. It may well be that the interference with the saccade to the visible target is due to both information intake processes and competitive saccade programming, with the relative contribution of each depending upon several factors such as the degree and type of information and the location of the stimulus in the visual field.

When subjects received a mixture of trials of varying directional information, interference equal to that found under the maximum interference condition present on those trials prevailed. Such carry-over or generalization of the interference effect suggests that there was a set or memory representation involved that resulted in a general interpretational delay. The strength of this effect isindicated by the fact that the delay with the arrow stimulus was as great as that with the informative digits, although the arrow condition alone produced no interference.

It is clear that there is much still to be learned about the processes involved in the interference effect and the factors that affect it. We do not know, for example, the conditions under which a stimulus will elicit the interference effect. A nonpredictive or a novel stimulus may be effective, or it may be necessary for a stimulus to have had some degree of temporal predictiveness with respect to the occurrence of the target. Also, a post-target presentation in combination with other paradigms, e.g., the various double-step sequences as investigated by Becker and Jurgens (1979), might provide information about the interference effect as it relates to the various stages of the programming sequence that occur following the appearance of the target stimulus.

ACKNOWLEDGEMENT

This research was funded in part by USPHS Grant HD 03352.

REFERENCES

Becker, W. & Jurgens, R. (1979). An analysis of the saccadic system by means of double step stimuli. Vision Research, 19, 967-983.

Cohen, M. E. & Ross, L.E. (1977). Saccade latency in children and adults: Effects of warning interval and target eccentricity. Journal of Experimental Child Psychology, 23, 539-549.

Cohen, M.E. & Ross, L.E. (1978). Latency and accuracy characteristics of saccades and corrective saccades in children and adults. Journal of Experimental Child Psychology, 26, 517-527.

Groll, S.L. & Ross, L.E. (1982). The saccadic eye movements of children and adults to double-step stimuli. Developmental Psychology, 18, 108-123.

Posner, M.I., Synder, C.R.R., & Davidson, B.J. (1980). Attention and the detection of signals. Journal of Experimental Psychology: General, 109, 160-174.

Potter, M.C. (1976). Short-term conceptual memory for pictures. Journal of Experimental Psychology: Human Learning and Memory, 2, 507-522.

Ross, L.E. & Ross, S.M. (1980). Saccade latency and warning signals: Stimulus onset, offset, and change as warning events. Perception & Psychophysics, 7, 251-257.

Ross, S.M. & Ross, L.E. (1981). Saccade latency and warning signals: Effects of auditory and visual stimulus onset and offset. Perception & Psychophysics, 29, 429-437.

Ross, S.M. & Ross, L.E. (1983). The effects of onset and offset warning and post-target stimuli on the saccadic latency of children and adults. Journal of Experimental Child Psychology, 36, 340-355.

Senders, J.W. (1976). Speculations and notions. In R.A. Monty & J.W. Senders (Eds.), Eye movements and psychological processes. Hillsdale, N.J.: Erlbaum.

Eye Movements and Human Information Processing
R. Groner, G.W. McConkie and C. Menz (eds.)

CONCEPTUAL MASKING OF BRIEFLY GLIMPSED PHOTOGRAPHS

Helene Intraub

University of Delaware
Newark, Delaware
U.S.A.

Conceptual masking is a term used by Potter (1976) to describe a specific type of interference that can occur during the early stages of picture processing. Potter's model and subsequent modifications (Intraub, 1984) have been based primarily upon research in which single fixations and some of the dynamic, sequential characteristics of visual scanning are mimicked through the use of tachistoscopic exposures and rapid sequential presentation of pictures. In addition to testing the early stages of picture processing, this type of research may provide insight into the processes initiated during the first fixation made on a new scene. The major focus of the paper will be the question of whether or not the type of masking discussed by Potter is actually conceptual in nature, or can be attributed either to visual masking or long-term memory effects.

INTRODUCTION

According to Potter's (1976) model of the early stages of picture memory, most pictures of common objects and scenes are rapidly understood -- perhaps within the first 100 msec of viewing. Once identification has occurred, a representation of the briefly glimpsed information is maintained for a few hundred milliseconds in a short-term conceptual memory while processes are initiated to store the information in a more permanent memory. Prior to conceptual identification, the visual information is vulnerable to visual masking. If a complex visual event is presented during this time it is likely that the picture will not be identified. Once identification occurs, however, the information becomes immune to visual masking, but is now vulnerable to conceptual masking caused by the presentation of new information that elicits the same processes (e.g., a new picture). This occurs because by eliciting conceptual processing itself, the new picture competes for space in the short-term conceptual store. Evidence for this view of picture memory comes from search experiments which support the contention that pictures may be momentarily understood and then forgotten and recognition memory experiments which support a distinction between visual and conceptual masking.

Rapid identification of sequentially presented pictures has been demonstrated in several search experiments in which pictures were presented at rates that mimicked or exceeded the average fixation frequency of 3 per second (Intraub, 1981a, 1981b; Potter, 1975, 1976). In these experiments, regardless of whether the target picture was specified in terms of a brief verbal title (e.g., "a road with cars"; Potter, 1975, 1976), a title indicating its superordinate category, or a negative cue (e.g., "report a picture that is not a type of transportation"; Intraub, 1981a, 1981b), subjects were very good at detecting it. Subjects in the detection group could detect and describe more pictures than subjects in the recognition memory group could recognize immediately following presentation of the sequence. For example, at a presentation rate of 258 msec per picture, subjects could detect and describe a target picture based on a negative cue 79% of the time, whereas subjects in the recognition memory condition recognized the same pictures only 58% of the time (Intraub, 1981b). The results of these experiments support Potter's (1976) claim that during rapid sequential presentation of pictures, many pictures are momentarily identified and then lost due to interference caused by the presentation of new pictures. Only those pictures that can be consolidated before the next picture is presented will be retained.

The search experiments suggest that visual masking cannot account for poor memory following rapid presentation because many of the pictures were at least momentarily identified during inspection. More direct evidence that a process other than visual masking is responsible, comes from recognition memory experiments with briefly glimpsed pictures. This research shows that although memory is poor following rapid continuous presentation of pictures, memory for briefly presented pictures is very good when the pictures are presented with interstimulus intervals (ISIs) that contain a colorful visual noise mask (Potter, 1976) or a familiar picture that repeats throughout the sequence (Intraub, 1980, 1984). For example, Intraub (1980) presented 150 color photographs for 110 msec each. In two conditions the interstimulus interval (ISI) was approximately 6 sec in duration. Depending on condition, it contained a blank field or a familiar picture that repeated throughout the sequence. In the remaining condition the pictures were presented continuously with no ISI. In spite of the presentation of a visual event (i.e., a potential visual mask) following each briefly presented picture, recognition memory in the repeating-ISI and blank-ISI conditions did not differ significantly. The proportion recognized was .73 and .77, respectively. When the pictures were presented with no ISI, and each picture was followed by a new picture, the proportion recognized dropped to .21. The argument is that neither a noise mask nor a familiar picture elicits the same identification processes as a new picture.

Consistent with this hypothesis, if a new picture is presented during a to-be-ignored ISI, recognition memory decreases as compared with conditions in which a blank or repeating picture are presented (Intraub, 1981a, 1984). For example, in one experiment, 16 pictures were presented for 112 msec each with a 1.5 sec ISI that contained a repeating picture (repeating-ISI) or a new picture each time (changing-ISI). The probability of recognizing a picture was .80 (SD = .14) and .64 (SD = .13), with false alarm rates of .08 and .05 for the repeating- and changing-ISI conditions, respectively (Intraub, 1984). Clearly, new pictures interfere with memory in some way. The question is whether or not the effect can be attributed to conceptual masking of information in the short-term conceptual store. In the next section we will consider some alternate explanations of the changing-ISI experiments and some other tests of the conceptual masking hypothesis.

IS THE INTERFERENCE "CONCEPTUAL"?

One alternate explanation of the relatively poor performance in the changing-ISI condition is a traditional explanation that focuses on long-term memory. Although subjects in the repeating- and changing-ISI conditions were faced with the task of remembering the same 16 briefly presented pictures, and were both instructed to ignore information presented during the ISI, subjects in the changing-ISI condition saw a total of 32 pictures (including the ISI pictures), whereas the other subjects saw a total of 17 pictures (including the ISI picture). The lower scores in the changing-

ISI condition may have been due to relatively greater difficulty in discriminating old from new pictures in the recognition test because these subjects had just seen a relatively large number of pictures. That is, the poor performance may not have been due to interference with the contents of a short-term buffer, but to interference with later recognition processes.

To test this hypothesis, a new step was added to the repeating-ISI condition so that like subjects in the changing-ISI condition, in addition to the 16 target pictures, these subjects would see 16 to-be-ignored pictures for 1.5 sec each. Immediately preceding the repeating-ISI condition, subjects were presented with a monitoring task. They were shown a picture and were told that it would appear briefly at some time during presentation of a continuous series of 16 pictures. The continuous series contained the 16 ISI pictures used in the changing-ISI condition, presented for 1.5 sec each. Subjects were instructed to think about the picture they were to search for while watching the sequence and to report its appearance. The picture they were searching for always appeared at the end of the continuous sequence. In this way, like the subjects in the changing-ISI condition, these subjects watched the 1.5 sec ISI-pictures while focusing attention on another task. The monitoring task was followed by the repeating-ISI condition, where subjects were instructed to focus attention on the briefly presented pictures in preparation for a recognition test.

A comparison of memory for the 16 briefly presented target pictures in the new repeating-ISI condition with memory for the same pictures in the changing-ISI condition, supported the conceptual masking hypothesis. Subjects in the new repeating-ISI condition recognized .90 (SD = .08) of the briefly presented pictures whereas subjects in the changing-ISI condition only recognized .73 (SD = .21) of the pictures (Intraub, 1984). The false alarm rates did not differ between the two conditions (they were .05 and .07, respectively). Apparently it is not the presentation of numerous to-be-ignored pictures per se that disrupts recognition memory for briefly presented pictures, but the placement of the to-be-ignored pictures within the sequence. Conceptual identification of a new picture may be automatic, occurring even when the subject tries to ignore the picture (e.g., Smith & Magee, 1980). If a briefly glimpsed target picture is in the short-term conceptual store when the ISI picture is presented, identification of that ISI picture will disrupt processing of the store's contents. If the same ISI picture is identified prior to viewing the brief target picture (as in the monitoring task condition), it will have no effect on processing of the target. The disruptive effect of conceptual identification may be due to its attentional demand. Indeed, if the status of the ISI pictures in the changing-ISI condition is changed from "pictures-to-be-ignored" to "pictures-to-be-remembered," this increases their disruptive effect. The next experiment was concerned with testing the hypothesis that automatic conceptual identification is the cause of poor memory in the changing-ISI condition.

The control conditions for experiments testing the conceptual masking hypothesis have been ones in which briefly presented pictures are followed by a single noise mask (Potter, 1976), a repeating gray field (Intraub, 1980), or a repeating familiar picture (Intraub, 1980, 1984). Besides differing from new pictures in terms of the necessity for new conceptual analysis, these items differ with respect to visual novelty and expectancy. Unlike a repeating picture or a repeating meaningless noise mask, each new ISI picture provides the subject with an unpredictable visual event. Maybe any novel stimulus, regardless of its conceptual content, would disrupt the contents of the unstable short-term store by drawing attention.

To test this hypothesis, a new changing-ISI condition was constructed and compared with the changing-ISI condition described above. In this case the pictures presented during the ISI were nonsense pictures. These were created by tracing the basic shapes of each of the ISI pictures used in the changing-ISI condition, and altering coloration and boundaries within the shape to disguise the picture's identity. Like the ISI pictures, the nonsense pictures provide a novel, unpredictable visual event following each target picture. They are object-like in that they present a colored shape against a gray background, just as the pictures do. The major difference between the two types of visual displays is that the nonsense pictures are not meaningful (i.e., do not readily map onto pre-existing concepts). If the conceptual masking hypothesis is correct, then presenting a new, nonsense picture during the ISI should not lead to as poor performance as presenting a new, meaningful picture. If, however, the memory disruption is the result of attention being drawn by any new visual stimulus, then nonsense pictures should disrupt memory as much as meaningful pictures.

The nonsense-ISI condition was conducted at the same time as the new repeating-ISI and changing-ISI conditions described above and will be compared to those conditions. The results supported the conceptual masking hypothesis. Memory for target pictures in the nonsense-ISI condition was significantly better than that obtained in the changing-ISI condition. Subjects in the nonsense-ISI condition recognized .87 (SD = .11) of the target pictures, with a false alarm rate of .07 (Intraub, 1984). This score was comparable to that obtained in the repeating-ISI condition (with the monitoring task) showing that subjects could ignore the colorful nonsense pictures about as easily as they could a familiar repeating picture. Presentation of a new, unpredictable visual mask did not disrupt memory as much as a new, meaningful picture. The good performance obtained when repeating pictures, noise masks, and nonsense pictures are presented during the ISI, argues against visual masking as the cause of poor memory following rapid presentation. Other converging evidence regarding this point has been reported by Loftus and Ginn (in press).

Loftus and Ginn (in press) tested the conceptual masking hypothesis by directly contrasting visual masking and conceptual masking. They presented target pictures for 50 msec, a briefer duration than that typically used in the recognition memory experiments described above. According to Potter's model, this would make the pictures susceptible to visual masking, because conceptual identification might not yet be complete. Depending on condition, subjects were presented with one of two types of masks (a meaningless visual noise mask or a new picture) at one of two levels of illumination. They postulated that if the mask was presented immediately at stimulus offset, the target picture would be subject to visual masking. This being the case, luminance would be expected to affect the power of the mask, but meaningful masks would not be expected to be any more effective than a meaningless noise mask. If the mask presentation was delayed for 300 msec, they predicted that luminance would have no effect on the effectiveness of the mask, but that meaningful pictures would be more effective masks than the visual noise mask. This is because by the time 300 msec has elapsed, subjects would be expected to have identified the picture. The picture at this stage would no longer be susceptible to visual masking but would be susceptible to conceptual masking.

The dependent measure in their experiment was the number of details subjects could report about a picture following the mask. The results followed the predictions, thus providing converging evidence for the contention that conceptual masking is a process that differs from visual masking and involves the conceptual content of the mask. Also, by showing an effect of mask type when memory for each picture is tested immediately following the mask, their results corroborate those obtained in the monitoring task/repeating-ISI condition, in showing that conceptual masking is not due to confusion in long-term memory.

INVERTED PICTURES AS CONCEPTUAL MASKS

One of the experiments in Intraub (1984) lead to the suggestion that inverting a picture might lessen its effectiveness as a conceptual mask by making the picture's concept less available. If this were the case, it was argued, inverted pictures would provide an excellent means of testing the conceptual masking hypothesis because the visual characteristics of inverted and upright pictures would be very similar, but their conceptual accessibility would differ. Research testing the effects of inverted versus upright ISI pictures, however, did not show any effect of this manipulation on recognition memory for target pictures. For example, in one experiment using the same pictures as Intraub (1984), target pictures were presented for 112 msec with a 1.5 sec ISI that contained a 250 msec ISI picture followed by a colorful visual noise mask. Subjects were instructed to focus attention on the target pictures which would be presented again in the recognition test. The proportion of pictures recognized in the upright and inverted ISI conditions respectively was .60 (SD = .21) and .65 (SD = .18). Similar experiments were conducted using more complex pictures (visual scenes), which might be expected to be more difficult to understand when inverted. These ISI pictures were presented for as little as 125 msec. Inverted pictures continued to disrupt memory as much as upright pictures.

Using a visual duration threshold method with the complex visual scenes, a pilot study has indicated that even at very brief durations (e.g., 30 msec), when subjects were capable of reporting something about the picture, although they could not provide a detailed description, they seemed to be able to report very general conceptual information about a scene regardless of whether it was inverted or upright. For example, subjects might not be able to report that the scene contained men and women folk dancers in traditional costumes, but they could report that the scene contained people. These results suggest that inverting a scene does not necessarily significantly retard or prevent conceptual identification. Extraction of this very general conceptual information is apparently enough to cause conceptual masking.

CAPACITY OF THE SHORT-TERM CONCEPTUAL STORE

According to Potter's (1976) original formulation of the conceptual short-term store, the buffer could hold one picture at a time. During rapid presentation, if a picture in the buffer could not be consolidated in memory before the onset of a new picture, it would be lost. Although memory in the changing ISI conditions described previously is worse than in conditions in which a blank field or repeating picture is presented during the ISI, memory does not approach the low level obtained during continuous rapid presentation where there is no ISI(e.g., Intraub, 1980, 1981b; Potter & Levy, 1969). This suggests that presentation of a new picture disrupts processing but may not necessarily terminate it. It seemed possible that the buffer might be able to hold more than one picture at a time.

To test this possibility, the capacity of the buffer was explored by comparing memory for 24 briefly presented visual scenes under conditions in which they were shown in groups of 1, 2, 3, or 4 pictures. In all conditions the same 24 pictures were used and the intergroup intervals (which contained a colorful visual noise mask) were adjusted so that the length of time from the beginning of each sequence to the test was the same. All pictures were presented for 250 msec each. The intergroup intervals for the single, double, triple, and quadruple grouping conditions was 1625, 3250, 4875, and 6500 msec, respectively. The control condition presented all 24 items in a continuous sequence followed by a 39 sec mask filled interval so that the time from the beginning of the sequence to the test was the same as in the other conditions. If the buffer can hold only one picture at a time, then memory in the double, triple and quadruple condition should be no better than memory following continuous presentation of all 24 pictures. Of course, to make the comparison it is necessary to disqualify the final picture in each grouping because this picture is the only one never followed by a conceptual mask. Only in the single picture condition, where each picture is immediately followed by a mask filled interval, should memory be superior to the continuous condition.

The results show that the buffer must hold more than one picture at a time. Recognition memory (excluding the final picture in each group) was superior to that obtained following rapid presentation in all but the quadruple grouping condition. The proportion recognized was .54, .56, and .37 in the double, triple, and quadruple conditions, respectively. The proportion of pictures recognized in the continuous condition was .29. In the single condition where no conceptual masking should have taken place, the proportion recognized was .90. Although presentation of additional conceptual masks causes more disruption of memory, the buffer can apparently hold up to three complex visual scenes.

SUMMARY AND IMPLICATIONS

These experiments provide support for a model of the early stages of picture processing proposed by Potter (1976). According to this view, pictures of objects and scenes are rapidly understood and stored in a short-term conceptual memory where they are no longer vulnerable to visual masking, but may have their processing disrupted by a conceptual mask. Conceptual masking is thought to occur when new conceptual information competes for space in the short-term conceptual store. The argument that conceptual processing rather than visual processing of a new stimulus is responsible for disruption of memory at this stage is supported by experiments showing that nonsense pictures and repeating pictures do not disrupt memory for briefly presented pictures as much as new pictures do (Intraub, 1984). The distinction between visual and conceptual masking was also supported in research showing differential effects of meaningless and meaningful masks on memory for a picture's details as a function of delay (Loftus & Ginn, in press).

Modifications of Potter's model have been based on experiments showing that, contrary to the initial formulation, the short-term conceptual buffer can maintain more than one picture at a time (Intraub, 1984; and the grouping experiment discussed above). As the buffer fills to its capacity of approximately three pictures, memory performance decreases as more attention is drawn by incoming information. Regarding attention and conceptual masking, there is a possible distinction that should be drawn. Experiments testing selective attention for pictures have shown that picture memory is affected by attention instruction (Graefe & Watkins, 1980; Intraub, 1980, 1981a, 1984; Weaver & Stanny, 1978). Some of the processes required to store a picture in a more stable memory are certainly under the subject's control. However, it may be the case that other processes are not. The research described here suggests that conceptual identification of a new picture may be automatic (see also, Smith & Magee, 1980), in the sense that the subject cannot terminate or bypass the process. Identification, however, may require allocation of attentional resources. For example, recall that memory for pictures dropped dramatically when each of the 16 briefly presented pictures was followed by a new ISI picture as compared with a colorful nonsense picture that retained the basic shape of each of the ISI pictures. When the subject is familiar with a picture through repeated exposure or if the picture does not contain meaningful features that readily map onto a concept, the identification processes either proceed rapidly (requiring little attention) or, in the latter case, may be terminated by the observer. This protects the contents of the short-term store, allowing the observer to process it further and store it in a more stable memory.

The implications of these processes for visual scanning (in which the average fixation frequency is no more than about three per second) are that the visual/cognitive system of the observer is set up to allow rapid comprehension of complex visual information. This information is stored briefly while decisions are made about further processing. New naturalistic information cannot be ignored and will impinge on processing. This latter point is quite reasonable when one considers that unlike the present experiments, during visual scanning, most fixations are probably highly redundant. The results of the experiments discussed, suggest that during normal visual activity subjects can rapidly assess the contents of each "scene" and adjust the extent of encoding and perhaps the location of the next fixation. These overlapping processes of identification and storage may also play a role in the integration of successive fixations during scanning.

REFERENCES

Graefe, T. M., & Watkins, M. J. (1980). Picture rehearsal: An effect of selectively attending to pictures no longer in view. Journal of Experimental Psychology: Human Learning and Memory, 6, 156-162.

Intraub, H. (1980). Presentation rate and the representation of briefly glimpsed pictures in memory. Journal of Experimental Psychology: Human Learning and Memory, 6, 1-12.

Intraub, H. (1981a). Identification and processing of briefly glimpsed visual scenes. In D. F. Fisher, R. A. Monty, & J. W. Senders (Eds.), _Eye movements: Cognition and visual perception_ (pp. 181-190). Hillsdale, NJ, Erlbaum.

Intraub, H. (1981b). Rapid conceptual identification of sequentially presented pictures. _Journal of Experimental Psychology: Human Perception and Performance_, _7_, 604-610.

Intraub, H. (1984). Conceptual masking: The effects of subsequent visual events on memory for pictures. _Journal of Experimental Psychology: Learning, Memory, & Cognition_, _10_, 115-125.

Loftus, G. R., & Ginn, M. (in press). Perceptual and conceptual masking of pictures. _Journal of Experimental Psychology: Learning, Memory, & Cognition_.

Potter, M. C. (1975). Meaning in visual search. _Science_, _187_, 965-966.

Potter, M. C. (1976). Short-term conceptual memory for pictures. _Journal of Experimental Psychology: Human Learning and Memory_, _2_, 509-522.

Potter, M. C., & Levy, E. I. (1969). Recognition memory for a rapid sequence of pictures. _Journal of Experimental Psychology_, _81_, 10-15.

Smith, M. C., & Magee, L. E. (1980). Tracing the time course of picture-word processing. _Journal of Experimental Psychology: General_, _4_, 373-392.

Weaver, G. E., & Stanny, C. J. (1978). Short-term retention of pictorial stimuli as assessed by a probe recognition technique. _Journal of Experimental Psychology: Human Learning and Memory_, _4_, 55-65.

Eye Movements and Human Information Processing
R. Groner, G.W. McConkie and C. Menz (eds.)

OCULOMOTOR CONTROL IN HUMAN INFANTS

Louise Hainline
Department of Psychology
Brooklyn College of CUNY
Brooklyn, New York 11210 USA

Abstract

The infant's capacity to control his eye movements must set limits on the ability to extract visual information from his environment. Recent work on the development of oculomotor control supports the conclusion that despite an immature visual system and, particularly, a highly immature fovea, many oculomotor systems are highly functional even in early infancy. Infants appear to be capable of some degree of smooth pursuit, although they revert to saccadic tracking at lower velocities than adults do. Infants' optokinetic nystagmus (OKN) also shows smooth slow phases and saccadic fast phases, but infants' OKN shows asymmetries not seen in normal adults. In addition to the developmental change in monocular horizontal OKN reported by other reseachers, we have found an age trend within binocular vertical OKN. Infants' saccades often show similar amplitudes and peak velocities to those of adults, although the characteristics of infants' saccades are highly related to the infant's state of attention. Young infants often show very good control of fixations, although they show greater fixational variability than adults; quality of fixational control may also depend on the infant's attentional state.

Until relatively recently, little was known about the development of oculomotor control systems. In fact, despite evidence that the vertebrate visual system is particularly susceptible to modification by environmental conditions early in life, oculomotor development in animals is only now beginning to be investigated. Studies of oculomotor development in human infants are also appearing with greater frequency, and this paper will describe some of the findings of this work.

Comparisons between the behaviors of infants and adults are not always straight-forward. In most studies of adults' eye movements, subjects are highly practiced and generally highly motivated to perform at the highest level of functioning of which they are capable. Instructions on how the subject should perform are made explicit. Sessions can be interspersed with rest breaks to insure that changes in attention or fatigue do not influence the oculomotor behavior being studied. To insure that an occasional unusual trial does not unduly influence the data, hundreds of trials can be run. If the task is demanding, these trials can be spaced at intervals of weeks or even months without a realistic concern that the subject will have undergone some change in the intervening time that would influence how eye movements are made. All of these experimental considerations are consistent with a motive to study the best, if not the most typical, level of performance for a given oculomotor system.

Those of us interested in understanding oculomotor control in young infants are dealing with a very different situation. Our subjects are not highly practiced, and are not amenable to direct instruction. Their motivation to perform a given behavior is unknown, and probably highly variable. The infant is subject to unpredictable, spontaneous changes in behavioral state or level of attention. Further, when infants get bored with a task that may require many trials, they express their feelings by fussing or falling asleep. Since infants are undergoing rapid developments in many areas, it is not always possible to compensate for the brief sessions necessitated by their short attention spans by spacing multiple sessions over some longer interval of time; the behavior in question may be qualitatively different at the end of the series of sessions than it was at the beginning, due to maturation and/or the greater opportunity for practice as the infant ages. All of these problems in working with infants do not mean that it is impossible to derive any useful information on oculomotor development from studies on infant eye movements; rather, these considerations determine that 1) knowledge about a given oculomotor system must be derived from the convergence of results from more than a few studies, ideally with each using slightly different methods and stimuli, and reasonably large numbers of subjects of different ages; 2) Knowledge about the infants' typical performance is going to be easier to get than knowledge of the best or optimal performance of a given system.

To rephrase the second point, if infants and adults show eye movement characteristics that are quantitatively similar, this similarity probably means that the infant system is capable (at least some of the time) of mature performance. If, however, one finds the not unexpected result that infants' eye movements are apparently less "mature", it is not logically correct to assume that this difference is necessarily caused by oculomotor immaturities. It is, of course, possible that developmental differences may actually be caused by neurologic immaturities in the sites in the nervous system responsible for oculomotor control. However, it is also possible that the infant's behavior is the result of differences in basic sensory abilities due to physiological immaturities at relatively peripheral (i.e., retinal) levels in the visual system; that is, performance may differ because the target is less visible for the infants. Alternatively, the task may be one which, while quite effective for adults, fails to engage the infants' attention or interest, the result being diminished performance. In typical studies with adult subjects, eye movements such as saccades or smooth pursuit are elicited by small targets presented under the control of the experimenter in settings in which other potential targets for eye movements have been removed. However, experiments which use small, silent targets that move unpredictably in an otherwise featureless field may not be the best method of enlisting an infant's cooperation.

A second problem with such a stimulus regime is that successful performance, for example localization of a target by a saccade, requires both the ability to know where the target is, and the capacity to make a saccade toward it. Infants might perform poorly either because of a system deficient in the ability to generate saccades or because of problems at what can be regarded as "higher" or cognitive levels; for example, they may lack good "maps" of space. Infants are known to be less capable than older children in localizing auditory and probably also visual targets in space (Muir, Abraham, Forbes, and Harris, 1979). Piaget has postulated that one of the achievements of the sensory motor period is the attainment of a well articulated and integrated system of spatial maps (Piaget, 1952). Still another factor that may cause differences in the oculomotor performance of infants and adults is that infants have slower reaction times than older children or adults. Whether this is due to basic neuromuscular immaturity or attentional factors is not clearly understood; infants probably respond more slowly to change around them because of differences in both factors. As a result, measures of latency and reaction times are not easy to interpret for infants. Thus, requiring that infants respond to the movement of a smooth pursuit target or the abrupt change in location of a saccadic target may result in "poorer" performance from infants, not necessarily because they are less developed from an oculomotor perspective, but because it simply takes them longer to respond to the change.

Infant Eye Movements

Infant eye movements have been recorded primarily with either EOG or corneal reflection. Other methods with greater precision (e.g., contact lens search coil, double Purkinje systems, etc.) are too intrusive to be used easily with infants. We favor an infrared corneal reflection system for recording infant eye movements since it does not require the application of electrodes to the infant. As an example of how corneal reflection can be used with infants, a schematic of the system we use in our laboratory is provided in Fig. 1. The oculomotor systems that we have been particularly interested in studying are those that are normally conjugate, i.e., saccades, smooth pursuit, optokinetic nystagmus (OKN) and fixation. Estimates of our system's measurement errors, and procedures for spatial and dynamic calibration of the device are provided elsewhere (Hainline, 1981; Harris, Hainline and Abramov, 1981; Harris, Abramov and Hainline, 1984).

The central retina, or fovea, and the peripheral retina serve different roles in oculomotor control. The fovea has the highest acuity, and is of major importance in fixational control, saccadic localization and smooth pursuit of small targets. The periphery is responsible for grosser localization of targets during the planning of saccades, and for smooth eye movements and nystagmus when large portions of the visual field are in motion. A major unresolved issue in studies of infant oculomotor control is whether the young infant has a functioning fovea, and if so, whether foveal immaturity is responsible for some of the reported deficits in certain oculomotor domains. We have recently confirmed some old and difficult to substantiate claims (Bach and Seefelder, 1914; also cited in Mann, 1964) that the human fovea is markedly immature in the early months of life (Abramov, Gordon, Hendrickson, Hainline, Dobson and LaBossiere, 1982). The peripheral retina, on the other hand, is at a more mature level of development. The fovea is thus undergoing substantial development throughout at least the first half year of life. It is likely that the significant improvements in acuity over this period result in large part from foveal developments (Dobson and Teller, 1978), but it is not known whether this foveal immaturity has oculomotor consequences, apart from those stemming directly from reduced target visibility.

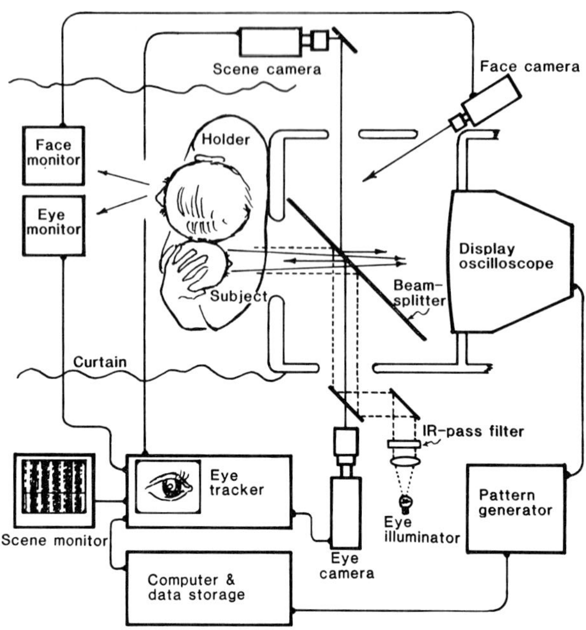

Fig. 1: A schematic representation of the elements of an infrared corneal reflection eye movement monitor for use with infants. The essential optical elements are the infrared sensitive "eye" camera and the dichroic beam splitter that transmits visible and reflects infrared wavelengths.

Smooth Pursuit in Infants

Many descriptions of eye movement control systems make a distinction between foveal and peripheral systems, as, for example, in a distinction made by some (Tauber and Atkin, 1968; Hood and Leech, 1974; Collewijn, 1981) between smooth pursuit and OKN. Some studies (Aslin, 1981; Atkinson and Braddick, 1981; Shea and Aslin, 1984) have reported that infants are not able to show smooth pursuit of small targets under 2-3 months of age. Rather, pursuit is reported to be completely saccadic. Other studies, however, report that even neonates can show smooth pursuit, but only for relatively low velocities (Kremenitzer, Vaughan, Kurtzberg, and Dowling, 1979; Roucoux, Culee, and Roucoux, 1983). Thus, since at least some studies find that pursuit exists at low velocities, the difference between infants and adults does not seem to be in the presence or absence of a "foveal" pursuit system, but in how well the system functions. This may be dependent on how large the target is; the studies reporting good pursuit in younger infants have, in general, used larger targets (12 deg. in Kreminitzer, et al., and 2-10 deg. in Roucoux, et al., versus a 2-2.5 deg. wide bar in Aslin, 1981 and Atkinson and Braddick, 1981). In the Roucoux, et al. study, the effect of varying target size on pursuit is not reported, but Shea and Aslin (1984) reported better pursuit at a given age for larger (6 deg.) versus smaller (2 deg.) targets. The observation that target size is important could be due to one or a combination of several factors; larger targets are easier for the infant to detect, given the limitations of acuity for younger infants. Larger targets also will cover a greater portion of the retina, so that parafoveal regions can contribute to the pursuit response. Large targets are probably easier for the infant to locate and are also more salient and thus likely to attract the infant's attention. If infants are alert and attentive, they may be able to pursue at higher velocities than when they are paying less attention to the target.

We have recently begun some studies in our laboratory (in collaboration with Johan de Bie) in which the infant's attention to the pursuit target is enhanced by computer-generated music ("Alouette" and "She'll be Coming Round the Mountain" are particular favorites). Since infants are sensitive to temporal correspondences between vision and audition, and prefer temporally synchronized events (Spelke, 1976), the 1.5 deg. target in these studies changes luminance slightly in time to the music. Fig. 2 shows some examples of smooth pursuit from subjects of different ages. The records support the finding that younger infants can show smooth pursuit, but to lower velocities than older infants. However, older infants sometimes show saccadic pursuit to targets moving rather slowly. Perhaps, for them, smooth pursuit requires greater concentration than saccadic pursuit.

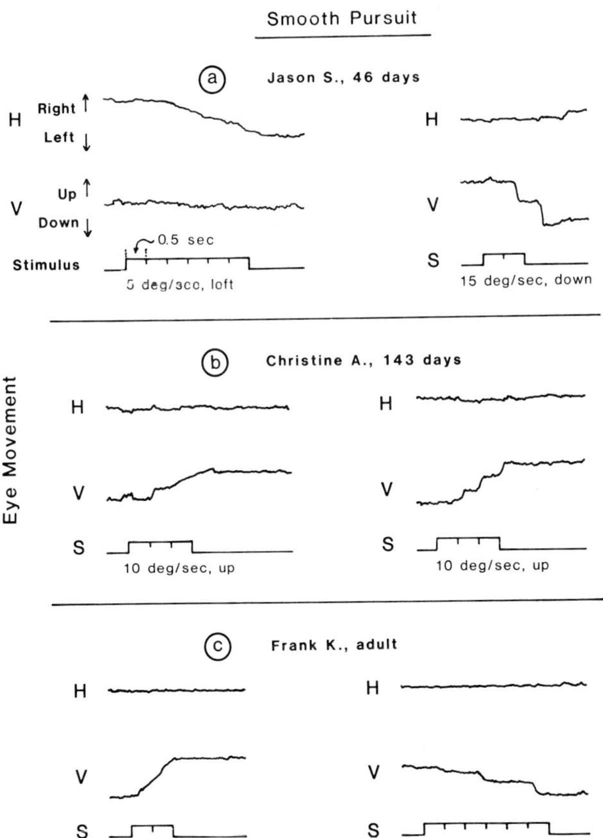

Fig. 2: Examples of smooth pursuit from infants of different ages and an adult. The target was a 1.5 deg. spot. The top trace for each example represents horizontal and the bottom trace vertical eye position, each plotted versus time. Note that the younger infant (Panel a) shows smooth pursuit at lower velocities but not higher velocities. The older infant (Panel b) is able to show smooth pursuit to higher velocities, but does not do so all the time. A naive adult subject (Panel c), capable of smooth pursuit at higher velocities, also shows saccadic pursuit to lower velocities on some trials.

Interestingly, we are also observing that naive adults who have been instructed only to "follow the target" in an unspecified way also, at times, show saccadic pursuit even for relatively low velocities. In these cases, however, we do not doubt that they have functionally mature smooth pursuit systems.

Optokinetic Nystagmus in Infants

Another form of eye movement to moving stimuli is optokinetic nystagmus (OKN), in which alternating episodes of slow and fast movements are elicited by movement of a large portion of the visual field. OKN can be elicited even in neonates, although most of the studies of infant OKN have not provided rigorous quantitative analysis of the properties of the two phases. Most of the existing studies have elicited OKN with full-field motion, but both horizontal and vertical OKN can be elicited for infants with stimuli subtending smaller angles (e.g., 20 to 30 deg.; Hainline, Lemerise, Abramov, and Turkel, 1984).

There have been few reports of marked changes in the characteristics of binocular OKN to horizontally moving stimuli (HOKN), but as indicated, most studies have restricted themselves to qualitative judgements about the presence or absence of the response. An asymmetry in monocular HOKN that decreases with increasing age has been reported in several laboratories (Atkinson, 1979; Naegele and Held, 1982; van-Hof-van Duin and Mohn, 1983); stimulus movement in the nasal to temporal direction initially fails to elicit good HOKN, while temporal to nasal stimulus movement usually is effective as an OKN elicitor. It has been claimed that the development of monocular HOKN symmetry is keyed to the development of binocular function, with the addition of an indirect cortical pathway through the nucleus of the optic tract to supplement an earlier direct pathway responsible for temporal/nasal OKN. However, there is apparently only a very rough correlation between the emergence of measured binocular function (stereopsis) and HOKN symmetry (Braddick and Atkinson, 1983). Whether the maturation of other structures such as the fovea (Tauber and Atkin, 1968) or interhemispheric transfer across the corpus callosum (Mehdorn, 1983) are more related to the emergence of symmetrical monocular HOKN is not at this point known. However, it is well established that individuals with significant problems of binocular vision continue to show, even as adults, a monocular HOKN asymmetry like that seen in normal infants (Schor, 1983).

We have recently completed a study of binocular OKN with both horizontal (HOKN) and vertical (VOKN) stimulus movement in young infants. Rather than filling the whole visual field, our stimuli were what would be classified as "small field" in the context of OKN studies, although the stimuli (30 x 22 deg.) filled a significant portion of the near periphery. Infants' OKN under these conditions showed smooth phases and saccadic fast phases. Their frequency, as measured by the number of slow and fast episodes, was lower than that for adults. While it is known that the frequency of adult OKN is sensitive to the instructions given to the subject, the infant subjects could not, of course, be instructed; this simple difference may account for the differences in OKN frequency for infants and adults, but it is possible, as has been reported for vestibular nystagmus (Eviatar, Miranda, Eviatar, Freeman, and Borkowsky, 1979), that OKN frequency is a measure of the subject's neurological maturity. We also discovered that within

VOKN (a response system that has not been well studied even in adults), infants show a developmental asymmetry such that, for the youngest infants, downward moving stimuli elicit relatively poor OKN, while for infants of all ages, upward moving stimuli elicit good OKN (see Fig. 3). OKN for downward moving targets improves gradually over the first few months of life. Unfortunately, most of our data were collected at only one relatively slow velocity (7 deg./sec); to understand the system better, it is important to use higher velocities.

Some animals, such as adult cat, show a natural VOKN asymmetry like that observed here for young infants (Darlot, Lopez-Barneo, and Tracey, 1981). A similar VOKN asymmetry can be created in adult monkeys, who do not naturally show such an asymmetry, by surgically sectioning interhemispheric connections (Pasik, Pasik, Valcuikas, and Bender, 1971). These observations, coupled with the renewed speculation about the neurological origins of the monocular HOKN asymmetry, support the conclusion that the developmental differences reported in OKN asymmetries are probably caused by real neurological changes in the relevant oculomotor control systems, rather than being the result of problems such as as fluctuations in attention or motivation, often encountered in infancy studies. These findings also imply that changes in OKN asymmetries over age may be of some utility in tracing the development of a number of visual system structures.

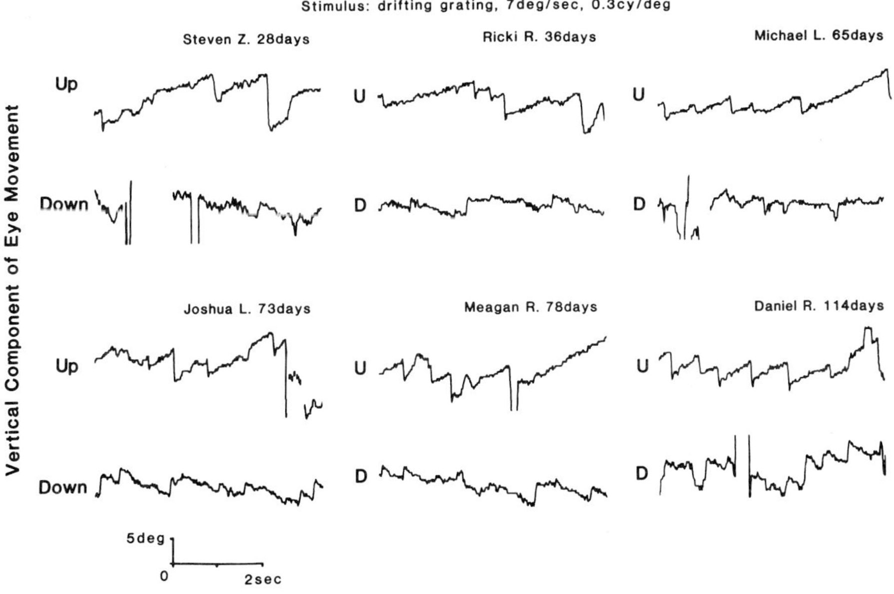

Fig. 3: Examples of binocular vertical OKN from infants of different ages. Only the vertical trace is shown, for trials on which the stimulus moved either up or down. Note that with increasing age, OKN for downward-drifting stimuli acquires the classic biphasic quality, while even at the youngest ages, OKN to upward-drifting stimuli has distinctive slow and fast phases. (From Hainline, Lemerise, Abramov, and Turkel, 1984)

Saccades in Infants

Different conclusions may be warranted from a brief review of the work on infant saccades. Several reports now exist that infants localize small targets by a series of successive small, extremely hypometric saccadic steps (Aslin and Salapatek, 1975; Salapatek, Aslin, Simonson, and Pulos, 1980; Roucoux, et al., 1983), rather than by a single large saccade, or a large saccade followed by a smaller corrective saccade as adults normally do. Infants often accompany their hypometric "steps" of the eye with coordinated "steps" of the head, if head movements are permitted (Regal, Ashmead, and Salapatek, 1983). Some investigators (Aslin, 1981; Shea and Aslin, 1984) have attributed the presence of "step" saccades to an immaturity of the saccadic system itself. We believe, on the contrary, that such behavior may be a very special case, and that in normal circumstances, the saccadic system in infants can be demonstrated to be quite mature. First of all, since it has now been demonstrated that both the eye and the head can be found to show the "step" pattern, it is difficult to regard the problem as being isolated to the saccadic generator. Also, the type of target and the infant's level of arousal may be especially important in influencing what kinds of saccades infants make.

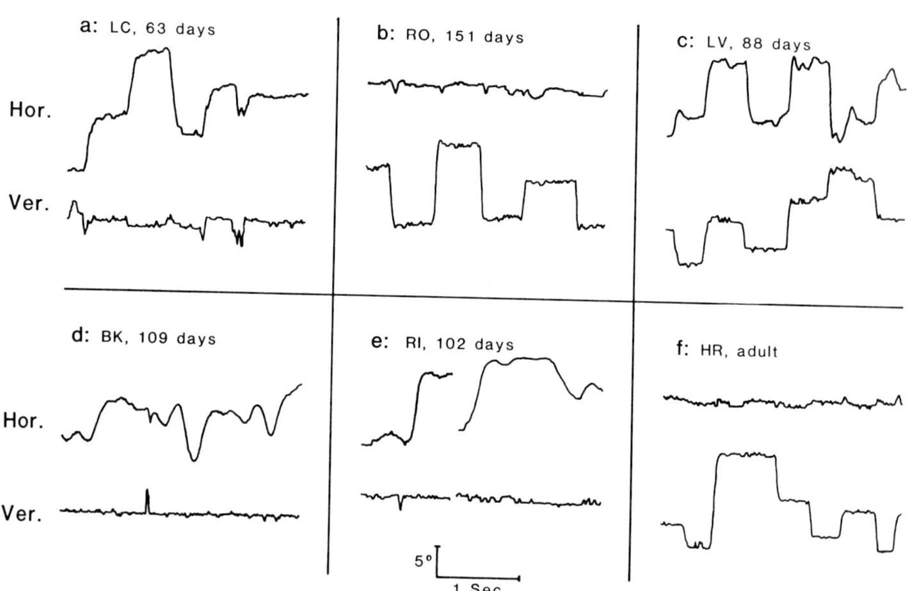

Fig. 4: Examples of saccades from infants and an adult. The top trace represents horizontal and the bottom trace vertical eye position, each plotted versus time. Examples show horizontal (Panel a), vertical (Panel b), and oblique (Panel c) movements from infants of different ages. Panel d illustrates infant saccadic oscillation, while Panel e shows an example of a slow saccade from an infant who also makes saccades with normal peak velocities. Panel f shows adult saccades for comparison. (From Hainline, Turkel, Abramov, Lemerise, and Harris, 1984).

In a recently completed study of infant saccades (Hainline, Turkel, Abramov, Lemerise, and Harris, 1984), we recorded scanning of simple visual stimuli that filled a significant portion of the central visual field. Stimuli were presented for a number of seconds, while spontaneous or "free-scanning" saccades were recorded. Unlike the earlier studies, no attempt was made to "elicit" eye movements to particular locations by flashing small targets. Two results of that study are of particular relevance here. First, the frequency of multiple "step" saccades, reported to be the norm in other studies, was so low as to neglible. Single saccades were the rule (see Fig. 4). Further, the saccades that infants made (at least for one type of stimulus) were adult-like, both in their peak velocity/amplitude (or main sequence, see Bahill, Clark and Stark, 1975) properties, and in the mean and distribution of their saccadic amplitudes (see Fig. 5). Although in this stimulus situation, it could not be determined what the intended target of any given saccade was, the fact that the adult and infant amplitudes are so similar suggests that the two groups had intended targets at similar eccentricities. These findings are consistent with a relatively mature saccadic system early in life.

We feel that the strong differences in saccade morphology in this as compared with earlier studies are due to two factors: first, we believe that the pattern of small steps toward a target in the periphery reflects not

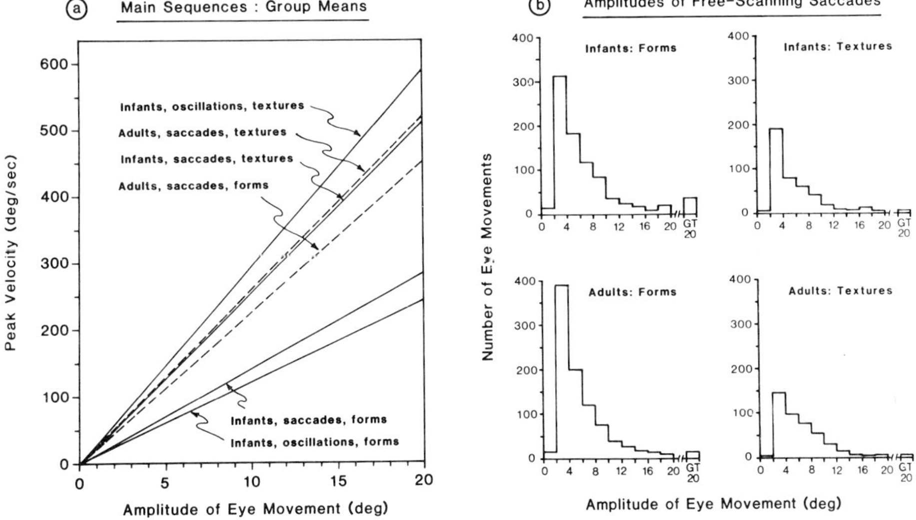

Fig. 5: Panel a shows average main sequence curves for infants and adults for two types of visual stimuli. For the infants, separate main sequence curves have been calculated for saccadic oscillations and non-oscillating saccades within a given stimulus set. It is clear that the oscillations are in fact back-to-back saccades. Infant saccades to simple geometric forms are significantly slower than saccades infants make to more highly textured stimuli or than adult saccades. Panel b contains amplitude histograms for infants and adults for the two stimulus types. Within a stimulus set, infants and adults show similar distributions of saccadic amplitudes.

saccadic immaturity, per se, but problems in correctly localizing small targets in the absence of visual details and contours extending from the present fixational target into the periphery; such cues may be important to allow a metrically correct judgement of target location. Since infants make directionally correct but metrically incorrect movements when the target appears in the periphery, they appear to "know", as it were, in what direction the target is, but not the distance of the target from their current fixation. If our hypothesis is correct, we predict that eliciting saccades with targets embedded in a background with some visible contours should result in more accurate saccadic localization than seen with targets on a featureless background; we plan to carry out such a study soon.

A second possible explanation for the unusual form of step saccadic localization involves attentional factors. In our studies of "free-scanning" saccades, we recorded saccades made by infants to two different types of stimuli: relatively austere geometric shapes (plane geometric triangles, squares and circles varying in angular subtense on an unpatterned background), and gradients of lines and textures filling most of the central visual field. The texture stimuli contained more pattern elements, and were of a type that would be predicted to elicit more attention from infants than the shapes would, based on the large literature on infant pattern preferences (see, e.g., Fantz, Fagan, and Miranda, 1975; Salapatek, 1975). While their saccades to the texture stimuli were in many ways adult-like (described above), for the simple geometric forms, infants made saccades that were both much slower and often of a very unusual form (Fig. 4c and d). While we did not notice an increase in "step" saccades for the geometric forms, we did note a high proportion of back-to-back saccades or saccadic oscillations to that type of stimulus, a pattern rare in the infants' texture data sets and in the adult records. We believe that these unusual properties were influenced by the lower level of arousal caused by the relatively boring geometric stimuli. Since both the mechanisms for basic arousal and saccade generation lie in the brain stem, it seems reasonable to posit some correlation between them. The small targets used in the previous work simply may not have elicited the most mature behaviors of which infants are capable because these stimuli were not sufficiently interesting.

Since it is necessary to keep infants interested in repetitive and rapidly boring stimuli in order to obtain a good gauge of their saccadic competence, in a recent study of elicited saccades (done in collaboration with Christopher Harris) we added sound effects located in a position to cause non-specific orienting to the stimulus screen on which the saccadic targets are presented. We are observing that while the frequency of multiple saccades is higher than we had seen in the studies of free-scanning saccades, their frequency is substantially lower than had previously been reported. Thus, some of the observed hypometria may be the product of attentional/motivational factors. More examples of saccades when infants are known to be very alert are needed to separate factors having to do with arousal from intrinsic oculomotor immaturities.

Fixational Control in Infants

We have suggested that as a result of foveal immaturities, oculomotor behaviors in the young infant may rely proportionally more on parafoveal and peripheral regions of the retina. We have yet to find, however, a clear demonstration that the immaturity of the central fovea adversely influences most oculomotor systems. Rather, when tested under conditions that maximize the infant's alertness and motivation to perform, most of the oculomotor systems that have been studied actually seem to have a surprising degree of functional maturity quite early in life. The asymmetries in monocular HOKN and binocular VOKN are, however, exceptions to the general observation that developments in oculomotor behaviors do not appear to be tied to basic neuromuscular immaturities. Another system in which the lack of a fully functioning fovea might be a major handicap is in the control of fixation, particularly of small targets. Good fixational control requires the ability to detect slippage of the retinal image over the photoreceptors and appropriate correctional strategies to compensate for this slippage.

On the basis of our previous work, we have hypothesized that for infants, fixational control may be both stimulus and arousal dependent. We are currently carrying out a rigorous quantitative analysis of infant fixational control for four types of stimuli: 1) 2 deg. "elicited" saccade targets presented on an unpatterned background, 2) simple 5 to 30 deg. geometric shapes, 3) more complex and highly contoured textures, and 4) several very complex colored slides of realistic scenes. The stimuli can be ordered on the amount of parafoveal and peripheral contour present, on the average, for each fixation. We are currently evaluating whether infants' fixations are in fact better for targets with a greater amount of parafoveal and peripheral contour that can facilitate the detection, by non-foveal areas, of retinal slip. At this point, we have observed that while the nature of the stimulus may exert some influence on the quality of fixations, even very young infants are capable of very stable fixations, with little drift or "wobble" although the same infants also show episodes of fixations with considerable drifts (see Fig. 6). Whether differences in behavioral state or

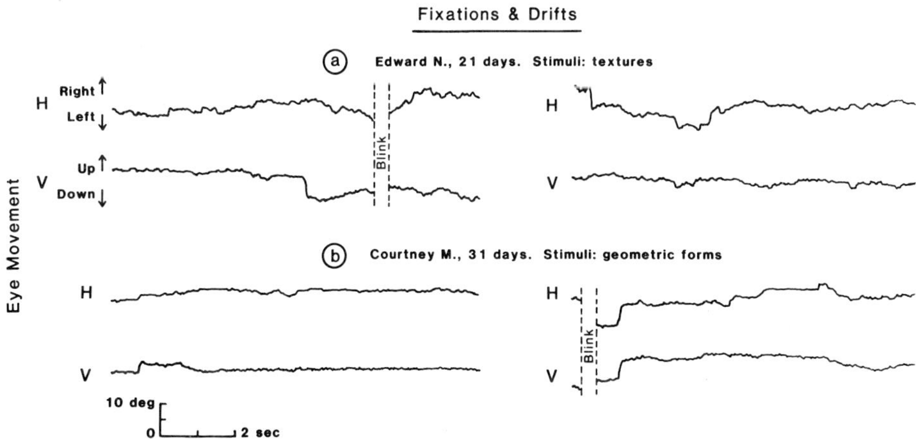

Fig. 6: Examples of fixations and drifts from young infants. The top trace shows horizontal and the bottom trace vertical eye position, each plotted versus time. Panel a shows two 10 second periods of data for a young infant viewing textured stimuli. Panel b shows two 10 second periods from a young infant viewing geometric shapes. In both cases, the infants show long periods of very stable fixation, but also large slow drifts in both horizontal and vertical position.

arousal can help explain these variations in behavior remains to be established. However, it is clear at this point that whatever foveal immaturities young infants may possess, their state of foveal development does not preclude reasonable fixational control much of the time.

To summarize: the special problems involved in studies of oculomotor control with infants require somewhat different research tactics than would be needed in comparable studies with adults. To control for possible confounds with level of arousal and behavioral state, the researcher must strive to make the experimental setting as interesting and varied as possible, often by literally adding "bells and whistles" to the stimulus display. Even so, it is going to be necessary to replicate the finding of unusual eye movement properties with a number of different stimuli or experimental paradigms, ideally across different laboratories, to establish the generality of a given behavior. At this point in the work on oculomotor development, we are surprised at how mature many infant behaviors are when tested under optimal conditions. While this is an interesting observation in its own right, we feel that it also opens possibilities for the early detection of oculomotor abnormalities accompanying visual disabilities that may be otherwise difficult to detect in infancy. Thus, increasingly, measures of oculomotor behavior may be added to the growing list of techniques for early visual assessment.

Acknowledgements

This work was supported in part by grant EY03957 from the Eye Institute of the National Institutes of Health and by Grants 661078, 662199, and 663127 from the PSC-CUNY Research Award Program of the City University of New York. Facilities for computer analysis were provided by the University Computer Center of the City University of New York. I wish to thank Dr. David Kliot and Downstate Medical Center for their assistance in recruiting subjects, and also the infants and their parents for participating in the research. I also gratefully acknowledge assistance of Elizabeth Lemerise, Israel Abramov, Christopher Harris, Johan de Bie, and Cheryl Camenzuli in what is necessarily a collaborative research effort.

References

[1] Abramov, I., Gordon, J., Hendrickson, A., Hainline, L., Dobson, V., and LaBossiere, E., The retina of the newborn human infant, Science 217 (1982) 265-267.

[2] Aslin, R.N., Development of smooth pursuit in human infants, in: Fisher, D.F., Monty, R.A., and Senders, J.W. (eds.), Eye Movements: Cognition and Visual Perception (Erlbaum, Hillsdale, N.J., 1981).

[3] Aslin, R.N. and Salapatek, P., Saccadic localization of visual targets by the very young human infant, Perc. & Psychophys. 17 (1975) 293-302.

[4] Atkinson, J., Development of optokinetic nystagmus in the human infant and monkey infant: an analogue to development in kittens, in: Freeman, R.D. (ed.), Developmental Neurobiology of Vision (Plenum Press, New York, 1979).

[5] Atkinson, J. and Braddick, O., Development of optokinetic nystagmus in infants: an indication of cortical binocularity?, in: Fisher, D.F., Monty, R.A., and Senders, J.W. (eds.), Eye Movements: Cognition and Visual Perception (Erlbaum, Hillsdale, N.J., 1981).

[6] Bach, L. and Seefelder, R., Atlas zur Entwicklungsgeschichte des menschlichen Auges (Engelmann, Leipzig, 1914).

[7] Bahill, A.T., Clark, M.R., and Stark, L., The main sequence, a tool for studying human eye movements, Math. Biosci. 24 (1975) 191-204.

[8] Braddick, O. and Atkinson, J., Some recent findings on the development of binocularity: a review, Behav. Brain Res. 10 (1983) 141-150.

[9] Collewijn, H., The optokinetic system, in: Zuber, B.L. (ed.), Models of Oculomotor Behavior and Control (CRC Press, Boca Raton, Florida, 1981).

[10] Darlot, C., Lopez-Barneo, J., and Tracey, D., Asymmetry of vertical vestibular nystagmus in the cat, Exp. Brain Res. 41 (1981) 420-426.

[11] Dobson, V. and Teller, D., Assessment of visual acuity in infants, in: Armington, J.C., Krauskopf, J., and Wooten, B.R. (eds.), Visual Psychophysics and Physiology (Academic Press, New York, 1978).

[12] Eviatar, L., Miranda, S., Eviatar, A., Freeman, K., and Borkowski, M., Development of nystagmus in response to vestibular stimulation in infants, Ann. Neurol. 5 (1979) 508-514.

[13] Fantz, R.L., Fagan, J.F., and Miranda, S.B., Early visual selectivity, in: Cohen, L.B. and Salapatek, P. (eds.), Infant Perception: From Sensation to Cognition, Vol. 1 (Academic Press, New York, 1975).

[14] Hainline, L., An automated eye movement recording system for use with human infants, Behav. Res. Meth. Instr. 13 (1981) 20-24.

[15] Hainline, L., Lemerise, E., Abramov, I., and Turkel, J., Orientational asymmetries in small-field optokinetic nystagmus in human infants, Behav. Brain Res. (in press, August, 1984).

[16] Hainline, L., Turkel, J., Abramov, I., Lemerise, E., and Harris, C.M., Characteristics of saccades in human infants, Vis. Res. (in press, August, 1984).

[17] Harris, C.M., Abramov, I., and Hainline, L., Instrument considerations in measuring fast eye movements, Behav. Res. Meth. Instr. (in press, August, 1984).

[18] Harris, C.M., Hainline, L., and Abramov, I., A method for calibrating an eye-monitoring system for use with human infants, Behav. Res. Meth. Instr. 13 (1981) 11-20.

[19] Hood, J.D. and Leech, J., The significance of peripheral vision in the perception of movement, Acta Otolaryng. 77 (1974) 72-79.

[20] Kremenitzer, J.P., Vaughan, H.G., Kurtzberg, D., and Dowling, K., Smooth-pursuit eye movements in the newborn infant, Child Dev. 50 (1979) 442-448.

[21] Mann, I., The Development of the Human Eye (British Medical Association, London, 1964).

[22] Mehdorn, E., Optokinetic asymmetries in split brain patient, Invest. Ophthal. Vis. Science Suppl. 24 (1983) 23.

[23] Muir, D., Abraham, W., Forbes, B., and Harris, L., The ontogenesis of an auditory localization response from birth to four months of age, Canadian J. Psychol. 33 (1979) 320-333.

[24] Naegele, J.R. and Held, R., The postnatal development of monocular optokinetic nystagmus in infants, Vis. Res. 22 (1982) 341-346.

[25] Pasik, P., Pasik, T., Valcuikas, J.A., and Bender, M.B., Vertical optokinetic nystagmus in the split-brain monkey, Exp. Neurol. 30 (1971) 162-171.

[26] Piaget, J., The Origins of Intelligence in the Child (International Universities Press, New York, 1952).

[27] Regal, D.M., Ashmead, D.H., and Salapatek, P., The coordination of eye and hand movements during early infancy: a selective review, Behav. Brain Res. 10 (1983) 125-132.

[28] Roucoux, A., Culee, C., and Roucoux, M., Development of fixation and pursuit eye movements in human infants, Behav. Brain Res. 10 (1983) 133-139.

[29] Salapatek, P., Pattern perception in early infancy, in: Cohen, L.B. and Salapatek, P. (eds.), Infant Perception: From Sensation to Cognition Vol. 1 (Academic Press, New York, 1975).

[30] Salapatek, P., Aslin, R.N., Simonson, J., and Pulos, E., Infant saccadic eye movements to visible and previously invisible targets, Child Dev. 51 (1980) 1090-1094.

[31] Schor, C.M., Directional anisotropia of pursuit tracking and optokinetic nystagmus in abnormal binocular vision, Amer. J. Opt. 60 (1983) 481-502.

[32] Shea, S. and Aslin, R.N., Development of horizontal and vertical pursuit in human infants, Invest. Ophthal. Vis. Science Suppl. 25 (1984) 263.

[33] Spelke, E., Infants' intermodal perception of events, Cog. Psychol. 8 (1976) 553-560.

[34] Tauber, E.S. and Atkin, A., Optomotor responses to monocular stimulation: relation to visual system organization, Science 160 (1968) 1365.

[35] van Hof-van Duin, J. and Mohn, G., Optokinetic and spontaneous nystagmus in children with neurological disorders, Behav. Brain Res. 10 (1983) 163-175.

Eye Movements and Human Information Processing
R. Groner, G.W. McConkie and C. Menz (eds.)

OPTOKINETIC NYSTAGMUS IN CHILDREN TREATED FOR BILATERAL CATARACTS

Terri L. Lewis, Daphne Maurer, & Henry P. Brent

Department of Ophthalmology
The Hospital for Sick Children
Toronto, Ontario, M5G 1X8
Canada

We found an asymmetry of optokinetic nystagmus (OKN) in children who had been binocularly deprived during early infancy because of dense central cataracts: OKN was easy to elicit when stripes moved from the temporal visual field toward the nasal visual field but difficult to elicit when stripes moved in the opposite direction. In contrast, there was no such marked asymmetry in normal subjects or in children who developed dense central cataracts after 18 months of age. We conclude that early binocular deprivation leads to asymmetrical OKN in humans as it does in cats (c.f. van Hof-van Duin, 1978). Possible mechanisms for this asymmetry are discussed.

Introduction

When normal adult cats are tested monocularly, optokinetic nystagmus (OKN) can be elicited easily when a repetitive pattern sweeps across the visual field. This is true whether the pattern moves from right to left or from left to right (c.f. Braun & Gault, 1969). In contrast, cats which were binocularly deprived shortly after birth show nearly normal OKN when a pattern moves from the temporal visual field toward the nasal visual field but little or no OKN when a pattern moves in the opposite direction (Harris, Leporé, Guillemot, & Cynader, 1980; van Hof-van Duin, 1978). Like previous studies (c.f. Atkinson, 1979; Maurer, Lewis, & Brent, 1983), we refer to this difference in the ease of eliciting OKN by patterns moving toward the temporal versus nasal fields as "asymmetrical OKN."

Recent studies in cats have shown that that the nucleus of the optic tract (NOT) in the pretectum is the main link between sensory input from the retina and motor output of OKN through the inferior olive (Hoffmann, Behrend, & Schoppmann, 1976; Hoffmann & Schoppmann, 1975). Single-cell recordings have shown that the left NOT is activated maximally by large patterns moving from right to left, and the right NOT is activated maximally by large patterns moving from left to right (Hoffmann, 1979,

1981, 1983). There are at least three pathways which project to each NOT, two from the contralateral eye and one from the ipsilateral eye (Hoffmann, 1979, 1981, 1983; Hoffmann & Schoppmann, 1975). Figure 1 shows the projections from the right eye to each NOT in the normal cat. Crossed

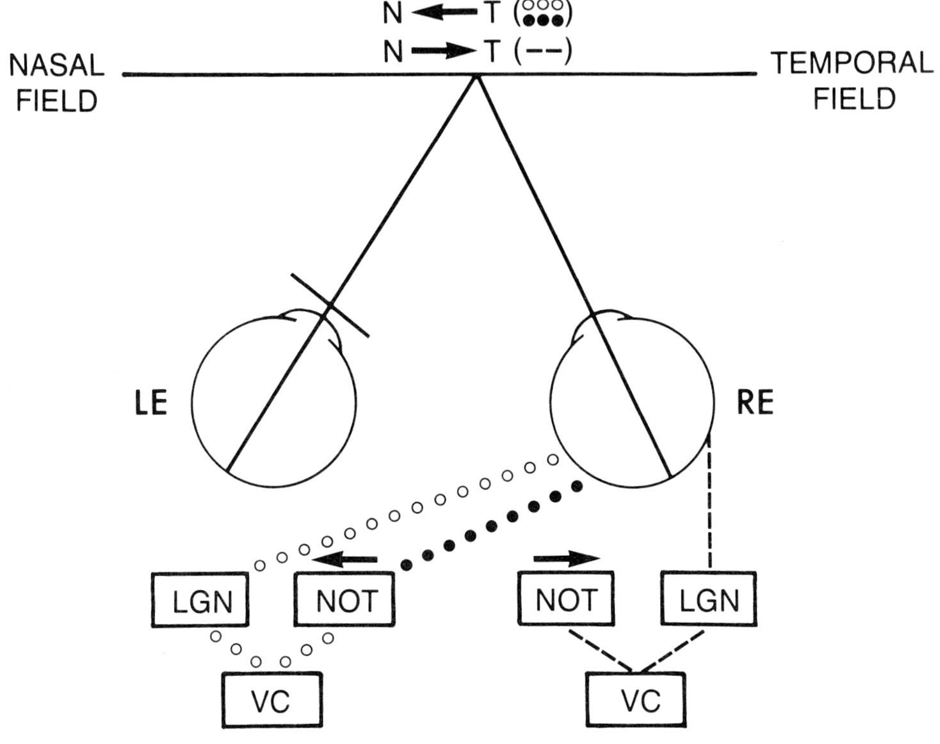

Figure 1
Pathways Projecting from the Right Eye (RE)
to the Nucleus of the Optic Tract (NOT) in the Normal Cat

fibres from the nasal retina of the right eye project directly to the left NOT (... in Figure 1) and indirectly to the left NOT via the left lateral geniculate nucleus (LGN) and binocular cells in Areas 17 and 18 of the left visual cortex (ooo in Figure 1). Uncrossed fibres from the temporal retina of the right eye project to the right NOT only indirectly via the right LGN and binocular cells in Areas 17 and 18 of the right visual cortex (--- in Figure 1). Similarly, the left eye projects to the right NOT both directly and indirectly via the cortex, and to the left NOT only indirectly via the cortex (projections from the left eye are not shown in Figure 1). Clinical evidence suggests that in humans OKN is mediated by similar pathways, with the addition of an interhemispheric connection via the corpus callosum

(Yee, Baloh, Honrubia, & Jenkins, 1982).

In cats, the direct pathway through the contralateral NOT (... in Figure 1) is sufficient to mediate nearly normal OKN when stripes move from the temporal visual field toward the nasal visual field, especially when the stripes move slowly. The indirect pathway through the ipsilateral LGN and visual cortex to the ipsilateral NOT (--- in Figure 1) is necessary for any consistent OKN when stripes move from the nasal visual field toward the temporal visual field (Harris et al., 1980; Hoffmann, 1979, 1981, 1983; Montarolo, Precht, & Strata, 1981). Consequently, in cats with lesions of the visual cortex, OKN can be elicited easily when stripes move from the temporal field toward the nasal field but hardly at all when stripes move in the opposite direction (Hoffmann, 1983; Montarolo et al., 1981; Strong, Malach, & Van Sluyters, 1981; Wood, Spear, & Braun, 1973). Normal kittens (Malach, Strong, & Van Sluyters, 1980, 1981; van Hof-van Duin, 1978), normal infant monkeys (Atkinson, 1979), and normal human infants (Atkinson, 1979; Atkinson & Braddick, 1981; Naegele & Held, 1982, 1983) show a similar asymmetry, presumably because the projection through the visual cortex to NOT is too immature to mediate consistent OKN when stripes move from the nasal field toward the temporal field (reviewed in Maurer & Lewis, 1979). In cats, binocular deprivation during a critical period shortly after birth renders NOT unresponsive to visual input from the cortex (Hoffmann, 1979, 1981, 1983) but leaves intact the direct pathway from the retina to the contralateral NOT (Harris et al., 1980; Hoffmann, 1979, 1981, 1983). As would be expected, such binocularly deprived cats show asymmetrical OKN (Harris et al., 1980; van Hof-van Duin, 1978).

Little is known about the effect of binocular deprivation in humans on the symmetry of OKN. Children treated for congenital cataracts provide an opportunity to study these effects because, like lid suture in cats, a dense central cataract permits only diffuse light to reach the retina. After the cataract is removed surgically and the aphakic eye is fitted with a suitable optical correction, nearly normal visual input is restored. We recently reported an asymmetry of OKN in children treated for monocular deprivation caused by a unilateral congenital cataract (Maurer et al., 1983). The purpose of the experiments described here was to examine the effects of binocular deprivation on the symmetry of OKN by studying children treated for dense, central cataracts in both eyes. The cataracts either were present from birth or developed after six months of age. For comparison, we also tested subjects who had no history of eye problems.

Experiment 1

Method

Subjects

Children treated for congenital cataracts. We tested 6 children aged 1 to 12 years (median age = 3.5 years) who had had congenital cataracts diagnosed by 6 months of age. Four children had had congenital cataracts in both eyes but the data from one of these eyes were excluded because of secondary glaucoma. The remaining two children had had a dense congenital cataract in one eye diagnosed before 6 months of age and then later developed a cataract in the other eye. The two eyes treated for developmental cataracts were included in the group described immediately below. Thus, the final sample of eyes treated for congenital cataracts consisted of 9 eyes of 6 children. The cataracts in these 9 eyes were diagnosed at a median age of 2 months (range birth to 6 months) and in all cases they were dense and central at the time of the first eye examination. The cataracts were removed at a median age of 6.5 months (range 4.5 to 16 months) and the aphakic eyes were first fitted with appropriate optical correction at a median age of 7.5 months (range 6 to 18 months). In all eyes, after surgery there was a clear view of the fundus and there were no abnormalities of the retina or optic disc. Both eyes of one child were microphthalmic.

All children had a history of strabismus and one child had had surgery to correct an esotropia of 40 prism dioptres. At the time of the asymmetry test, the amount of strabismus ranged from 6 to 18 prism dioptres. The median refractive error (spherical equivalent) at the time of the asymmetry test was +20.0 D (range +10.5 to +29.75). Because most of the children were young, linear acuities were available for only two eyes. At the time of the asymmetry test, their acuities were 6/7.5 and 6/15.

Children treated for developmental cataracts. We also tested 9 children aged 2 to 17 years (median age = 7.5 years) who had developed cataracts after 6 months of age. In all cases, the eyes with developmental cataracts had shown no evidence of any ocular abnormality during the first 6 months. Seven children then developed cataracts in both eyes; the remaining two children had had a congenital cataract in one eye (see above) but only later developed a cataract in the other eye. Thus, the final sample of eyes treated for developmental cataracts consisted of 16 eyes of 9 children. The cataracts in these 16 eyes were diagnosed as dense and central at a median age of 30 months (range 7.5 months to 10 years). The cataracts were removed surgically at a median age of 34.5 months (range 9 months to 10 years) and the aphakic eyes were first fitted with an appropriate optical correction at a median age of 35 months (range 13 months to 10 years). In every case, after surgery there was a clear view of the fundus, and there were no abnormalities of the retina or optic disc.

All children had a history of strabismus and one child had had strabismus surgery for an esotropia of 40 prism dioptres at near and 16 prism dioptres at far. At the time of the asymmetry test, the amount of strabismus ranged from 4 to 25 prism dioptres. The median refractive error (spherical equivalent) at the time of the asymmetry test was +13.25 D (range +11.0 to +18.5). Seven children were old enough to read a Snellen eye chart and their median linear acuity at the time of the asymmetry test was 6/10.5 (range 6/6 to 6/120).

Normal controls. The normal control subjects (n=46) ranged in age from 1 year to adulthood (median age = 4 years) and had no history of eye problems. We tested the right eye of half the subjects and the left eye of the other half.

Apparatus and procedure

The apparatus and procedure have been described elsewhere (Maurer et al., 1983). Briefly, the child wore a patch over one eye and sat 50 cm. from a 90° x 90° rear projection screen surrounded by black plywood. Black-and-white vertical stripes (square wave gratings of 0.6 cycles/deg) were swept across the screen horizontally at a velocity of 13 deg/sec by a 35 mm slide projector projecting through a rotating mirror. Shielded peepholes on either side of the screen permitted an observer to see the child's unoccluded eye but not the stimuli. The test included 39 randomly ordered 7-sec trials: 15 trials with stripes moving from the temporal field toward the nasal field, 15 trials with stripes moving from the nasal field toward the temporal field, and 9 control trials during which no stripes were presented. The observer decided during each trial whether OKN definitely occurred, possibly occurred, or definitely did not occur.

Results

On control trials, when no stripes were presented, the observer never reported definite OKN for any subject in any group. To analyze the data from experimental trials, we used a two-tailed X^2 test for each eye to compare the frequency of trials on which OKN was judged definitely to occur when stripes moved from the temporal visual field toward the nasal visual field versus the frequency when stripes moved in the opposite direction.

Figure 2 shows the difference between these two frequencies for each eye tested. A positive difference score means that definite OKN was observed on a greater proportion of trials when stripes moved from the temporal field toward the nasal field than when they moved in the opposite direction. Conversely, a negative difference score means that OKN was observed on a greater proportion of trials when stripes moved from the nasal field toward the temporal field than when they moved in the opposite direction. An asterisk indicates that a difference was significant in that eye by the X^2 test (i.e. asymmetrical OKN) and a dot indicates that a difference was not significant (i.e. symmetrical OKN).

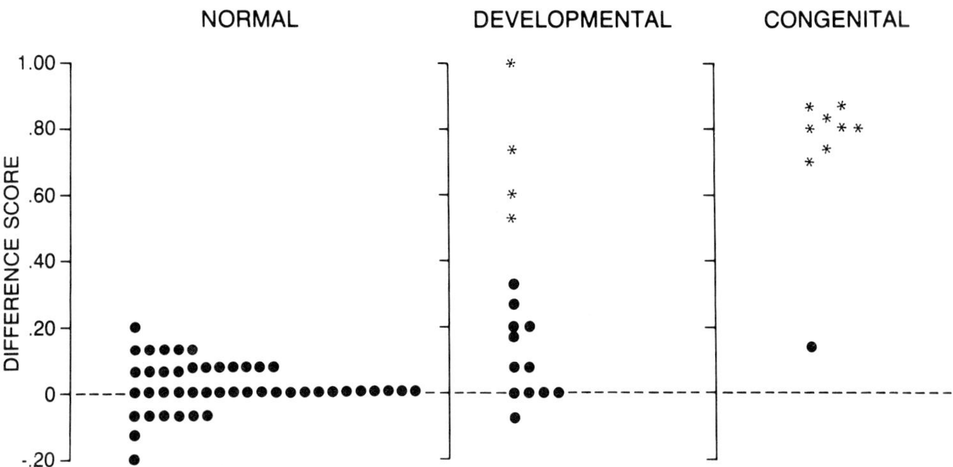

Figure 2
Differences in the Proportion of Trials with OKN for Stripes Moving Temporally to Nasally versus Nasally to Temporally

For normal subjects, OKN was observed on most experimental trials. When stripes moved from the temporal field toward the nasal field, OKN was observed on a median of 100% of the trials (range = 73 to 100%) and when stripes moved from the nasal field toward the temporal field, OKN was observed on a median of 93% of the trials (range = 73 to 100%). The difference scores for individual subjects tended to cluster around zero and in no individual case was there a significant asymmetry by the X^2 test (see Figure 2). To test whether, nevertheless, a small asymmetry might be significant in the group as a whole, we used a Wilcoxon test to compare the mean proportion of trials with OKN when stripes moved temporally to nasally versus the mean proportion of trials with OKN when stripes moved nasally to temporally. The test was not significant, $\underline{T}(25) = 94.0$, $\underline{p} > .1$.

In contrast, eyes treated for congenital cataracts showed OKN more frequently when stripes moved from the temporal field toward the nasal field than when they moved in the opposite direction: OKN was observed on a median of 87% of the trials (range = 67 to 100%) when stripes moved temporally to nasally but only on a median of 11.5% of the trials (range = 6 to 53%) when stripes moved nasally to temporally. In this group all of the difference scores were positive and X^2 tests revealed a significant asymmetry in 8 of the 9 individual eyes tested (see Figure 2).

Eyes treated for developmental cataracts fell between these two extremes. When stripes moved from the temporal field toward the nasal field, OKN was observed on a median of 93% of the trials (range = 30 to 100%) and when stripes moved from the nasal field toward the temporal field, OKN was observed on a median of 75% of the trials (range = 0 to

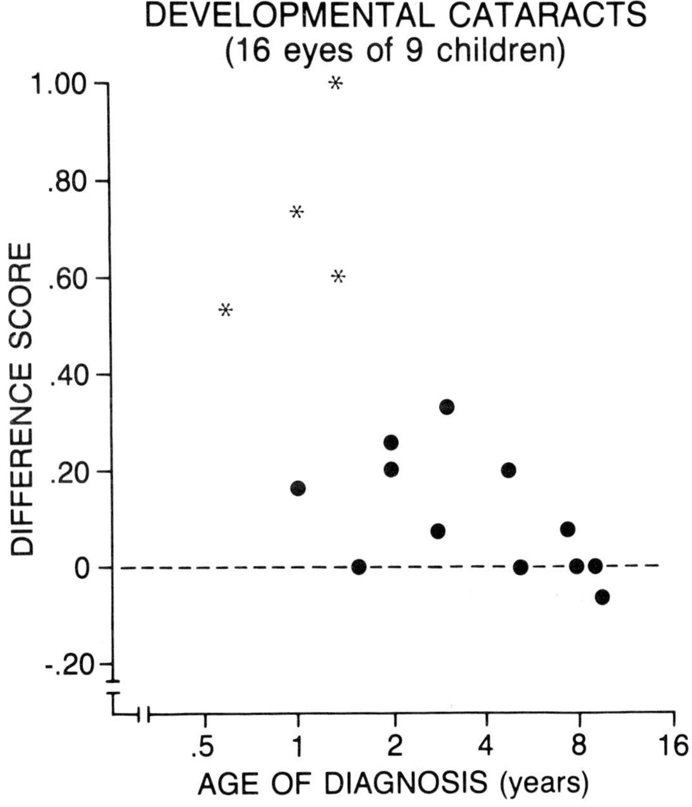

Figure 3
Symmetry of OKN for the Developmental Group Plotted as a Function of Age of Diagnosis of a Dense Central Cataract

100%). The difference scores for individual eyes ranged from below zero to 100% and X^2 tests showed that there was a significant asymmetry in 4 of the 16 individual eyes (see Figure 2). However, for this group, the age at which a dense cataract was first detected varied from 7.5 months to 10 years. Figure 3 shows the difference score for each child plotted as a function of the age at which a dense cataract was diagnosed. As in Figure 2, an asterisk indicates a significant asymmetry in an individual eye and a dot indicates no asymmetry. As shown in Figure 3, children who developed cataracts at a younger age were more likely to show asymmetrical OKN than children who developed cataracts at an older age. In fact, there was a significant asymmetry in 4 of the 5 eyes which developed cataracts before 18 months of age but in none of the 11 eyes which developed cataracts after 18 months of age.

To examine further the effects of deprivation on the symmetry of OKN, we located each eye on a plot of the age at which a dense, central cataract was diagnosed versus the length of deprivation. (We defined length of deprivation as the time from the diagnosis of a dense, central cataract until the cataract was removed surgically and the aphakic eye fitted with an appropriate optical correction.) Figure 4 includes each eye of the congenital group (_N_= 9) and of the developmental group (_N_ = 16). An eye is plotted with an asterisk if it showed a significant asymmetry of OKN by χ^2 tests but with a dot if it showed no significant asymmetry. The vertical dashed line separates eyes which had cataracts diagnosed before and after 18 months of age.

Figure 4 suggests that there was no effect of the length of deprivation on the symmetry of OKN. Most of the 14 eyes which had cataracts diagnosed before 18 months of age showed asymmetrical OKN regardless of the length of deprivation (see Figure 4). Moreover, the size of the asymmetry (not shown in Figure 4) was as large in the 5 eyes with 5 to 6 months of deprivation as in the 4 eyes with 12 to 18 months of deprivation. In contrast, none of the 11 eyes which developed cataracts after 18 months of age showed asymmetrical OKN even though 6 of these eyes were deprived for more than 5 months (see Figure 4). However, since the 3 eyes in which a dense cataract was first diagnosed between 18 months and 3 years all had relatively short periods of deprivation (see Figure 4), it is possible that longer deprivation might have an effect on the symmetry of OKN up to 3 years of age. Clearly after 3 years of age, 5 to 14 months of

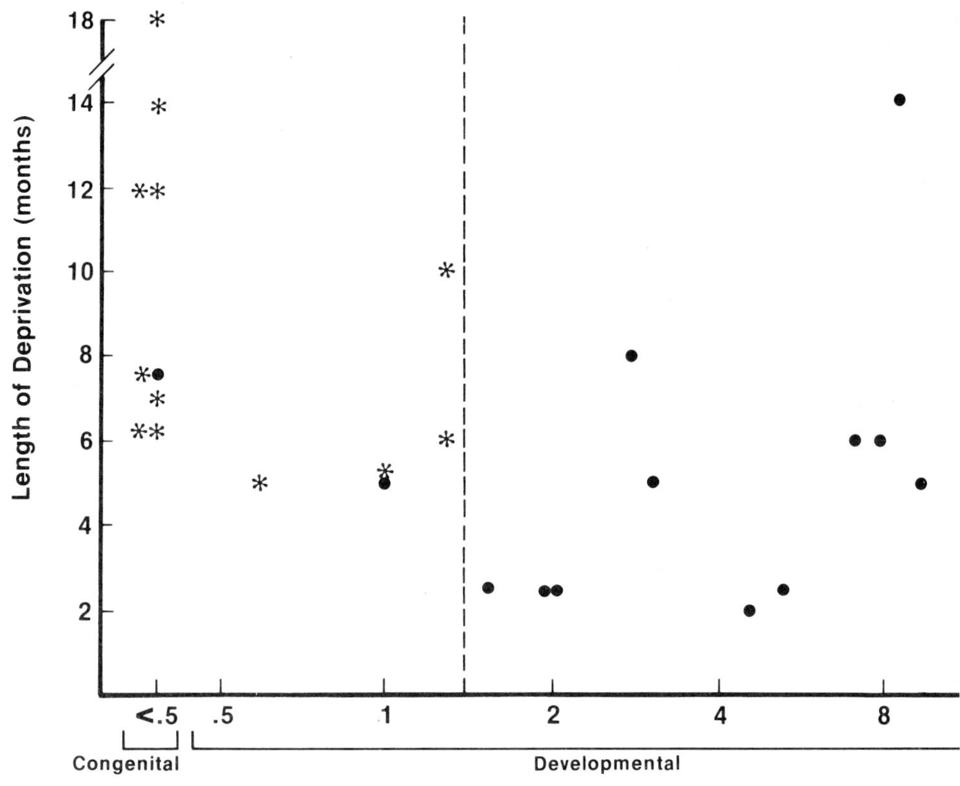

Figure 4
Length of Deprivation Plotted as a Function of Age of Diagnosis of a Dense Central Cataract

deprivation has no effect on the symmetry of OKN as measured in this experiment.

Discussion

Most children treated for bilateral cataracts showed asymmetrical OKN when a dense, central cataract had been diagnosed by 18 months of age. Thus, they showed OKN significantly more often when stripes moved from the temporal visual field toward the nasal visual field than when stripes moved in the opposite direction. This was true for 8 of 9 eyes which had been deprived from birth (congenital group) and for 4 of 5 eyes in the developmental group which had a normal early history and then developed a dense cataract between 7 and 17 months of age. In contrast, subjects with no history of eye disorders (normal group) and children in the developmental groups who had a normal early history and then developed dense cataracts after 18 months of age showed no such gross asymmetry. Thus, the timing of deprivation appears to be important for determining whether or not OKN is symmetrical.

In contrast, we found no effects of length of deprivation on the symmetry of OKN: Most eyes which suffered deprivation before 18 months showed asymmetrical OKN following as little as 6 months of deprivation and the asymmetry was as large after 6 months of deprivation as after 12 to 18 months of deprivation. Of course, it is possible that periods of deprivation shorter than 6 months might have less effect. Similarly, eyes which were deprived later might show asymmetrical OKN after longer periods of deprivation.

Another limitation on our conclusions is that the measure of asymmetry in Experiment 1 was fairly insensitive: On each trial we recorded only whether or not OKN had occurred and then, for each child, determined whether OKN occurred on more trials when stripes moved temporally to nasally than when they moved in the opposite direction. A more sensitive test might reveal gradations in asymmetry for eyes with different lengths of deprivation or for eyes with cataracts diagnosed at birth versus diagnosed between 6 and 18 months. A more sensitive test also might reveal a subtle asymmetry in eyes with cataracts diagnosed after 18 months of age. Consequently, in Experiment 2, we timed the duration of OKN during each trial and retested a subsample of the children from Experiment 1.

Experiment 2

Method

Subjects

The subjects were a subsample of the subjects tested in Experiment 1. The congenital group consisted of 4 eyes (from 3 children) in which cataracts had been diagnosed as dense and central before 6 months of age. The developmental group consisted of 6 eyes (from 4 children) which had developed cataracts after 6 months of age. The normal control group consisted of 20 subjects ranging in age from 3 years to adulthood (median = 4 years).

Apparatus and procedure

The apparatus and procedure were identical to that described in Experiment 1 except that during each 7-sec trial, the observer pushed a timer whenever she observed definite OKN.

Results

For no subject was OKN ever observed on control trials, when no stripes were presented. To analyze the data from the experimental trials, we used a two-tailed Mann-Whitney U test for each eye to compare the duration of OKN when stripes moved from the temporal field toward the nasal field versus the duration when stripes moved from the nasal field toward the temporal field. Figure 5 shows the difference between these two durations for each eye tested. A positive difference score means that the

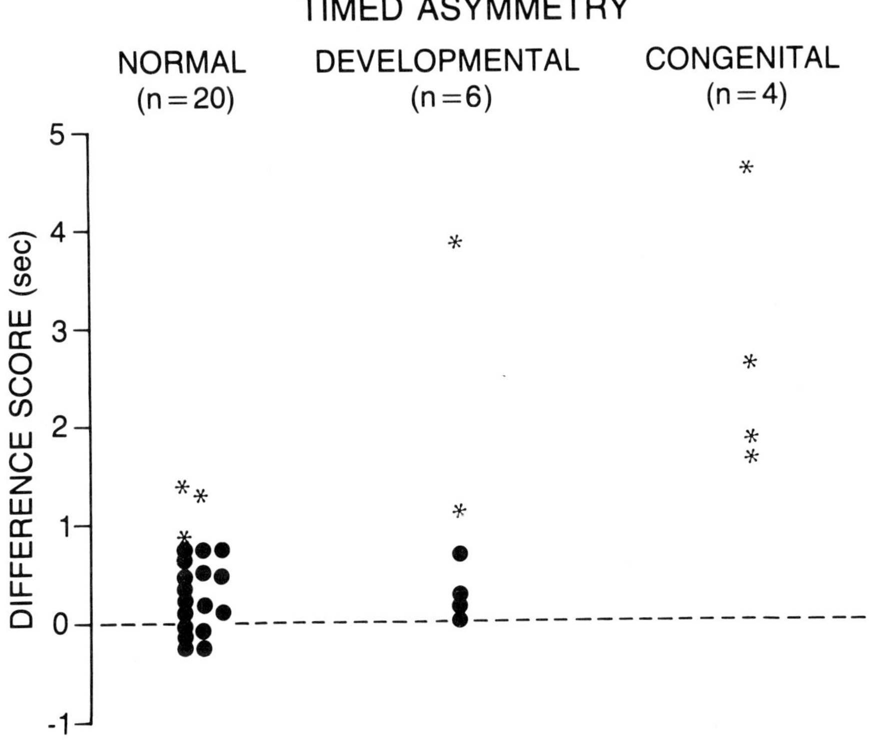

Figure 5
Differences in the Duration of OKN for Stripes Moving Temporally to Nasally versus Nasally to Temporally

duration of OKN was longer when stripes moved temporally to nasally than when they moved nasally to temporally. Conversely, a negative difference score means that the duration of OKN was longer when stripes moved nasally to temporally than when they moved temporally to nasally. An asterisk indicates that the difference in that eye was significant by the

Mann-Whitney U test (i.e. asymmetrical OKN) and a dot indicates that the difference was not significant (i.e. symmetrical OKN).

Normal group. For the 20 normal subjects, the mean duration of OKN during the 7-sec trials was 4.07 sec (range 2.59 to 5.40 sec) when stripes moved from the temporal field toward the nasal field and 3.69 sec (range = 2.47 to 5.43 sec) when stripes moved from the nasal field toward the temporal field. The difference scores for individual subjects ranged from -0.24 to +1.37 sec (M = +0.38 sec) and in only 3 of the 20 eyes was there a significant asymmetry (see Figure 5). To see whether there was a significant asymmetry in the group as a whole, we used a Wilcoxon T-test to compare the mean duration of OKN when stripes moved temporally to nasally versus the mean duration of OKN when stripes moved nasally to temporally. The test revealed a significant asymmetry of OKN in the normal group $T(20) = 26.5$, $p < .01$.

Congenital group. All 4 eyes treated for congenital cataracts showed longer durations of OKN when stripes moved from the temporal field toward the nasal field than when they moved in the opposite direction: When stripes moved temporally to nasally, the mean duration of OKN was 3.03 sec (range 2.06 to 4.88 sec) but when stripes moved nasally to temporally, the mean duration of OKN was only 0.39 sec (range 0.27 to 0.72 sec). All of the difference scores were positive and there was a significant asymmetry in each of the 4 eyes tested. The asymmetries observed in the 4 eyes from the congenital group were all larger than any observed in an eye from the normal control group (see Figure 5). Each of the 4 eyes from the congenital group had also shown a significant asymmetry of OKN in Experiment 1, and eyes showing larger difference scores calculated from proportion of trials with OKN (Experiment 1) also tended to have larger difference scores calculated from duration of OKN (Experiment 2).

Developmental group. For the developmental group, the mean duration of OKN was 4.19 sec (range 2.31 to 5.59 sec) when stripes moved from the temporal field toward the nasal field and 3.19 sec (range 0.43 to 5.37 sec) when stripes moved from the nasal field toward the temporal field. The difference scores ranged from 0 to 3.83 sec and there was a significant asymmetry in 2 of the 6 eyes tested. As seen in the congenital group, eyes showing larger difference scores comparing proportion of trials with OKN (Experiment 1) also tended to have larger difference scores comparing duration of OKN (Experiment 2). For 5 of 6 eyes, the presence or absence of an asymmetry was the same whether the asymmetry was calculated from the proportion of trials with OKN (Experiment 1) or from the duration of OKN (Experiment 2). For the remaining eye, an asymmetry of OKN was revealed only by measuring the duration of OKN. However, the difference in mean duration of OKN for stripes moving temporally to nasally versus nasally to temporally was only 1.16 sec in this eye, well within the range of differences observed in our normal group (see Figure 5).

Discussion

The duration of OKN (Experiment 2) proved to be a more sensitive measure of asymmetrical OKN than the proportion of trials on which OKN occurred (Experiment 1). Timing the duration of OKN (Experiment 2) revealed a significant asymmetry in 3 individual eyes of normal subjects and in the normal control group as a whole. In contrast, determining the proportion of trials with OKN revealed no such asymmetries either in the entire normal sample tested in Experiment 1 nor in the subsample also tested in Experiment 2.

Our finding of some asymmetry in the normal control group is not surprising. Electrophysiological studies in normal cats have shown that when stripes are viewed monocularly, all cells in the NOT contralateral to the open eye respond to movement from the temporal visual field toward the nasal visual field, but only about half the cells in the NOT ipsilateral to the open eye respond to movement from the nasal visual field toward the temporal visual field (Hoffmann, 1981, 1983). Thus, tests of normal cats sometimes reveal a small asymmetry of OKN (Cynader & Harris, 1980; Hoffmann, 1981, 1983; Malach et al., 1981) but sometimes do not (Braun & Gault, 1969; Hoffmann, 1983; Malach et al., 1980, 1981).

Although the duration of OKN proved a more sensitive measure of asymmetry than the proportion of trials with OKN, Experiment 2 confirmed the main conclusions drawn in Experiment 1. Specifically, eyes with dense cataracts early in life showed more frequent and larger asymmetries of OKN than did eyes in the normal control group. In contrast, eyes which developed dense cataracts after 18 months of age showed asymmetries of OKN no different from those observed in the normal control group.

General Discussion

We found an asymmetry of OKN in most eyes of bilateral aphakes treated for congenital cataracts. This was true both when we compared the proportion of trials with definite OKN for stripes moving from the temporal field toward the nasal field versus from the nasal field toward the temporal field (Experiment 1) and when we compared the duration of OKN for stripes moving in the two directions (Experiment 2). There have been no previously published studies of the asymmetry of OKN in humans who had been deprived binocularly of pattern vision. However, unpublished findings by C.M. Schor (personal communication, November 14, 1980) revealed an asymmetry of OKN in three children who had bilateral congenital cataracts removed at about 8 years of age. Our results show that when children are deprived of pattern vision from birth, asymmetrical OKN is evident even when the cataracts are removed as early as 4.5 months of age and even when nearly normal visual experience is restored by optical correction as early as 6 months of age. Moreover, the size of the asymmetry appears to be as large when deprivation lasts 6 months as when deprivation lasts 12 to 18 months. Previously we reported a similar asymmetry in both eyes of children who had been treated for a unilateral congenital cataract as early as 3 months of age (Maurer et al., 1983). Note, however, that even shorter periods of deprivation might have less effect on the symmetry of OKN.

Even children who had normal visual experience early in life showed asymmetrical OKN if they had developed a dense, central cataract between 6 and 18 months of age. Deprivation beginning after 18 months of age had little or no effect on the symmetry of OKN. Note, however, that most of the children treated for developmental cataracts had had relatively short periods of pattern deprivation (usually no more than 6 months). Thus, it is possible that asymmetrical OKN could result from very long periods of pattern deprivation beginning even after the second year of life. We previously reported a similar symmetry of OKN in the deprived eye of children who had normal early histories and then developed a dense, central cataract in one eye because of an injury after 3 years of age (Maurer et al., 1983).

Our findings of an asymmetry of OKN in children binocularly deprived of pattern vision early in life are similar to those reported for cats binocularly deprived shortly after birth (Harris et al., 1980; van Hof-van Duin, 1978): In both species OKN is easily elicited when stripes move from the temporal visual field toward the nasal visual field, but rarely elicited when stripes move in the opposite direction; and in both species, the asymmetry observed following binocular deprivation early in life is larger than that observed in normal subjects. To our knowledge, there have been no studies of the symmetry of OKN in cats deprived later in life.

Factors other than pattern deprivation per se might account for the asymmetry we observed. Providing the abnormality began early in life, asymmetrical OKN is shown frequently by amblyopes both with and without strabismus (Atkinson & Braddick, 1981; Schor & Levi, 1980), strabismics both with and without amblyopia (Atkinson & Braddick, 1981; Naegele & Held, 1983; Crone, 1977; Loewer-Sieger, cited in Crone, 1977; Schor & Levi, 1980; Rosenberg, Pritchard, & Flynn, 1981), and subjects with reduced stereopsis for whatever reason (Schor & Levi, 1980). Other visual disorders early in life also result frequently in an asymmetry of OKN. For example, such asymmetries have been observed in patients with "congenital occlusion" of one eye (Atkinson & Braddick, 1981) or with a latent nystagmus (Schor & Levi, 1980; van Hof-van Duin & Mohn, 1983). Note that cats deprived of pattern vision early in life also show many of these complications, e.g. reduced visual acuity, strabismus, and poor stereopsis (c.f. Kaye, Mitchell, & Cynader, 1982; Mitchell, 1981; Timney, 1983). Hence, asymmetrical OKN in cats also could result not from pattern deprivation per se but from one of these complications.

Although some of these visual problems likely contributed to our results, none is likely to be the sole factor. First, half of the aphakic children in our study who were old enough for traditional tests of linear acuity had amblyopia in one or both eyes (acuities worse than 6/12). Amblyopia might have contributed to our results since 3 of 4 eyes in the developmental group which showed an asymmetry had acuities worse than 6/12, and since some children in the congenital group, although too young for traditional tests of linear acuity, likely had amblyopia. Yet, amblyopia cannot account entirely for our results since one child in the congenital group showed an asymmetry of OKN even though her acuity in that eye was as good as 6/7.5 and some children in the developmental group showed no asymmetry of OKN with acuities as poor as 6/18. Moreover, in this study, as in previous studies (Maurer et al., 1983; Nagele & Held, 1983; Shor & Levi, 1980), the size of the asymmetry was not related to acuity. Other studies have also shown that amblyopia per se cannot account for asymmetrical OKN because the asymmetry is often present even in the <u>normal</u> eye of patients with a history from birth of strabismus or of unilateral cataract (Loewer-Sieger, 1962, cited in Crone, 1977; Maurer et al., 1983; Schor & Levi, 1980).

Second, strabismus might have contributed to our results since children who showed an asymmetry in both eyes tended to have strabismus at a younger age (median age of onset = 19 months, range 7.5 months to 5.5 years) than children who showed no asymmetry in either eye (median age of onset = 5 years, range 3.5 to 9 years). Little is known about the relationship between the age of onset of strabismus and the development of symmetrical OKN except that congenital esotropes usually show an asymmetry of OKN in both eyes (Atkinson & Braddick, 1981; Schor & Levi, 1980) and those who develop strabismus in late childhood show no asymmetry in either eye (Schor & Levi, 1980). Thus, it is possible that the earlier a child develops strabismus, the more likely he is to show asymmetrical OKN. Nonetheless, strabismus cannot account entirely for our results since some children who developed strabismus as late as 5.5 years of age showed an asymmetry of OKN in both eyes while others who developed an even larger strabismus at 3.5 years showed no asymmetry of OKN in either eye. Moreover, the degree of ocular deviation did not differ between children who showed an asymmetry and those who did not: Both groups had deviations ranging from 6 to 40 prism dioptres of esotropia and the median deviation was similar in both groups. Nor was there any relationship between the size of the asymmetry and the age of onset of strabismus or the degree of ocular deviation.

Third, reduced stereopsis cannot account for the asymmetry because we found no relationship between stereoacuity and symmetry of OKN in children old enough to do the Titmus test. For example, two children with no evidence of stereopsis showed symmetrical OKN in both eyes. In addition, if stereopsis were the only relevant factor, then a child always should show symmetrical OKN in both eyes or in neither eye. Yet, 3 children in our sample showed asymmetrical OKN in one eye but not in the other. Nor was fusion as measured by the Worth Four Dot Test related to the symmetry of OKN. For example, children who showed no evidence of fusion were as likely to have symmetrical as asymmetrical OKN. Others have also argued that poor binocularity alone cannot account for asymmetrical OKN since subjects with reduced stereopsis who became strabismic in late childhood show normal OKN (Schor & Levi, 1980). Thus, the binocular mechanisms mediating symmetrical OKN must be different, at least in part, from those mediating stereopsis and fusion (Wolfe, Held, & Bauer, 1981). Finally, latent nystagmus cannot account for our results since only one child had this complication.

Thus, the most plausible explanation for our results is that binocular deprivation early in life causes asymmetrical OKN in humans. These findings complement our previous findings of a similar asymmetry of OKN in children monocularly deprived from birth because of a dense cataract in one eye (Maurer et al., 1983). This asymmetry in visually deprived humans is similar to that observed in cats visually deprived from birth either in both eyes (Harris et al., 1980, van Hof-van Duin, 1978) or in one eye (van Hof-van Duin, 1976, 1979). It is also similar to that observed in normal human infants (Atkinson, 1979; Atkinson & Braddick, 1981; Naegele & Held, 1982, 1983), normal kittens (Malach et al., 1980, 1981; van Hof-van Duin, 1978) and cats with lesions of the visual cortex (Hoffmann, 1983; Montarolo et al., 1981; Strong et al., 1981; Wood et al., 1973). Studies of cats suggest that pattern deprivation leads to these deficits by disrupting input from binocular neurons in Areas 17 and 18 of the visual cortex to the nucleus of the optic tract (Harris et al., 1980; Hoffmann, 1979, 1981, 1983). The similarities in asymmetrical OKN between visually deprived cats and children treated for cataracts suggest that in humans, deprivation early in life might also affect the development of cortical control over the midbrain.

Of course, other explanations are plausible, particularly in light of possible differences between cats and humans in the pathways which mediate OKN. First, in addition to the pathways involved in the mediation of OKN in cats (see Figure 1), humans might have pathways which have input to each NOT via cortical commissures (Yee et al., 1982). Second, humans might depend entirely on pathways through the cortex for the mediation of OKN both when stripes move from the temporal field toward the nasal field and when they move in the opposite direction (Braddick & Atkinson, 1983). Both these alternatives still suggest that asymmetrical OKN results from nonfunctional projections from the ipsilateral visual cortex through NOT. A third possibility is that, unlike the cat, the human might have a direct pathway from the temporal retina to the ipsilateral NOT which is sufficient to mediate OKN when stripes move from the nasal field toward the temporal field (van Hof-van Duin & Mohn, 1983). This possibility does not explain why normal human infants show asymmetrical OKN (Atkinson, 1979; Atkinson & Braddick, 1981; Naegele & Held, 1982, 1983) because ipsilateral projections appear to develop simultaneously with contralateral projections, at least in monkeys (Rakic, 1976). However, ipsilateral projections might be more vulnerable to deprivation than contralateral projections. If that were so, asymmetrical OKN in visually deprived humans might be due to a selective loss of direct projections from the temporal retina to the ipsilateral NOT.

Regardless of the physiological basis of asymmetrical OKN, this study complements previous work in demonstrating striking similarities in behaviour between humans and cats. In both species, OKN is symmetrical, or nearly so, in the normal adult. Moreover, in both species, OKN is asymmetrical during early infancy and following either monocular or binocular deprivation early in life.

References

Atkinson, J. (1979). Development of optokinetic nystagmus in the human infant and monkey infant: An analogue to development in kittens. In R.D. Freeman (Ed.), Developmental neurobiology of vision (pp. 277-287). New York: Plenum.

Atkinson, J., & Braddick, O. (1981). Development of optokinetic nystagmus in infants: An indicator of cortical binocularity? In D.F. Fisher, R.A. Monty, & J.W. Senders (Eds.), Eye movements: Cognition and visual perception (pp. 53-64). Hillsdale, New Jersey: Lawrence Erlbaum.

Braddick, O.J., & Atkinson, J. (1983). Some recent findings on the development of human binocularity: A review. Behavioural Brain Research, 10, 141-150.

Braun, J.J., & Gault, F.P. (1969). Monocular and binocular control of horizontal optokinetic nystagmus in cats and rabbits. Journal of Comparative and Physiological Psychology, 69, 12-16.

Crone, R.A. (1977). Amblyopia: The pathology of motor disorders in amblyopic eyes. Documenta Ophthalmologica, 45, 9-17.

Cynader, M., & Harris, L. (1980). Eye movement in strabismic cats. Nature, 286, 64-65.

Harris, L.R., Lepore, F., Guillemot, J.P., & Cynader, M. (1980). Abolition of optokinetic nystagmus in the cat. Science, 210, 91-92.

Hoffmann, K.P. (1979). Optokinetic nystagmus and single-cell responses in the nucleus tractus after early mnocular deprivation in the cat. In R.D. Freeman (Ed.), Developmental neurobiology of vision (pp. 63-72). New York: Plenum.

Hoffmann, K.P. (1981). Neuronal responses related to optokinetic nystagmus in the cat's nucleus of the optic tract. In A. Fuchs & W. Becker (Eds.), Progress in oculomotor research (pp. 443-454). New York: Elsevier.

Hoffmann, K.P. (1983). Control of the optokinetic reflex by the nucleus of the optic tract in the cat. In A. Hein & M. Jeannerod (Eds.), Spatially oriented behavior (pp. 135-153). New York: Springer-Verlag.

Hoffmann, K.P., Behrend, K., & Schoppmann, A. (1976). A direct afferent visual pathway from the nucleus of the optic tract to the inferior olive in the cat. Brain Research, 115, 150-153.

Hoffmann, K.P., & Schoppmann, A. (1975). Retinal input to direction selective cells in the nucleus tractus opticus of the cat. Brain Research, 99, 359-366.

Kaye, M., Mitchell, D.E., & Cynader, M. (1982). Depth perception, eye alignment and cortical ocular dominance of dark-reared cats. Brain Research, 254, 37-53.

Malach, R., Strong, N., & Van Sluyters, R.C. (1980). OKN and cortical neurophysiology in visually deprived cats. Investigative Ophthalmology & Visual Science, (Supp. April), 270. (Abstract)

Malach, R., Strong, M., & Van Sluyters, R.C. (1981). Analysis of monocular optokinetic nystagmus in normal and visually deprived kittens. Brain Research, 210, 367-372.

Maurer, D., & Lewis, T.L. (1979). A physiological explanation of infants' early visual development. Canadian Journal of Psychology, 33, 232-252.

Maurer, D., Lewis, T.L., & Brent, H.P. (1983). Peripheral vision and optokinetic nystagmus in children with unilateral congenital cataract. Behavioural Brain Research, 10, 151-161.

Mitchell, D.E. (1981). Sensitive periods in visual development. In R.N. Aslin, J.R. Alberts, & M.R. Petersen (Eds.), Development of perception: Vol. 2. The visual system (pp. 3-39). New York: Academic Press.

Montarolo, P.G., Precht, W., & Strata, P. (1981). Functional organization of the mechanisms subserving the optokinetic nystagmus in the cat. Neuroscience, 6, 231-246.

Naegele, J., & Held, R. (1982). The postnatal development of monocular optokinetic nystagmus in infants. Vision Research, 22, 341-346.

Naegele, J.R., & Held, R. (1983). Development of optokinetic nystagmus and effects of abnormal visual experience during infancy. In M. Jeannerod & A. Hein (Eds.), Spatially oriented behavior (pp. 155-174). New York: Springer-Verlag.

Rakic, P. (1976). Prenatal genesis of connections subserving ocular dominance in the rhesus monkey. Nature, 261, 467-471.

Rosenberg, M.L., Pritchard, C., & Flynn, J. (1981). Asymmetry of the optokinetic response and of visual suppression of the vestibulo-ocular reflex in strabismic patients. Investigative Ophthalmology & Visual Science, 20, 26. (Abstract)

Timney, B. (1983). The effects of early and late monocular deprivation on binocular depth perception in cats. Developmental Brain Research, 7, 235-243.

Schor, C.M., & Levi, D.M. (1980). Disturbances of small-field horizontal and vertical optokinetic nystagmus in amblyopia. Investigative Ophthalmology & Visual Science, 19, 668-683.

Strong, R., Malach, R., & Van Sluyters, R.C. (1981). Cortical and sub-cortical pathways subserving OKN in the cat. Investigative Ophthalmology & Visual Science, 20, 56. (Abstract)

Van Hof-van Duin, J. (1976). Early and permanent effects of monocular deprivation on pattern discrimination and visuomotor behavior in cats. Brain Research, 111, 261-276.

Van Hof-van Duin, J. (1978). Direction preference of optokinetic responses in monocularly tested normal kittens and light deprived cats. Archives Italiennes de Biologie, 116, 471-477.

Van Hof-van Duin, J. (1979). Development of visuomotor behavior in normal and light-deprived cats. In V. Smith & J. Keen (Eds.), Clinics in developmental medicine (Vol. 73, pp. 112-123). London: Spastics International Medical Publications.

Van Hof-van Duin, J., & Mohn, G. (1983). Optokinetic and spontaneous nystagmus in children with neurological disorders. Behavioural Brain Research, 10, 163-175.

Wolfe, J.M., Held, R., & Bauer, J.A. (1981). A binocular contribution to the production of optokinetic nystagmus in normal and stereoblind subjects. Vision Research, 21, 587-590.

Wood, C., Spear, P., & Braun, J. (1973). Direction-specific deficits in horizontal optokinetic nystagmus following removal of visual cortex in the cat. Brain Research, 60, 231-237.

Yee, R.D., Baloh, R.W., Honrubia, V., & Jenkins, H.A. (1982). Pathophysiology of optokinetic nystagmus. In V. Honrubia & M.A.B. Brazier (Eds.), Nystagmus and vertigo: Clinical approaches to the patient with dizziness (pp. 251-275). New York: Academic Press.

Acknowledgements

We thank Dr. J. Donald Morin, Ophthalmologist-in-Chief, for his encouragement and support. We also thank Adrienne Richardson, Donna Stewart, Kelly Johnson, and Janet Warren for helping to collect and analyze the data, and our subjects for volunteering their time.

This research was supported by grants from the National Eye Institute (NIH 5-R01-EY03475), from the Ontario Ministry of Health (PR 928), and from the Medical Research Council of Canada (MA-8894).

II.

STUDIES USING EYE MOVEMENTS TO INVESTIGATE PERCEPTUAL AND COGNITIVE TASKS

A. Word Perception and Reading

Eye Movements and Human Information Processing
R. Groner, G.W. McConkie and C. Menz (eds.)

WORD PERCEPTION AND READING

INTRODUCTION

Some of the earliest research on the relation of eye movements to psychological processes dealt with reading. The observation that the eyes execute a series of brief saccadic movements separated by fixation pauses contradicted introspective experience and raised questions about how perception was actually taking place. Once techniques were developed to record the movements of the eyes, the great within-subject variability in fixation times and saccade lengths became apparent, as well as the eye movement pattern differences between readers. Attempts were made to relate these differences to text characteristics and reading ability differences.

The focus of much of this early research was on eye movements as the *object* of study. However, most of the recent eye movement research on reading has shifted focus to using eye movements as a *means* of study. The object of these studies is typically to understand some aspect of the perceptual or language processing taking place during reading, or factors that affect the general fluency of reading. Eye movement recording is part of the method by which the study is conducted. Eye movement data are used for a variety of purposes: to indicate where the eyes were centered and hence what region of the text was attended during certain fixations of interest; as an indicator of the occurrance of certain processing events or characteristics; as an indicator of the general fluency of reading; as a basis for becoming more analytic about differences in reading time, whether they occur at certain text locations, or are associated with differences in fixation time, saccade length, or frequency of regressing; or making real-time display changes contingent upon some aspect of the eyes' behavior.

While using eye movements as the object vs. the means of study may sound like a clean distinction, these often become entangled, even within the same study. This is expected because our ability to use eye movements as indicators of other processes depends on the degree to which we understand the basis of eye movement control itself and of the perceptual processes associated with the fixations and saccades. Thus, research reports in this area often move back and forth between asking what the eye movement data indicate about processing during reading, and asking what the outcomes of the study indicate about eye movement control. The papers in this section employ eye movement data primarily as a means of studying questions about aspects of reading other than eye movements themselves.

In the first chapter, Dunn-Rankin, who cleverly studies eye movements without the benefit of eye movement monitoring equipment, examines where the eyes are centered in reading a word. He finds that they tend to go to a different place in the word "desert" when it refers to a dry region than when it refers to the act of deserting.

The next chapter deals with a methodological issue. Frequently, the result of an experiment is to observe a difference in the means between the experimental and the control conditions. However, this difference does not indicate the proportion of the scores in the experimental condition that have been influenced by the experimental manipulation. McConkie, Underwood, Wolverton and Zola propose a method for estimating the frequency with which a manipulation produced its effect, and the size of that effect when it occurred.

Two of the chapters investigate word perception during fixations. Fisher & Shebilske tested Just & Carpenter's (1980) eye-mind assumption, that the time spent fixating a word during reading indicates the amount of time spent in processing that word. A corollary is that words that are not fixated receive zero processing time; hence, are not processed. Fisher & Shebilske have demonstrated that, contrary to the assumption, unfixated words are processed during reading. McConkie & Hogaboam used eye movement contingent control of the text display to investigate what words are read during a fixation in reading. Immediately following selected fixations the text was masked and removed from the screen and subjects reported what words they had just read.

The next two chapters report studies of the effects of typographic variables on reading. Heller & Heinisch had children, mostly poorer readers, read passages in which the letter spacing and letter size were manipulated. Larger print and wider spacing, up to a limit, facilitated reading. Menz & Groner, working with older subjects, used several methods of breaking up the normal image presented by the words: adding blanks or slashes between letters or displacing letters vertically so the line of text was "bumpy." Each of these slowed reading. One contrast between these two studies is that the same manipulation that facilitated children's reading interfered with that of adults. These studies remind us that most of the research concerning typography's effects on reading, used as a guide by the publishing industry, is now several decades old. It is time for someone to update this work, conducting a thorough analysis of the effects of these variables on the reading fluency of people of different ages and reading ability levels.

Kerr & Underwood report studies that investigated whether the phenomenon of priming occurs during reading as it does in tasks involving perception of individual words. They demonstrated that readers do fixate a word for less time when an associate of that word has appeared earlier in the passage. The next issue, of course, is whether this facilitation occurs during perception or only later. If it is due to spreading activation (Meyer & Schvaneveldt, 1976) then the lexical structure onto which perception maps its input during reading must be in constant ferment, with new waves rolling forth from one or more nodes in the structure on each new fixation, typically four times per second. The alternative is that, at least in reading, the facilitation is post-lexical in nature.

In the final chapter, Vonk uses eye movement data to examine the process of resolving referents for pronouns during reading. She finds that referent assignment is made quickly, and that the information used for this varies with the reading task. Vonk's chapter represents the increasingly popular use of eye movement data as a means of studying language processing during reading.

References

Just, M. A. & Carpenter, P. A. (1980), A theory of reading: From eye fixations to comprehension. Psychological Bulletin, 87, 329-354.

Meyer, D. E. & Schvaneveldt, R. W. (1976), Meaning, memory structure, and mental processes. In C. N. Cofer (Ed). The Structure of Human Memory, San Francisco, W. H. Freeman.

Eye Movements and Human Information Processing
R. Groner, G.W. McConkie and C. Menz (eds.)

PERCEPTUAL CHARACTERISTICS OF WORDS

Peter Dunn-Rankin

Department of Educational Psychology
University of Hawaii at Manoa
Honolulu, HI
U.S.A.

This paper reports the results of a series of studies related to word recognition. These experiments (1) look at the efficacy of syllables as primary units of recognition, (2) explore the measurement of word similarity by measuring the similarity of their phonemes, (3) use homonym passages and EMG recordings of labial muscles to predict reading age, (4) test whether word recognition is idiosyncratic, (5) analyze the effect of context on focal point placement, and (6) defend word length as an important word recognition feature. These studies indicate that strategies and features used in word recognition are task dependent.

After a decade of research in analyzing some of the visual characteristics of words (Scientific American, 1978) my colleagues and I have turned our attention to a series of experiments designed to illuminate other important dimensions of standard English words. These new studies were intended to increase our understanding of how the meaning, the sound, and the shape of a word relates to its perception.

Syllables as a Basic Unit?

Some researchers have been struck by the reasonableness of using syllables as a basic unit of perception. It is generally concluded that it is functionally useful to group letters into larger but more compact units which are then processed as wholes. This is suggested because an increase in unit size apparently reduces the number of elements a subject must process. Syllables appear suited to represent both the visual and phonetic aspects of speech. This is because syllables and syllable-like units are compact (can be easily seen in one focalization) and their graphic representation has a definite sound. It is conjectured that less than 1500 short groups of letters (a hidden phonetic alphabet) would have to be learned in order to pronounce 95 percent of all standard English words. Letters, it is argued, make only rudimentary phonetic sense and are too prolific to process independently.

Cognitive judgments are syllabically based. One experiment seemed to support the vision of an unstated phonetic alphabet based on syllables. In this study (Dunn-Rankin et al., 1979) a set of target words was selected and each word was divided into two parts. The division occurred in three ways for each word. A target word like WIZARD, for example, was divided syllabically (WI_ ZARD); in a phonetic blend (WIZ__ZARD); and vocalically (WIZ__ARD). A blend occurs when a single consonant carries the ending and beginning sound of the syllables in a longer word. GOLDEN is a good example in which D ends GOLD and begins DEN. It has been demonstrated that letter units that contain vowels, such as syllables, reduce verbal processing (Spoehr and Smith, 1975). Spoehr and Smith have called such groups, "vocalic center" groups. PAINT contains one vocalic group while PAPER contains two vocalic center groups, for example.

Using paired comparisons, ninth graders and college students ranked segmented words in order of their similarity to a true target word. There were 44 target words and three different separations for each target. In this cognitive appraisal the syllabic representation was generally selected as most like the target. Subjects were sometimes influenced in their selection, however, by whether the first or second unit of the segmented broken word was itself a word. In a word like PARENT, for example, the word units PA, PAR or RENT influenced the choice of vocalic rather than a syllabic representation.

Timed tasks are not syllabically based. In a follow up study, however, a timed task was used to test the syllabic hypothesis. Thirty-two two-syllable words and 20 two-syllable nonwords containing blend units were selected as stimuli (see Table 1). Equal numbers of stimuli were selected so that four categories (word-word, word-nonword, nonword-word and nonword-nonword) could be created with the blend. Table 1 presents the words and nonwords used as stimuli.

Table 1

Words and Non-words Used as Stimuli

Word-Word	Word-Non-word	Non-word-Word	Non-word-Nonword
	Words		
golden	hostess	honest	leopard
nearest	speaker	sustain	wizard
lagoon	armies	present	travel
parent	graphic	measure	danger
clothing	manure	liking	peevish
mistress	spinal	respite	filing
piping	sneaker	despite	money
parole	hinder	record	famous
	Non-words		
gildim	hurtiss	hanote	prestane
mostruss	westirn	rogel	wozerd
popang	graphac	degreat	treval
lagene	spanol	respate	dangur
clothong	meanere	poreal	faleng

A segmentation of the stimuli in the three ways previously described produced a total of 156 segmented stimuli. This time each broken word was hidden behind a shutter. When the experimenter electrically rotated the shutter exposing the segmented word a timing clock was started. Students were asked to press one of two switches indicating whether the broken parts would form a true word. The non-words were included in the set to act as distractors. Length of time to respond was taken as a measure of how easily the parts could be combined.

In addition, the spacing was varied. One-third of the words were segmented with one space between units (GOLD_EN, MEA_NERE) and one-third were segmented with two spaces (SPEA__KER, ROG__EL). The last third, the blends, contained one space (HOST_TESS, SPAN_NOL).

A number of word characteristics were used to predict response speed. Among these were: (1) word familiarity or frequency, (2) type of break,

(3) whether the beginning or ending units were words, (4) familiarity of the beginning and ending units, (5) length of the units, (6) spacing between the words, and (7) relative position of the stimulus in the task. In the analysis only four predictors made significant contributions to prediction. These variables were (1) word frequency, (2) relative position in the task, (3) spacing between the units, and (4) length of the ending unit. Forty-two percent of the variance in response time was accounted for by these four variables with twenty-three percent of the variance due to word familiarity alone.

The results of this experiment are interesting because they fail to confirm an auditory bias in word recognition under speeded conditions. Specifically, strategies for word recognition appear to be time and task dependent. Under speeded conditions the task becomes more perceptual than cognitive. In latency studies familiarity with the words was paramount to recognition and word features were subordinated.

Using words as syllables is predictive. The influence of single syllables, which were also common words, on the recognition of two syllable words has, however, been clearly demonstrated (Dunn-Rankin & Freese, 1980). A carefully selected set of two syllable words was made. The syllables in this set were either words or nonwords as shown in Table 1.

	Examples	
Stimulus Type	Words	Nonwords
word-word	breakfast	quakefast
word-nonword	inferred	inbured
nonword-word	delight	deplight
nonword-nonword	scalpel	sorpel

Subjects were asked to indicate whether 32 two-syllable stimuli were words or nonwords by pressing a switch following stimulus exposure. Time to respond was used as a criterion for ease of recognition. A direct but inverse relationship occurred between the time to respond for words and nonwords. If both syllables were words and the entire stimulus was a word the SHORTEST latency occurred. If, however, the stimulus was not a word and both syllables were words the LONGEST latency occurred. The importance of "word-syllable" familiarity to the recognition of longer words was strongly suggested.

Pseudowords are not syllabically based. Suggesting syllables as primary units in reading was not supported by Bennett (1979). She had subjects cluster specially constructed pseudowords of seven letters (knatlem or knatram, for example). Bennett was interested in subject's representations of similarity within groups of pronounceable non-words. Her conclusions were that large beginning or ending sets of letters, found to be the same, among groups of 30 pseudowords, were the primary basis for estimating similarity. The first four letters or the last three letters of the seven letter pseudowords were used 80 percent of the time. The units selected, however, did not create or constitute specific syllabic breaks. Bennett concluded that, when familiarity and meaning are removed from word-like stimuli, similarity is largely based on graphic characteristics.

Discussion. It is surprising that word familiarity is such a definitive a predictor of recognition time. It is surprising because most of the words used in these studies are a familiar part of a graduate student's lexicon. That is, they are all moderately frequent. Even frequency of usage or exposure to the stimulus words in the task (words appearing later in the tasks are recognized more quickly) is predictive of recognition and supports the importance of familiarity in recognition. It has been argued that letters and words gain relative equality after a given amount of meaningful exposure. Two words which differ in their frequency but which are fairly common should be recognized in relatively equal amounts of time without conscious thought. Some authors have referred to this acquisition as automaticity. Automaticity, however, can not be a true dichotomy but must reflect a continuum of skill maintained above a particular level. This conclusion is drawn because the relative frequency of common words is such a powerful predictor of recognition speed.

It has been argued that judging similarity appears to make perceptual rather than cognitive demands. This appears to be correct but time dependent. Since a great many demands are made in reading, the process cannot be considered perceptual unless the text is highly familiar. We are therefore left with the problem of how to interpret the studies testing the efficacy of syllables as the phonetic unit. If one considers the reading task to be largely perceptual and non-cognitive (that is, quickly recognizing familiar material) then syllabic representations are probably _not_ greatly utilized. In this case it is suggested that familiarity triggers perceptual generality in which only brief glimpses determine global recognition. In the case of highly familiar text it is supposed that the recognition of the word _rat_ is accomplished as fast as recognizing a color such as orange. Words that are consciously pronounced, however, probably demand vocalic or syllabic representation.

Phonemes

Similarity Estimates. Maeda (1980) explored the subjective similarity between isolated phonemes. She obtained similarity estimates between 780 pairs of (40) phonemes. She then mapped the similarities into a four dimensional space and obtained the distances between each pair of phonemes. These distances are presented in Table 2 and Table 2a. According to expectation, most vowels and consonants were clearly defined as not similar. Maeda was able to show, however, that some vowel-consonant correspondences were more similar than vowel-vowel or consonant-consonant pairs.

Table 2

Interphonemic Distances in the Four-Dimensional Solution

	p	b	t	d	ch	dʒ	k	g	f	v	θ	ð	s	z	ʃ	w	r	l	j	h
p																				
b	.43																			
t	.50	.47																		
d	.80	.27	.55																	
ch	.83	.66	.40	.59																
dʒ	.91	.57	.61	.34	.47															
k	.46	.64	.35	.46	.67	.64														
g	.67	.30	.62	.24	.76	.48	.39													
f	.38	.58	.35	.75	.60	.86	.58	.83												
v	.35	.30	.38	.46	.63	.67	.33	.44	.46											
θ	.56	.67	.40	.77	.48	.80	.70	.89	.22	.54										
ð	.47	.31	.40	.39	.51	.48	.43	.45	.48	.18	.48									
s	1.47	1.25	1.13	1.10	.75	.84	1.36	1.29	1.23	1.23	1.04	1.06								
z	.98	.66	.64	.46	.39	.16	.74	.62	.87	.69	.77	.54	.69							
ʃ	1.22	.95	.98	.94	.68	.74	1.20	1.25	1.02	1.00	.83	.83	.36	.63						
w	.63	.60	.81	.71	.86	.84	.86	.79	.68	.58	.67	.50	1.18	.87	1.03					
r	.56	.59	.85	.75	1.00	.92	.80	.73	.74	.51	.80	.52	1.40	.99	1.08	.31				
l	.56	.40	.74	.50	.84	.67	.67	.51	.73	.42	.76	.38	1.24	.76	.94	.32	.28			
j	1.10	.45	1.13	.76	1.03	.78	1.13	.85	1.15	.91	1.09	.78	1.45	.81	.78	.58	.72	.56		
h	.83	.86	.87	.93	.81	.98	1.07	1.08	.67	.81	.55	.70	1.00	.88	.69	.44	.72	.72	.82	
m	.78	.62	1.03	.71	1.18	.92	.84	.61	1.05	.68	1.12	.71	1.57	1.04	1.28	.64	.44	.38	.70	1.07
n	.97	.62	.99	.50	1.00	.61	.83	.45	1.12	.73	1.14	.68	1.29	.74	1.08	.77	.72	.49	.55	1.12
ŋ	1.74	1.44	1.88	1.36	1.93	1.56	1.64	1.30	2.00	1.65	2.06	1.64	2.18	1.68	2.01	1.60	1.55	1.44	1.33	1.97
ʍ	.44	.62	.71	.81	.87	.96	.80	.87	.47	.52	.52	.52	1.31	.99	1.00	.32	.39	.50	.90	.47
ʒ	1.09	.78	.83	.90	.56	.36	.95	.77	.98	.82	.86	.64	.56	.28	.44	.81	.98	.76	.62	.85
i	2.06	1.80	2.14	1.75	2.15	1.98	2.00	1.82	2.20	2.10	2.27	2.09	2.42	2.05	2.33	2.04	2.11	2.00	1.92	2.20
I	1.89	1.58	1.84	1.46	1.76	1.62	1.76	1.58	1.96	1.87	1.97	1.80	1.96	1.65	1.94	1.83	1.96	1.74	1.66	1.93
e	2.12	1.85	2.10	1.74	1.96	1.87	2.09	1.91	2.17	2.09	2.11	2.02	1.98	1.93	1.95	1.92	2.11	1.92	1.73	1.93
ɛ	1.91	1.65	1.87	1.55	1.75	1.69	1.87	1.72	1.92	1.92	1.90	1.83	1.85	1.69	1.82	1.77	1.95	1.76	1.63	1.77
æ	1.88	1.60	1.84	1.37	1.67	1.56	1.87	1.66	1.87	1.84	1.82	1.75	1.60	1.55	1.55	1.58	1.79	1.61	1.34	1.57
ɑ	1.34	1.15	1.50	1.16	1.52	1.42	1.42	1.27	1.47	1.42	1.52	1.38	1.82	1.48	1.65	1.23	1.34	1.21	1.23	1.37
ɔ	1.47	1.37	1.62	1.41	1.64	1.66	1.60	1.55	1.60	1.62	1.59	1.58	1.95	1.69	1.80	1.43	1.58	1.48	1.54	1.45
o	2.08	1.96	2.24	1.96	2.17	2.14	2.26	2.11	2.12	2.17	2.12	2.08	2.21	2.14	2.04	1.76	1.96	1.89	1.71	1.75
U	1.51	1.39	1.77	1.43	1.81	1.68	1.69	1.51	1.68	1.60	1.72	1.56	2.03	1.74	1.78	1.25	1.33	1.28	1.23	1.43
u	1.91	1.82	2.16	1.86	1.83	2.07	1.38	1.96	2.02	2.01	2.04	1.95	2.26	2.11	2.02	1.58	1.71	1.69	1.55	1.66
ʌ	1.02	.84	1.34	.86	1.16	1.10	1.14	1.00	1.10	1.07	1.12	1.00	1.45	1.14	1.24	.82	.98	.85	.89	.94
ɜ	1.71	1.66	1.97	1.76	2.16	2.09	1.78	1.76	1.94	1.91	2.09	1.96	2.68	2.18	2.50	1.93	1.90	1.84	2.08	2.13
ɑI	1.92	1.83	1.89	1.84	1.86	2.01	1.95	2.00	1.86	2.06	1.89	2.01	2.17	2.00	2.14	2.02	2.20	2.07	2.16	1.92
oI	1.99	1.96	2.14	2.02	2.18	2.24	2.18	2.17	2.00	2.18	2.03	2.13	2.37	2.24	2.24	1.93	2.11	2.05	2.08	1.82
ɑU	1.94	1.86	2.02	1.88	2.18	2.02	2.13	2.07	1.87	2.04	1.84	1.95	1.94	1.99	1.81	1.67	1.92	1.85	1.73	1.51

Table 2--Continued

Interphonemic Distances in the Four-Dimensional Solution

	m	n	ŋ	ʍ	ʒ	i	I	e	ɛ	æ	ɑ	ɔ	o	U	u	ʌ	3	ɑI	oI	ɑU
p																				
b																				
t																				
d																				
ch																				
dʒ																				
k																				
g																				
f																				
v																				
θ																				
ð																				
s																				
z																				
ʃ																				
w																				
r																				
l																				
j																				
h																				
m																				
n	.46																			
ŋ	1.14	1.05																		
ʍ	.79	.99	1.82																	
ʒ	1.04	.73	1.65	1.00																
i	1.89	1.80	1.30	1.80	2.05															
I	1.78	1.58	1.37	1.98	1.65	.58														
e	2.01	1.84	1.70	2.08	1.79	.89	.63													
ɛ	1.87	1.71	1.64	1.91	1.64	.84	.50	.27												
æ	1.73	1.54	1.58	1.78	1.42	1.82	.83	.46	.50											
ɑ	1.23	1.25	1.22	1.34	1.44	.88	.87	.95	.81	1.07										
ɔ	1.57	1.61	1.66	1.47	1.66	1.13	1.01	.97	.81	.99	.55									
o	1.95	1.98	1.90	1.91	2.00	1.40	1.43	1.00	1.07	.93	.98	.92								
U	1.23	1.36	1.25	1.40	1.64	1.22	1.33	1.25	1.21	1.10	.56	.81	.83							
u	1.68	1.80	1.68	1.73	1.97	1.46	1.59	1.31	1.34	1.18	.93	1.00	.49	.51						
ʌ	.98	1.00	1.33	.95	1.08	1.28	1.12	1.17	1.01	.94	.44	.66	1.12	.68	1.05					
3	1.75	1.89	1.60	1.91	2.25	1.05	1.40	1.70	1.54	1.83	1.04	1.05	1.73	1.28	1.62	1.34				
ɑI	2.24	2.19	2.34	2.00	2.04	1.40	1.23	1.22	1.02	1.39	1.25	.89	1.54	1.70	1.81	1.37	1.49			
oI	2.17	2.24	2.28	1.94	2.20	1.44	1.49	1.22	1.14	1.33	1.09	.67	.91	1.25	1.16	1.04	1.43	.88		
ɑU	2.03	2.12	2.24	1.75	1.86	1.67	1.55	1.12	1.10	1.01	1.13	.88	.65	1.18	.99	1.11	1.89	1.23	.71	

Table 2a

KYST-2 Coordinates for the
40 Phonemes of English in Four Dimensions

	Dimension 1	Dimension 2	Dimension 3	Dimension 4
p	-0.597	0.141	-0.496	-0.203
b	-0.478	0.210	-0.093	-0.175
t	-0.741	-0.084	-0.133	-0.424
d	-0.461	0.180	0.172	-0.172
ch	-0.696	-0.335	0.158	-0.335
d3	-0.658	0.015	0.399	-0.148
k	-0.690	0.264	-0.126	-0.423
g	-0.566	0.393	0.125	-0.178
f	-0.675	-0.212	-0.421	-0.278
v	-0.749	0.145	-0.188	-0.125
θ	-0.711	-0.374	-0.298	-0.204
ð	-0.705	0.029	-0.071	-0.066
s	-0.709	-0.765	0.618	0.076
z	-0.673	-0.136	0.435	-0.151
ʃ	-0.682	-0.604	0.351	0.256
w	-0.483	-0.059	-0.259	0.337
r	-0.615	0.205	-0.357	0.332
l	-0.536	0.202	-0.117	0.224
j	-0.378	0.038	0.262	0.561
h	-0.466	-0.493	-0.292	0.277
m	-0.482	0.565	-0.136	0.337
n	-0.490	0.459	0.302	0.227
ŋ	0.258	1.165	0.483	0.350
ʍ	-0.570	-0.105	-0.503	0.161
ʒ	-0.589	-0.232	0.484	0.094
i	1.221	0.617	0.337	-0.324
I	0.901	0.242	0.634	-0.413
e	1.187	-0.193	0.593	-0.056
ε	1.016	-0.175	0.481	-0.227
æ	0.821	-0.304	0.582	0.207
ɑ	0.657	0.219	-0.081	0.015
ɔ	0.848	-0.071	-0.301	-0.181
o	1.241	-0.313	-0.151	0.595
U	0.698	0.295	-0.274	0.530
u	1.023	0.018	-0.360	0.800
ʌ	0.285	0.005	-0.113	0.099
3	0.916	0.854	-0.613	-0.555
ɑI	1.024	-0.523	-0.179	-0.921
oI	1.296	-0.476	-0.585	-0.191
ɑU	1.008	-0.809	-0.268	0.270

Using phonemes to predict word similarity. Atkins (1983) used the distances of Figure 1 and tested the validity of using discrete phonemes to measure the phonemic similarity between words. A computer program was written to compare the phonemic distance between any two words (See Table 3). The comparison is accomplished by sliding the phonemes of each word back and forth (while maintaining their order but varying their spacing) until the minimum summed distance is achieved. This sum is then averaged by the total number of phonemes in both words, resulting in a Phonemic Similarity Index (PSI).

Scores on the Wepman Auditory Discrimination Test (1973) were used to test the utility of the Phonemic Similarity Index (PSI). Atkins found that when word familiarity is taken into account the prediction of the error scores on the Wepman using the PSI were reasonably high. The importance of familiarity can be understood by comparing two word pairs from the Wepman. Even though the words CLOVE and CLOTHE (two unfamiliar words) are as similar as LEG and LED in PSI units people are less able to distinguish the difference between the unfamiliar words when spoken orally. Possible uses for the PSI include the creation of more effective measures of auditory discrimination, creating a phonemic similarity index for testing trade names, and building a phonemic similarity index for text materials.

Internal Speech

Freese (1982) studied lip movements during silent reading. She composed paragraphs consisting largely of homonyms such as "hour knew made" for "our new maid," (see Figure 1). While subjects read these and regular passages their labial muscles were monitored at 15 second intervals. By comparing electromyographic activity levels when reading the homonym and regular passages; noting the time taken to read each passage, and using the interaction of these two variables, Freese was able to account for 74 per cent of the variance in the reading age of the responding children.

Table 3

Interphonemic Distances and Familiarities of Wepman and IDT Items

Item Number	Item Word Pair	Phonemic Similarity Index (PSI)	Rinsland Word Freq. Counts	Familiarity Category
1	tub-tug	.30	22-1	2
3	web-wed	.27	0-1	1
4	leg-led	.24	108-5	3
6	gum-dumb	.24	14-7	2
7	bale-gale	.30	6-0	1
8	sought-fought	1.23	0-2	1
9	vow-thou	.18	0-0	0
10	shake-shape	.46	24-6	2
13	thread-shred	.83	7-0	1
15	bass-bath	1.04	1-74	3
16	tin-pin	.50	28-33	2
17	pat-pack	.35	19-20	2
18	dim-din	.46	0-0	0
19	coast-toast	.35	8-63	3
20	thimble-symbol	1.04	0-0	0
21	cat-cap	.50	1492-182	5
22	din-bin	.27	0-2	1
23	lath-lash	.83	0-0	0
24	bum-bomb	.44	1-5	1
25	clothe-clove	.18	0-0	0
26	moon-noon	.46	44-19	2
27	shack-sack	.36	1-22	2
28	sheaf-sheath	.22	0-0	0
31	pork-cork	.46	1-0	1
32	fie-thigh	.22	0-0	0
33	shoal-shawl	.92	0-0	0
36	pat-pet	.50	18-387	4
37	muff-muss	1.23	0-0	0
39	lease-leash	.36	0-0	0
40	pen-pin	.50	54-33	3
41	jack-pack	.91	9-20	2
44	bath-bat	.40	74-61	3
45	tong-tall	1.44	0-41	2
46	such-sung	1.93	29-1	2
47	age-ate	.61	12-157	4
48	late-let	.27	65-751	5
49	suit-sit	1.59	133-160	4
52	see-zee	.69	2971-***	5
53	king-kick	1.64	30-20	2
54	tail-tool	1.31	88-40	3
55	pint-point	.88	0-0	0
56	hat-heat	1.82	228-2	4
58	put-putt	.68	1131-0	5
60	foot-fat	1.10	48-78	3

IDT item (Interphonemic Distance Test, Atkins, 1983)

*** Does not appear in Rinsland word frequency count.

Hour knew made was called Gene. She was two bee at hour house bye ate that mourning. Wear mite she bee? Had she mist the write tern onto hour rowed? Eye tolled her two go past the mane gait reel sloe and tern wear the sine reeds, "Hoarse four rent." Eye could knot weight four her past won that afternoon. Eye had two meat my sun and his socker teem. After fore ours had past eye said allowed, "She mist her chants. Eye can knot weight any longer."

Eye called her later and tolled her eye wood meat her at the tern inn the rode the next mourning. Eye tolled her too weight close two the mane rowed ware she will sea a blew gait. At ate wee met at the gait.

Gene's first week did knot work out sew well. Four won thing she did knot clothes the gait sew hour hoarse got aweight. Also, she eight sew much of hour food, the shelves were bear. Knot even a peace of bred was left. She spilled a hole bag of flower all over the floor. What a site!

Wee decided Gene did knot have much common cents. She did knot seam too bee the write made four us. Wee new it wood knot bee whys two keep her. Wee had two tell her that wee did knot knead her anymore.

Questions:

1. Who was Gene in the story?
2. What time was Gene supposed to be at the house?
3. Where was Gene supposed to turn?
4. What did the sign on the road say?
5. Who did the person in the story have to meet?
6. How long did the person in the story wait for Gene before deciding to leave?
7. Where did the person in the story tell Gene to wait for her the next morning?
8. What happened to the horse in the story?
9. What did Gene spill?
10. How did Gene do on the job the first week?
11. What happened to Gene at the end of the story?
12. Did the person in the story have any children?

Figure 1. Homonym passage used to predict reading age following the measurement of labial muscle activity.

It is interesting that essentially non-cognitive measures predicted reading level so adequately. This finding suggests that phonemic sensitivity (the sound and flow of the text language) may be an important ingredient in reading skill along with persistent effort (motivation). The ramifications of this exploration are made tentatively. The findings suggest, however, extensive reading to children so that they can mimic the sound and syntax of text materials. Articulation training may also be important so that internalized speech patterns are accurate surrogates of overt speech.

Word Potency.

Gima (1981) was able to show that word potency influences recognition in the periphery of the focal point. He used potent four letter words as stimuli. He was also able to show that when recognition thresholds were minimal (about 20 ms) the effects of standard English readers being able to see more to the right of the focal point no longer held. This finding is contrary to many studies which find that the ability to see more to the right of the focal point is greater than to the left of the focal point. In the other studies (Bouma, 1973), however, more time was given to recognize the stimulus.

Idiosyncratic Perception.

It has long been felt that word recognition may be idiosyncratic. The strategy that one person uses in word recognition may be different from someone else's strategy. In an initial study, four sophisticated readers responded to 61 three letter words and nonwords that were presented on a video terminal in capital letters. The subjects responded by pressing a key to indicate whether the stimuli were words or nonwords and the latency of the response was measured in cycles of 4 milliseconds each. The subjects repeated this task as many as 15 times and the medians of their response times were used as the latency criterion. A step-wise linear regression was then used to predict each subjects latencies using the unique characteristics of the words as predictors.

Characteristics of the words were determined as follows:

Word Frequency: Word frequency was ranked by three of the subjects and the median of these scores was taken.

Word Potency: Word potency was ranked by three of the subjects and the median taken.

Time to Pronounce: A separate study was conducted to determine this variable. 12 adult subjects read each word ten times and each reading time was determined with a stop watch. The mean reading time for each subject was subtracted from his set of scores and the median corrected time for all 12 subjects was used as the value for this variable.

Unique letters: Two letters, O and I, were used as variables. They were scored as follows: 1 if the word contained the letter, 0 otherwise.

Vowel-Consonant Combinations: Consonant-vowel-consonant arrangements were scored 1 if the combination was CVC and 0 otherwise.

Beginning A: If the word began with an A it was scored 1 and zero otherwise.

These variables served as predictors of latency for each subject. The weights of the variables following linear regression were analyzed and the results are provided in Table 4.

Table 4

Beta Weights of the Predictors of Subject's Latency, R^2 and Mean Latency of Subjects. For the 1st 3 Variables a + Sign Indicates a Positive Predictor of Shorter Latency. For All Other Variables a Negative Sign Predicts Shorter Latency.

Subj.	Freq.	Ptncy	Time to Pron.	Vowel O	Vowel I	Cons. Vowel Cons.	Beginning A	R^2	Mean Latency in cycles
P	.236	.088	-.215	-.346	.183	.124	.262	.359	109.67
S	.503	.407	-.053	-.220	.479	.414	.095	.398	98.91
K	.221	-.052	.364	-.450	-.167	.127	.156	.426	99.79
E	.403	.275	.058	-.227	.088	-.001	.134	.312	94.91
Mean	.341	.180	.039	-.311	.146	.166	.162	.374	100.82

Table 4 reveals that a substantial amount of variance ($\bar{R}^2$=.374) can be accounted for by the predictor variables chosen. It also indicates that Word Frequency and the letter "O" were consistent predictors of word recognition speed. The four subjects varied, however, in the use of the other predictor variables. For two of the subjects potency was an important predictor while for two others the time to pronounce was a differentially effective predictor of response latency. Since many of the words used began with the letter A it is not surprising that it was, in general, a negative predictor of response time. Within some bounds, however, word perception appears to be idiosyncratic.

One surprising result of this study was that the individual estimates of frequency and potency did not predict those individuals latency as effectively as the median values. This suggests that one's psychological perception of word potency is less dominant under perceptual than it is under cognitive appraisal. That is, perceptual processing is not strongly influenced by apparent extremes in frequency or potency.

Context.

Dunn-Rankin et al. (1983) used homographs (words that look alike but can be pronounced more than one way, such as desert, refuse, project, etc.) to test the impact of context on eye-movement patterns. Strong context sentences or short paragraphs ending in a homograph were used as the stimuli. "He saw the oasis in the middle of the dry sandy desert." and "The army private was depressed and that night he decided to desert." are examples (See Figure 2). Results indicate significant differences in focal point placement in the two words which are graphically congruent. It is argued that the reader has some general conception of the shape of the words in order to utilize context in focal point placement. In this case length would be one characteristic of shape.

Using strong point after-images, marked on the homographs, the focal point positions were determined. Professors and beginning art students were used as subjects.

Age_____ Sex_____ Name ______________________________

Estimation of reading ability: Poor Reader______Super Reader

In art class there are always many assignments. At the end of class a big project is due.

John was late to Joan's birthday party. He had forgotten to buy her a present.

Ann wanted to make the best impression. She wore her finest dress in order to present herself effectively.

She told him that they should go to her apartment; it was an offer he couldn't refuse.

The oasis was a pleasant find since water is scarce in the dry sandy desert.

On the billy goat's head were two buttons of bone. His horns had begun to project.

Why was the soldier AWOL? The officer knew that Pvt. Brown wasn't the type to desert.

"You want to continue to hike but it's getting dark and I'm tired. Don't desert me, please."

They had lived many years in the ghetto but are now moving to a new housing project.

The camel is unique since he can go without water for a long time in the desert.

Lord Mears took Tom by arm and guided him to the lady. He said, "May I present a friend of mine?"
Little Mike's parents were gone all that day and the next. I hope they didn't desert him.

Old newspapers, letters, rags, and all manner of junk were thrown away in the refuse bin.

No one knew when the rocket would be launched. The exact date was difficult to project.

After the prosecutor had talked to the jury the defense lawyer was ready to present his case.

Figure 2. Passage used to detect focal point positioning on differently stressed homographs.

The semantic context was hypothesized to influence how the homograph was stressed. It was found that the context did influence focal point positioning. In addition, word length and word frequency also appeared to influence all 23 subjects in similar ways. That is, if the context suggested early stress, if the word was relatively short, and if the word was relatively familiar, the tendency was to look earlier in the word. All the subjects, however, were generally divided into early and late focal point positioners. The effects of above variables are, therefore, relative to this tendency. Both professors and art students could be divided into relatively early or late focal point positioners. The difference in the two groups (professors and art students) is dramatic. The difference for the art students is 2.5 units or a little more than one letter whereas the professors' difference is almost three letters. This suggests that an early or late strategy has become solidified in the more able readers.

The ramifications of such studies are dependent on confirming such idiosyncratic skills. Are there differences between exploratory and confirmatory readers? Does text difficulty change one's strategy? And finally, are the focal point positions for skilled and unskilled readers similar in mean position and in variance?

Length.

My bias is that word length is an important contributor to the reading process but I have been examining this bias more carefully in light of the experiments that have been reported to the contrary.

Many type fonts have character widths that are constant. In these cases words like "hill" and "wood" take up the same physical space. Notice that in the word "hill" spacing between the letters is greater. It has been shown (Gima, 1982) that such words are easier to identify in the periphery presumably because there is less lateral masking. Magazine publishers take advantage of spacing within words or sometimes between words in order to right justify margins or eliminate hyphenation or both. Presumably, these variations cause little difficulty in reading although this has not been tested. A quick perusal of the latest Time magazine shows most variations in the millimeter length of words with the same number of characters to be small.

These points are made to indicate that, with easy material, most readers probably adjust to small variations in word length, measured in millimeters, even though character length may be slightly different. In most texts physical word length and character length will be highly correlated.

Aside from these observations the argument for the importance of length has been based on focal point studies (Dunn-Rankin, 1978 and Rayner, 1979). As words increase in length the focal point moves to centralize the stimulus unless it gets so large that the initial letter moves out of clear vision. The focal point is the point of clearest vision and it is usually placed at the area of greatest ambiguity. What does the mind use to direct the eye to these central locations if it is not word length?

Word length measured in millimeters or in characters cannot by itself be an effective contributor to word recognition. Take for example the following sentence:

____ ________ __ _____ __ _____.

This sentence is hard to read. In almost any text most standard English words are of limited length (4 to 8 letters). While there are fewer one-, two-, and three-letter words even these words are difficult to determine just by their length. Length, if it is functional, must interact with some aspects of word shape. It has been argued (Dunn-Rankin, 1982) that initial and final letters can combine with length to reduce ambiguity. This argument is made more plausible when one realizes that less than 1 percent of the word pairs in any body of text will contain both the same initial letter and the same length.

It is unreasonable to allow straight lines to solely represent word length because a word appears as a bar when clarity is obscured. We therefore make the following substitutions for the sentence above:

Txxx sxxxxxxx ix hxxx tx rxxx.

or Txxs sxxxxxxe is hxxd to rxxd.

This sentence is still hard to read. Not all words, however, will be as completely obscured as those in the sentence above. Perhaps lateral masking makes it difficult to determine only a single word in the periphery of the focal point. For example:

This sentence is hxxd to read.

In this case the contextual constraints (semantic, syntactic, and graphic) also interact to force the obscured word to be read as "hard".

Look at the following sentences.

The man had a bxxxxxr named Harry.

It is reasonable that the missing word could be; brother, boxer, burner or buzzer but not bird or bud.

The man had a bxy named Harry.

The missing word could be boy, buy or bay but not buzzard.

The man had a dxg named Harry.

The missing word could be dog, dug, or day but probably not dachshund.

Given some context the following sentences should be fairly easy to read.

Txx mxx hxd x dxg nxxxx Hxxxy. Txx dxg wxx bxxxx xxx txn. Txx dxg rxn wxxn ix sxx txx mxn.

These sentences should read: The man had a dog named Harry. The dog was brown and tan. The dog ran when it saw the man.

If it is true that lateral masking occurs within words then length should have some confirmatory value for our expectations. In a recent study (Haber, Haber and Furlin, 1983) length is seen as a positive contributor to recognition and comprehension. I have also studied the interaction of length and word frequency on speed of recognition by having students read lists of three-, six-, and nine-letter words which were quite frequent and quite infrequent. Infrequent long words took a dramatically longer time to read.

Man, however, is an adaptable animal. He or she will use available clues to solve reading problems. If one reduces some of the advantages of length by making a text with all words of uniform length then shape, initial letter, context, etc. will assume greater prominence in the reading process. Because metric length may be held constant does not rule out its use in normal text. It may also be true that character length replaces metric length in texts of variable font.

In order to study this idea further I created a set of words which are all very similar in length but which vary in character width. The text is taken from a recent Time magazine article and the fonts were created by using an OKIDATA printer (see Figure 3).

Body builder Lisa Lyon is too busy these
days to pump much iron. The U.C.L.A.
anthropology graduate who can dead lift
225 lbs. has written and appeared in two
pictorial bestsellers that feature
muscle bulging poses she calls body
sculpture. Now she has left her duties
as hostess of a Playboy Network talk
show to develop a fashion modeling
career. The unscrawny mannequin
currently appears on six pages of the
German edition of Vogue. Her physique
may soon grace rag trade magazines.

Figure 3. Passage with words of approximately equal length.

Strong point after-images were created and I dotted my focal points as I read the passage. As Rayner and others have found fixation span is constant over a range of font widths. For this experimental text the number of characters per span appears to be utilized versus a change in visual angle when recognizing words.

Since focalization appears to depend on the number of characters and because men and women appear to be able to effect a "zoom lens" with regard to stimuli of varying font the use of length could be independent of a linear metric. There may be a generalized map against which the specific stimuli are reduced or expanded in order to be recognized. When the letters in a word are of mixed font such an adjustment may take more time and is therefore one reason for reduced reading speed. In general readers are extremely tolerant and flexible with regard to font differences. While characters like "&" are easily recognized few people can remember how to draw such stimuli. This suggests a mechanism that subdues or dulls our memory of images until the stimuli is reintroduced. Then, like a wave wetting a dull stone, the lines and colors spring to new life. It is quite possible to create font types in which every word occupies the same space, like reading kanji or hiragana. This would require, however, early instruction to be efficient. Its benefits would enhance printing but would we be better readers if we didn't have word length as a variable to aid recognition?

Discussion. These excursions into perception as it relates to reading reveal the difficulty of studying the sophisticated adult reader and relating their success to curriculum development. The conclusion is that our measures are invariably task dependent. Prediction depends on how similar the task is to one's reading behavior.

The studies reported here have led to a number of interesting questions. We know from eye-movement studies that adults focus on almost every word. What is the nature of this glance? Is it confirmatory or exploratory? Are strategies of focal point positioning equally beneficial or is it just important to have a strategy that is consistent? How idiosyncratic are strategies of word recognition? Are there unrecognized basic capabilities that can account for the success of word frequency as a predictor of word recognition? What is true role of internal speech in reading skill and acquisition? And finally, can other functional uses be made of the perceptual map of phoneme similarity?

References

Atkins, C. S. (1983). Auditory discrimination based on interphonemic distances. Unpublished Master's Thesis, University of Hawaii at Manoa, Honolulu.

Atkins, C. S., Dunn-Rankin, P., & Wong, E. K. (1982, January). Distances between phoneme contrasts as a criterion for auditory discrimination tests. Paper presented at the annual meeting of the Hawaii Educational Association, Honolulu, HI.

Bennett, D. E. (1978). An examination of the use of letter units in the visual recognition of words. Unpublished Master's Thesis, University of Hawaii at Manoa, Honolulu.

Bennett, D., & Dunn-Rankin, P. (1978, May). A study of the perceived similarity among words. A paper presented at the annual meeting of the Hawaii Psychological Association, Honolulu, HI.

Bouma, H. (1971). Visual recognition of isolated lower-case letters. Vision Research, 11, 459-474.

Bouma, H. (1973). Visual interference in the parafoveal recognition of initial and final letters of words. Vision Research, 13, 767-782.

Dunn-Rankin, P. (1977). Using after images in the analysis of letter and word focalization. Journal of Reading Behavior, 9(2), 113-122.

Dunn-Rankin, P. (1977). The importance of length in word perception. Unpublished paper.

Dunn-Rankin, P. (1978). The visual characteristics of words. Scientific American, 238(1), 122-130.

Dunn-Rankin, P., Abe-Sullivan, C. S., Gima, S., Hirata, G. T., & Loui, B. C. (1979, January). Word recognition in peripheral vision. Paper presented at the annual meeting of the Hawaii Educational Research Association, Honolulu, HI.

Dunn-Rankin, P., et al. (1979, January). Word Recognition in Periphereal Vision. A paper presented at the 1st annual meeting of the Hawaii Educational Research Association, Honolulu, HI.

Dunn-Rankin, P., et al. (1979, January). Is what we say what we see? The influence of vocalic segmentation on the visual perception of words. A paper presented at the Hawaii Psychological Association meeting, Honolulu, ; (1980, April). American Educational Research Association Convention, Boston, MA.

Dunn-Rankin, P., & Freese, A. (1980, August). Studies in Word Recognition. A paper presented at the Fourth Far West Regional Conference, International Reading Association, Honolulu, HI.

Dunn-Rankin, P., et al. (1981,January). The lack of relationship between phonological coding and word recognition in a latency task. A paper presented at the Hawaii Educational Research Association Meeting, Honolulu, HI.

Dunn-Rankin, P., et al. (1982, January). Predicting eye movements in reading. A paper presented at the Hawaii Educational Research Association 4th Annual Conference, Honolulu, HI.

Freese, A. R. (1982). The relation of phonological coding to reading proficiency. Unpublished doctoral dissertation, University of Hawaii at Manoa, Honolulu.

Freese, A., & Dunn-Rankin, P. (April, 1983). The relation of phonological coding to reading proficiency. A paper presented at the American Educational Research Association Annual Meeting, Montreal, Canada.

Gima, S. (1982). The effects of word potency, frequency, and graphic characteristics on word recognition in the parafoveal field. Unpublished doctoral dissertation, University of Hawaii at Manoa, Honolulu.

Gleitman, L. R., & Rozin, P. (1973). Teaching reading by use of a syllabary. Reading Research Quarterly, 8, 447-483.

Haber, L. R., Haber, R. N., & Furlin, R. R. (1983). Word length and word shape as sources of information in reading. Reading Research Quarterly, 2, 165-190.

LaBerge, D.,& Samuels, J. (1974). Towarda theory of automatic information processing in reading. Cognitive Psychology, 6, 293-323.

Maeda, A. R. T. (1981). A multidimensional map of the phonemes of English: A perceptual study. Unpublished doctoral dissertation, University of Hawaii at Manoa, Honolulu.

Rayner, K. (1979). Eye guidance in reading: Fixation locations within words. Perception, 8, 21-30.

Sperling, G. (1960). The information available in brief visual presentations. Psychological Monographs, 74, (11, Whole No. 498).

Spoehr, K. T., & Smith, E. E. (1973). The role of syllables in perceptual processing. Cognitive Psychology, 5, 71-89.

Thorndike, E. L., & Lorge, I. (1944). The teacher's wordbook of 30,000 words. New York: Teachers College, Bureau of Publications.

Wepman, J. M. (1973). Auditory Discrimination Test (rev. ed.). Chicago: Language Research Associates, 1958.

Yumori, W. H. (1983). The semantic representation of abstract concepts: Mapping intensional and extensional definitions. Unpublished doctoral dissertation, University of Hawaii at Manoa, Honolulu.

Eye Movements and Human Information Processing
R. Groner, G.W. McConkie and C. Menz (eds.)

ESTIMATING FREQUENCY AND SIZE OF EFFECTS DUE TO EXPERIMENTAL MANIPULATIONS IN EYE MOVEMENT RESEARCH

George W. McConkie, David Zola & Gary S. Wolverton

Center for the Study of Reading
University of Illinois at Urbana-Champaign
U.S.A.

In studies of eye movement behavior, once it has been demonstrated that an experimental manipulation has produced a reliable effect, it is often useful to try to estimate the frequency with which the effect occurred. This paper describes the Frequency of Effects Analysis and illustrates its use with data from a study on characteristics of the perceptual span of adult readers. The results of the analysis indicated that, in one instance, a manipulation which produced a 21 msec increase in fixation duration was actually producing a 151 msec increase in only 21% of the instances, and was having no effect in the remaining 79% of the cases.

This paper describes a problem which we have encountered several times recently in our studies of the eye movements of readers, and proposes a direction to take in its solution. We suspect that it is a problem that occurs quite frequently in eye movement research, as well as experimental research in other areas. It is referred to as the frequency of effects problem.

When conducting an experimental study, researchers typically make some stimulus manipulation in one condition, and compare the results with another condition in which the manipulation was not made. In each condition, data are obtained on at least one dependent variable for each trial, which can be represented as frequency distributions of the scores for the two conditions. Statistical techniques are used to determine the likelihood that these two distributions represent samples from two different populations, indicating whether the experimental manipulation produced a difference in the dependent variable. The most frequently used techniques involve calculating the statistical significance of the difference between the means of the two sets of scores. In some cases the difference in the variance of the two distributions is tested, or, through the use of something like the Kolmogorov-Smirnov test, the shapes of the distributions themselves are compared. A variety of other non-parametric tests can also be used. All these are aimed at determining whether the experimental manipulation produced an effect on the dependent variable.

The Frequency of Effects problem arises when, in order to answer some theoretical question, it is necessary to know more than just whether there was an effect, or the average size of that effect. For example, suppose that a study were conducted from which it was determined that an experimental manipulation produced a 20 msec increase in the duration of the next fixation. That is, the frequency distributions of these particular fixations had a mean that was 20 msec greater in the experimental condition than in the control condition. It is tempting to conclude that the response to that manipulation was to increase fixation duration by 20 msec, perhaps as a result of extra processing. Such a conclusion is based on the assumption that the experimental manipulation had an effect on 100% of its occurrences, and that the size of that effect, while perhaps variable, averaged 20 msec. In fact, this assumption has not been tested, and may actually be false. It is equally possible that the manipulation produced an effect on the dependent variable on only 25% of its occurrences, and on those instances the fixation duration was increased by an average of 80 msec. At the same time, there was no effect at all on 75% of the instances. These two possibilities and many others are equally harmonious with the original finding of a 20 msec average effect. But which of these is an accurate description of the data may make a great difference in the theoretical conclusions an investigator would draw from the study.

The Frequency of Effects problem arises once it has been established that an experimental manipulation has produced an effect, and consists of trying to determine the frequency with which the effect occurred and the size of the effect when it occurred.

In order to illustrate one possible solution to this problem, we will, first, briefly describe an eye movement experiment in which the problem arises, second, describe a Frequency of Effects Analysis procedure, third, present the results of using the analysis in the study described, and finally, comment on some of the problems and uses of the analysis.

The Study: Variability in the Perceptual Span

There are a number of studies which have used eye movement contingent display control techniques to study the size of the visual region within which certain aspects of the text are perceived during a fixation in reading (McConkie & Rayner, 1976; Rayner, Inhoff, Morrison, Slowiaczek, & Bertera, 1981; Rayner, Well, & Pollatsek, 1980; Rayner, Well, Pollatsek, & Bertera, 1982). In these studies, subjects read from text displayed on a cathode ray tube (CRT) under computer control as their eye position was monitored. On selected fixations or on all fixations, depending upon the study, erroneous letters or masking stimuli occurred in selected areas of the text, with these areas defined with respect to the letter that was directly fixated during the fixation. The eye movement patterns were then examined to determine whether this change in the stimulus pattern in a particular visual region caused a disruption in reading. If it did not, it was assumed that the type of information manipulated must not normally be used from that visual region during reading. These studies have agreed in finding that letter distinctions are perceived within a relatively small area, perhaps four character positions or less to the left of the fixated letter, and eight or fewer to the right, with lengths of words being perceived somewhat farther to the right.

The question studied in the experiment to be described here was this: Are these regions perceived in their entirety on each fixation, or does the actual region perceived vary from fixation to fixation, though always being within the perceptual spans observed in the earlier studies? The strategy used was similar to that just described: During selected fixations the letters at certain locations, defined with respect to the location of the fixated letter, were replaced by other letters, thus resulting in erroneous letters being present at specific retinal locations on those fixations. The eye movement data were then analyzed to determine whether the errors produced an effect, and if they did, to estimate the frequency with which this occurred.

The experimental manipulation was produced in the following manner. Text was displayed on the CRT, refreshed every 3 msec. The subject's eyes were monitored during reading, with sampling of eye position every msec. During the reading of each line, two fixations were selected as critical fixations. As soon as the location of the eyes on such a fixation could be determined, the display was changed in the manner proscribed for that fixation.

Three of the conditions used will be described here, one control and two experimental. In the control condition, no change was made in the text, thus no errors were present during those selected fixations. In the Left-0 condition, all letters to the left of the fixated letter were replaced by other letters, with each letter being replaced by the letter least visually similar to it which did not change the external shape of the word. In the Right-3 condition, all letters more than 3 to the left of the fixated letter were replaced by other letters in the same manner. These erroneous letters remained in the text until the following eye movement began, at which time the normal text was returned to the screen. Thus, the erroneous letters were present in the text only during occasional single fixations. In the experimental conditions, these erroneous letters appeared at locations previously shown to be within the region in which letters are perceived during fixations in reading (Underwood & McConkie, in press). The question to be investigated was whether these erroneous letters would produce an effect on reading every time they occurred or only on some occasions. Were the retinal areas where these letters appeared being attended during all fixations, or only during some of them?

Twelve college students served as subjects in the study, all having good reading skills. Each subject read 16 short passages of about 200 words each. This yielded over 1000 fixations in each condition on which the erroneous letters were present. The subjects were aware of the occasional occurrence of the errors, but reported that they were not bothered much by them. In fact, some of the subjects went a quarter or half of the way through the experiment before becoming aware of the errors.

The dependent variables to be discussed here were the duration of the fixation on which the errors were present (fixation F0), the duration of the following fixation (fixation F1), and the length and direction of the intervening eye movement (saccade S1).

Initial analyses indicated that all three variables showed significant effects of the manipulations. Condition Left-0 increased the duration of fixation F0 by 21 msec, increased the duration of fixation F1 by 13 msec, and increased the likelihood of a regression on saccade S1 from 17% to 34%. Condition Right-3 had no effect on the duration of fixation F0 but increased the duration of fixation F1 by 21 msec and reduced the length of S1 forward saccades by .6 character position. While these differences indicated that effects were occurring, they did not indicate their frequency. This required an additional analysis.

Frequency of Effects Analysis

It is assumed that, had it not been for the experimental manipulation, the frequency distribution of the data from the experimental condition would be very similar to that from the control condition. The difference between the two distributions is assumed to be due to the fact that on a certain proportion *P* of the occurrences of the experimental manipulation an effect was produced on the dependent variable. The size of this effect is assumed to be normally distributed, with a mean of *e* and a standard deviation of *v*. To simplify the model, the values of these parameters are treated as constant across subjects and across the frequency distribution intervals.

Estimates of these parameters can be obtained through an iterative procedure in which different possible values are tried and their effects observed. This procedure involves selecting a value for each parameter, then modifying the frequency distribution from the control condition according to these parameters; that is, taking *P* of the instances for each score or interval and increasing their value such that these instances are now normally distributed with a mean that is *e* greater than their original value and a standard deviation of *v*. This is done for each score or interval. When completed, a new frequency distribution is created by grouping the resulting instances, including both those that were not modified and those that were. This new distribution is then compared to the actual frequency distribution obtained from the experimental condition by obtaining a sum of squared differences (SS_d) index. The combination of values for the three parameters which results in the lowest SS_d index is taken to be the best estimate of these parameters.

For our analyses we used the following procedures.

(1) Decide on intervals to use in the frequency distribution. (We divided the range of fixation duration values into 20 msec intervals, with larger intervals at the extremes.) Obtain the frequencies for each interval for both distributions, (i.e., that from the experimental condition and that from the control condition).

(2) Select a value for each of the parameters, *P*, *e*, and *v*. Values chosen on different iterations can either be selected for the purpose of sampling a wide range of combinations, or obtained by hill-climbing techniques to more efficiently seek the optimal combination.

(3) Begin the creation of a third, hypothesized distribution by letting the frequency within each interval be equal to (1 - *P*) times the frequency of the corresponding interval in the control group distribution. This indicates the number of instances in each interval that are hypothesized to have remained unaffected by the experimental manipulation.

(4) A certain proportion *P* of the instances in each interval are assumed to have been affected by the manipulation. Thus, the scores for these instances must be increased as hypothesized. This was done by taking *P* times the number of instances receiving each score in the control condition, and then distributing these instances as a normal curve with a mean that was *e* msec greater than the original score with a standard deviation of *v*. The number of these instances that now fell within each of the intervals was calculated, and was added to the intervals in the new distribution being created. This was done for each score present in the data, creating a new hypothesized distribution.

(5) The hypothesized distribution was compared to the distribution actually obtained from the experimental condition by using the SS_d index. The difference was obtained between the frequencies of the hypothesized and experimental distributions for each interval, and these values were squared and summed. The resulting SS_d index was taken as an index of the degree of similarity between the two distributions.

(6) This process was repeated with other combinations of values for the parameters until the combination which yielded the lowest SS_d index value was obtained. These values were taken as the best estimate of the frequency with which the experimental manipulation produced an effect, and the nature of that effect when it occurred (i.e., its average size and variance).

We found that the simplest approach was to begin by assuming that $v = 0$, that is, that the effect size does not vary. This makes the calculations much more rapid. Once the optimal values are found for the other two parameters, it is possible to explore the effects of manipulating *v*. In our analyses, adding the third parameter to the model made little difference to the optimal values obtained for *P* and *e*, though it did lead to a better fit as indicated by a reduced SS_d value.

Application of the Frequency of Effects Analysis to the Current Data

The Frequency of Effects Analysis was carried out with the F0 fixation duration data, where the experimental manipulation had been found to produce an average increase in duration of 21 msec. The frequency distributions for these fixation durations are shown in Figure 1. The best fit to the data was obtained with values of .21 for *P*, 151 for *e* and 31 for *v*. Thus, it is estimated that the experimental manipulation actually influenced the F0 fixation duration in 21% of the cases, while the size of the effect, when it occurred, averaged 151 msec with a standard deviation of 31 msec. By this estimate, in 79% of the cases no effect was produced in the Left-0 condition.

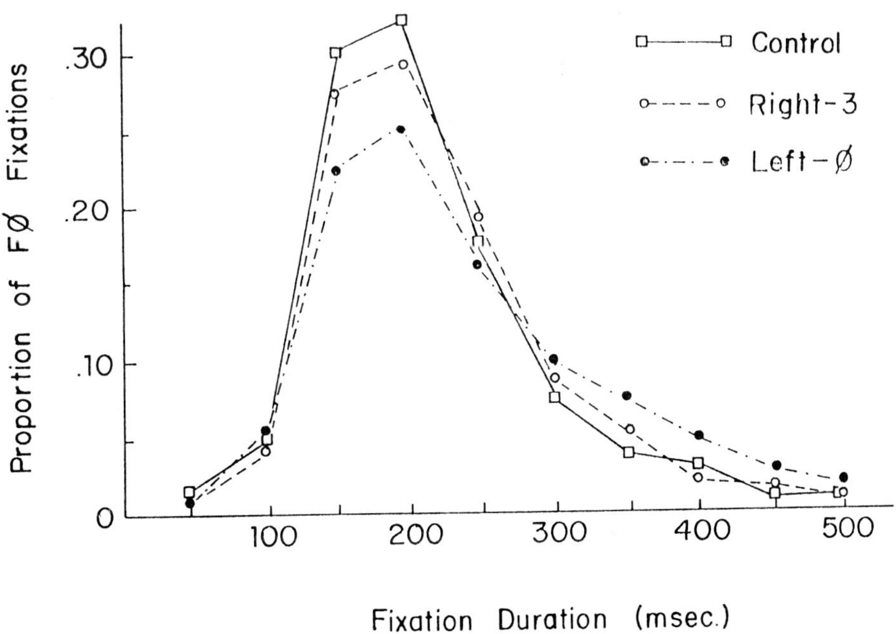

Figure 1

Frequency Distributions for the Duration of Fixation F0, the Critical Fixation, in Control, Left-0 and Right-3 Conditions

Some confirmation of the accuracy of this estimate of the frequency of the effect was obtained when it was found that an effect occurred only for those fixations which were followed by a regressive eye movement. The mean duration of fixations which were followed by a forward eye movement was within 5 msec of the corresponding mean for the control condition. Furthermore, there was a 20% reduction in the number of forward saccades in the experimental condition compared to the control. If 20% of the eye movements in the experimental condition were regressions induced by the presence of erroneous letters, and it was these instances which resulted in longer fixations, then these data suggest a pattern similar to the estimate obtained through the Frequency of Effects Analysis.

Figure 2 presents additional detail concerning the results of the Frequency of Effects Analysis showing the SS_d index for different values of the parameters *P* and *e*. The graph on the left plots the sum obtained for different values of *e*, the effect size parameter, given the optimal value of *P* for each value. The graph on the right is a similar plot, showing SS_d for different values of *P*, the frequency of effect parameter, when *e* was optimized for each. It is clear that there is a certain region within which each parameter minimizes the SS_d index. The effect of varying the third parameter, *v*, was to reduce the sum of squared deviations, but it had little effect on the shapes of the curves shown in Figure 2.

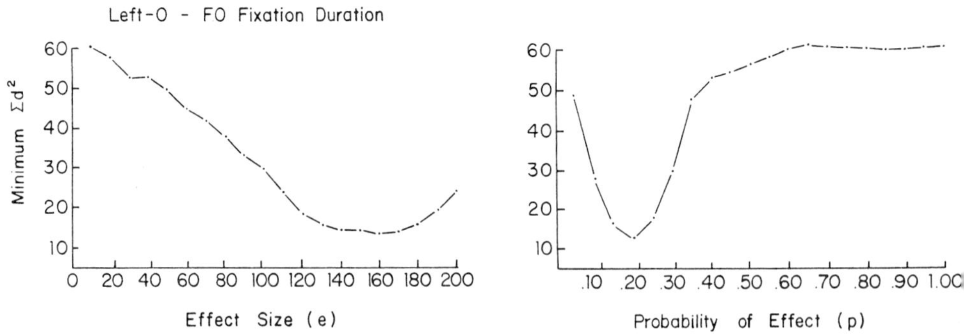

Figure 2

SS_d Values from Frequency of Effects Analysis of Fixation F0 Duration for Condition Left-0

Using the data from durations of F1 fixations following forward saccades, a second application of the Frequency of Effects Analysis involved the data from the Rigth-3 condition. In this case, no effects were found on fixation F0, but a significant difference of 21 msec was found on fixation F1. The analysis yielded estimates of .36 for P, 54 for e, and 30 for v. Thus, it was concluded that, in the cases where the F0 fixation showed no effect of the errors in the text, 36% of the F1 fixations showed an effect of an average 54 msec increase in the duration, with a 30 msec standard deviation.

Figure 3 presents the graphs of the sum of squared deviations as the parameters P and e were varied. Again, the graphs show clear regions where the index was minimized.

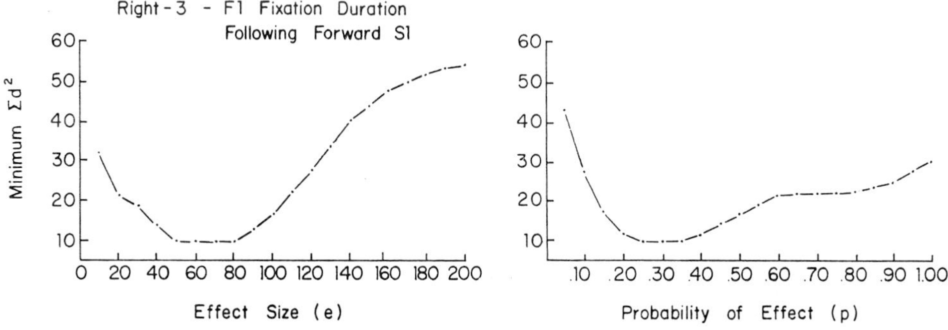

Figure 3

SS_d Values from Frequency of Effects Analysis
of Fixation F1 Durations for Condition Rigth-3

In the study described, other effects of the Rigth-3 experimental manipulations were also identified, leading to the conclusion that readers seldom, if ever, fail to perceive letters in the regions manipulated.

A third application of the Frequency of Effects Analysis was carried out with the S1 forward saccade length data from condition Right-3. In this condition, the duration of fixation F0 showed no effect, but saccade S1 was shortened by an average of .6 character position. This analysis yielded an estimate of 1.0 for P, of .7 for e and .2 for v. These parameters suggest that all saccades were shortened by about .7 character positions. Thus, again there is no indication of some instances in which erroneous letters in this region went undetected.

The application of the Frequency of Effects Analysis to these data appeared successful. It yielded quite different results for different sets of data, and the plots of the sum of squared deviations showed clear areas where the SS_d index was minimized. The results suggested quite a different picture of the effects produced by the experimental manipulation than might have been assumed without its use. Finally, in one case, independent data confirmed the frequency of effect estimate given by the analysis.

Comments on the Frequency of Effects Analysis

Knowledge of the characteristics of the Frequency of Effects Analysis is limited at the present time. Monte Carlo investigation is required in order to estimate the sampling characteristics of the parameters, to determine the sample size needed to yield stable parameter estimates, and to establish how robust the Frequency of Effects Analysis is to violations of its assumptions. In the meantime, the analysis should probably be used only with large data sets (in the data reported, sample sizes ranged from 700 to over 1000 for each condition) and the assumptions should be noted carefully.

It should be recognized that the particular model used in this analysis is only one of many possible models. It may be necessary to modify the model in certain cases to bring it in harmony with known or suspected characteristics of the data.

In spite of the limitations and concerns that exist at the present time, the general technique appears to be useful in revealing characteristics of experimental data which are not apparent from techniques typically used. There are many circumstances in which it would be useful to be able to estimate the frequency of effects in eye movement research. This analysis would be appropriate for use with various eye movement measures, including fixation durations, saccade lengths, and viewing time indices such as gaze duration and reading time. In addition, it would sometimes be appropriate to use the Frequency of Effects Analysis in studies where the time to accomplish certain tasks, such as finding a target in a complex display, serves as the dependent variable. Finally, it should be useful whenever a researcher needs to know the frequency with which an effect occurred.

References

McConkie, G. W., & Rayner, K. (1976). Asymmetry of the perceptual span in reading. Bulletin of the Psychonomic Society, 8, 365-368.

Rayner, K., Inhoff, A. W., Morrison, R. E., Slowiaczek, M. L., & Bertera, J. H. (1981). Masking of foveal and parafoveal vision during eye fixations in reading. Journal of Experimental Psychology: Human Perception and Performance, 7, 167-179.

Rayner, K., Well, A. D., & Pollatsek, A. (1980). Asymmetry of the effective visual field in reading. Perception & Psychophysics, 27, 537-544.

Rayner, K., Well, A. D., Pollatsek, A., & Bertera, J. H. (1982). The availability of useful information to the right of fixation in reading. Perception & Psychophysics, 31, 537-550.

Underwood, N. R., & McConkie, G. W. (in press). Perceptual span for letter distinctions during reading. Reading Research Quarterly.

Eye Movements and Human Information Processing
R. Groner, G.W. McConkie and C. Menz (eds.)

THERE IS MORE THAT MEETS THE EYE THAN THE EYEMIND ASSUMPTION

Dennis F. Fisher* and Wayne L. Shebilske**

*U.S. Army Human Engineering Laboratory
Aberdeen Proving Ground, MD 21005-5001 USA
**National Academy of Science, Vision Committee
Washington, D.C. 20418 USA

Evidence is presented that shows that processing of unfixated words is an integral part of reading semantically rich words in connected discourse. Unfixated words are processed when they are read in isolated sentences or when they are read in short essays. The reading of unfixated words is shown to be more ubiquitous than had been suggested by those who assume a tight link between the eye and mind during reading. This assumption, which has been called the eye-mind assumption, is central to some current models of reading. These models are contrasted with other models that are more compatible with the facts of reading unfixated words.

In order to understand the notions we are conveying in this chapter, as reader all you have to do is read. After reading a few more words pause and note how many words you may have skipped. How many did you fixate? Eyemovement data from the past and present help us answer this question. For example, in the 17 records published by Judd and Buswell (1922) we have found that less than two-thirds of the words were fixated in eight of the records and no more than three-fourths in any of those remaining. Figure 1 shows typical Buswell records.

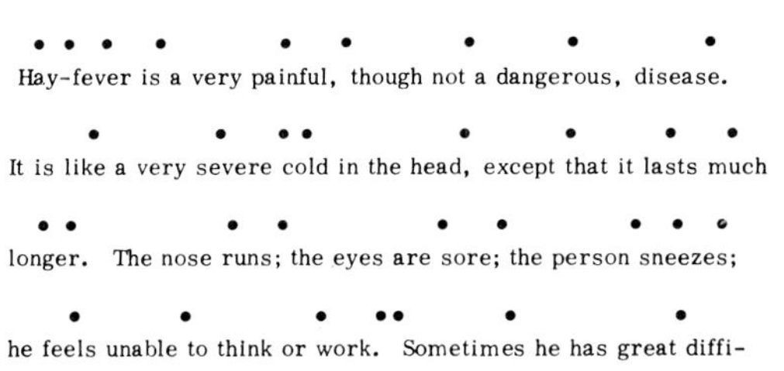

Hay-fever is a very painful, though not a dangerous, disease.
It is like a very severe cold in the head, except that it lasts much
longer. The nose runs; the eyes are sore; the person sneezes;
he feels unable to think or work. Sometimes he has great diffi-

Hay-fever is a very painful, though not a dangerous, disease.
It is like a very severe cold in the head, except that it lasts much
longer. The nose runs; the eyes are sore; the person sneezes;
he feels unable to think or work. Sometimes he has great diffi-

FIG. 1. Data adapted from Judd and Buswell (1922: Plates 16 and 17). Each dot shows the position of a fixation.

Now it would be a little too simplistic to assume that efficient reading depends very heavily on skipping words, and surely the wide range of individual variation among readers and content difficulty among passages makes measurement and assessment difficult. Still, recent data from Just and Carpenter (1980) and further elaborations by Carpenter and Just (1983) and Thibadeau, Just and Carpenter (1982) raise important questions about the processing of skipped words. While they found that readers skipped 62% of the function words like conjunctions, articles, and prepositions and skipped 17% of the content words like nouns, adjectives, adverbs, verbs and pronouns, they argued that only words not skipped are processed.

You as reader are undoubtedly skipping words as you read this chapter. Obviously you must not skip too many words or you will not get any meaning from this text. However, the question at hand is this: Did you read, that is, process the words that you did not fixate?

Unfortunately, eyemovement data do not answer this question directly. However, experimental methodology allows for direct inferences to be made. For example, Ehrlich and Rayner (1981) manipulated the extent to which context constrains the perception of certain words in text. Eyemovements for their special passages and special displays revealed that readers identify words parafoveally and then skip them when constraints are high. Such a conclusion can in itself raise some problems for notions of Carpenter and Just who have been quite explicit in specifying the relationship between the time spent gazing at a word and the amount of processing taking place. In fact, the Ehrlich and Rayner findings of parafoveal identification would be considered an exceptional case.

It must be understood that we are not criticising the Just and Carpenter model and reading simulation directly. That has been done recently by Hogaboam and McConkie (1981), Kliegl, Olson and Davidson (1983), Shebilske and Fisher (1983b), Slowiaczek (1983). Most recently Carrithers and Bever (1984), who reanalyzed the Just and Carpenter data, surprisingly enough were able to reduce the number of variables in their model to 4 from the Just and Carpenter revised list of 11 and account for more (82% vs 78%) of the variance with the most potent variable being word length. While Carrithers and Bever go so far as to say that the Just and Carpenter model does not involve comprehension or the acquisition of new knowledge, our concern is with the major tenants of their model which we do not believe to be exclusionary. They are:

> The IMMEDIACY ASSUMPTION: The assumption that the reader tries to interpret each word upon encountering it; and the EYEMIND ASSUMPTION: The reader continues to fixate a word until all cognitive processes initiated by that word have been completed to some criterion.

According to Carpenter and Just (1983), these assumptions are supported by evidence that the time spent looking at a word (1) is strongly influenced by the characteristics of that word (the word <u>n</u> effect) and (2) is not influenced by the length or frequency of the preceeding word (the word (<u>n</u>-1) null result). These results suggest to them that encoding and lexical access "begin on the word that enables them, as immediacy posits, and that they tend to be completed before the next word is fixated, as the eye-mind assumption posits" (Carpenter and Just, 1983, p. 280).

While these results are indeed consistent with these assumptions, they are also consistent with an important alternative. The alternative is that readers routinely divide their processing time between the fixated word and the following parafoveal words (cf. Hochberg, 1970; Fisher, 1975; Fisher and Lefton, 1976 among others). We call this the "parafoveal processing hypothesis" and it implies that the gaze duration alone does not indicate how processing time is distributed between adjacent words.

Neither the word (n-1) null result nor the word n effect is contrary to the parafoveal processing hypothesis. With respect to the word (n-1) null result, the hypothesis does not imply a requirement that gaze duration of a word should be related to the length or frequency of the preceding word. In fact, neither the existence of a word (n-1) effect nor a word (n-1) null result would contradict the parafoveal processing hypothesis since that hypothesis makes no claims about whether or not the processing of a word fixated during one fixation continues on into the next fixation. With respect to the word n effect, the fact that characteristics of a word influences gaze duration on that word suggests that some processing of a word occurs while the word is fixated. But it does not indicate the proportion of gaze time spent processing the fixated word. Thus, neither the word (n-1) null result nor the word n effect is a strong test of the eye-mind assumption vs. the alternative parafoveal processing hypothesis.

A stronger test is enabled by the fact that readers typically do not fixate every word as mentioned earlier. The eye-mind assumption claims that these words are not processed; in contrast, the parafoveal processing hypothesis claims that; they are processed parafoveally. Evidence for processing is therefore a diacritical test of these two alternatives. To make this test as strong as possible the critical target words selected were important content words and they were not flanked by short function words.

This test, which is so simple in the abstract, is in fact rather difficult to operationalize. One difficulty is determining which words are not fixated. Another difficulty is determining whether the unfixated words were processed. This second difficulty arises because the production of a word on a recall test is not necessarily evidence of processing since the word might be inferred from the context. We overcame the first difficulty by precisely measuring eye position as an experimental group was reading; we overcame the second difficulty by employing a yoked-control group. Subjects in the latter group saw the same context as the experimental subjects, but they did not see the target words that their yoked counterpart did not fixate. That is, each subject in the experimental group had a counterpart in the yoked control group who was presented text containing blanks in place of the target words that the experimental subject did not fixate. Both groups were tested for retention of the target words after reading. They were presented the reading material with blanks in place of the target words, and they were asked to fill in the blanks.

The experimental group was asked to give the exact word that was in the material they read; the yoked-control group was told to guess from the context the exact word or the most likely word at that position. According to the eye-mind assumption, the experimental group and yoked-control group should have equivalent performance on the unfixed (or blank) words since unfixated words are not being processed. In contrast, the parafoveal processing hypothesis predicts that the experimental group should perform significantly better on the unfixated (or blank) words than the yoked-control group since these words are being perceived parafoveally.

METHOD

SUBJECTS: Sixty (60) freshman and sophomore undergraduate students participated in the experiment. Of these, 26 read sentences and 34 read paragraphs.

APPARATUS: One-half of the subjects participating in each of the sentence and paragraph readings had their eyemovements recorded. The eyemovement system was developed by Applied Science Lab. It is an infra-red TV based monitoring system which samples data every 16.7 msec. Subjects sat in a comfortable chair totally unencumbered by biteboards or headrest so that a most natural reading posture can be maintained. In fact, the majority of the time subjects did not even know their eyemovements were being recorded. The display was 40 deg. by 25 deg. where 4 letters/deg. with a resolution of < .9 deg. The subjects sat approx. 3 meters from the screen. Further information about this totally unobtrusive monitoring system can be found in Karsh and Breitenbach (1983).

The remaining subjects in each group were yoked to the eyemovement (E-M) subjects. The following example shows a typical sentence shown to an E-M subject.

Pets have funny names such as my favorite dog, Jingles.
If the E-M subjects "skipped" words 'funny' and 'dog', the yoked subject would see the sentence as:

Pets have _____ names such as my favorite ___, Jingles.

Those subjects yoked to each of the paragraph readers read paragraphs with blanks corresponding to the words that were skipped as detected during eyemovement monitoring. In order to impose a conservative criterion for establishing that a word was unfixated, a word was classified as unfixated only if there were no fixations on it or on the two letter spaces (1/2 deg.) on either side of it.

RESULTS

The data examined were percent of target words skipped, percent of these words that could be reported, and percent of the fixated words that could be reported. The data for subjects reading sentences are presented in Figure 2 and that for subjects reading paragraphs are presented in Figure 3.

Reading vertically these figures indicate the number of subjects in each group and the percent of meaningful content words skipped during reading. They next indicate the percent of skipped or omitted words

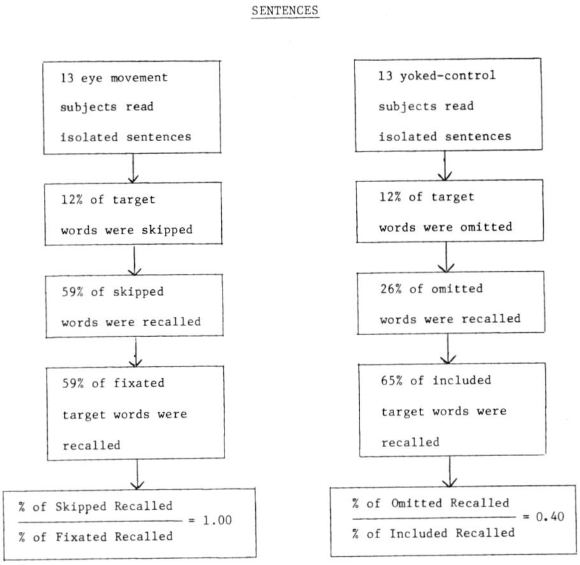

SENTENCES
13 eye movement subjects read isolated sentences
12% of target words were skipped
59% of skipped words were recalled
59% of fixated target words were recalled
% of Skipped Recalled / % of Fixated Recalled = 1.00
13 yoked-control subjects read isolated sentences
12% of target words were omitted
26% of omitted words were recalled
65% of included target words were recalled
% of Omitted Recalled / % of Included Recalled = 0.40

FIG. 2. Comparison of eye movement subjects and yoked controls on filling in words in sentences.

SHORT ESSAYS
17 eye movement subjects read short essays
21% of target words were skipped
59% of skipped words were recalled
61% of fixated target words were recalled
% of Skipped Recalled / % of Fixated Recalled = 0.97
17 yoked-control subjects read short essays
21% of target words were omitted
30% of omitted words were recalled
67% of included target words were recalled
% of Omitted Recalled / % of Included Recalled = 0.45

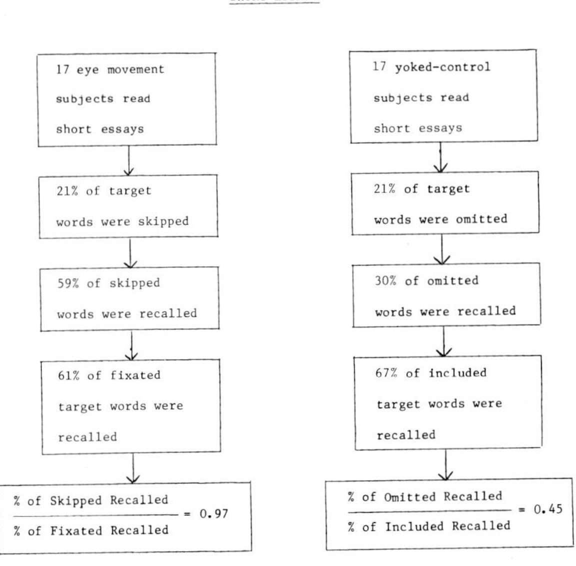

FIG. 3. Comparison of eye movement subjects and yoked controls on filling in words in short essays.

reported and the percent of fixated or non-omitted words reported. Whereas the eye movement group could report the fixated and non-fixated words equally well, the yoked control group was much poorer at reporting the omitted words than those that were not omitted. The ratio of reporting skipped or omitted words to fixated or included words is given at the bottom of the figures. This ratio is 1.0 and .97 for the eye movement groups, and only .40 and .45 for the yoked control groups. The percent of report of omitted words by the yoked control group indicates the extent to which these words could be inferred from the context. The fact that the eye movement group showed a much higher percent of report of these words indicates that they were reading the words even though the words were not fixated. Such a result is incompatible with the EYEMIND ASSUMPTION.

DISCUSSION

The proportion of target words skipped for sentences (12%) and essays (21%) is consistent with previous results for this kind of material. For example, 17 records published by Judd & Buswell (1922) indicated that as many as one-third of the words were skipped on eight of the records, and between 18% and 30% of the words were skipped on the remaining records. Furthermore,these results indicated that readers skipped content words as frequently as they skipped function words (cf. Shebilske, 1975; Shebilske & Fisher, 1983).

More importantly, after knowing for more than 50 years that readers do not fixate every word, we can finally say on the basis of empirical evidence that the unfixated words are read. That is, performance on recall tests of unfixated words exceeds levels that can be accounted for on the basis of inferences from context. These results oppose the eye-mind assumption and support the parafoveal processing assumption

Accordingly, these results have important implications for defining an appropriate unit of analysis for relating reading eye movements to language processes. Specifically, they call into question the unit of "gaze duration per word" or any other unit that is based on the eye-mind assumption (e.g., Just & Carpenter, 1980; Kliegl, Olson, & Davidson, 1983). While this conclusion implies that the more elaborate Thibadeau, Just & Carpenter's (1982) computer simulation model does not represent real time characteristics of reading behavior, it does not undermine many of the important contributions made by Just & Carpenter (1980) although Carrithers and Bever (1984) may have done that. As we noted in an earlier review paper (Shebilske & Fisher, 1983), Carpenter and Just (1977) were pioneers in using larger units of analysis such as gaze duration per sentence to reveal influences of a text's thematic structure on reading eye movements.

Another positive implication of the present results is that they support the importance of extensive efforts that are being made to understand reading at the level of fixations as opposed to gazes. This research on the guidance of fixations includes investigations of temporal decisions about the duration of fixations and spatial decisions about the location of fixations (e.g. cf. Rayner, 1983, chaps. 1-11; Hochberg, 1970).

More specifically, the present results support the generality of the hypothesis that expectations based on contextual constraints can interact with parafoveal information to determine the guidance of fixations. This hypothesis was supported in earlier experiments (e.g. Ehrlich & Rayner, 1981; Ehrlich, 1983), but the design of those experiments raised questions about the generality of the conclusions. For example, Ehrlich & Rayner found that readers fixated target words less frequently when the preceding context highly constrained the meaning of the word. They concluded that "the quality of information picked up from parafoveal vision is constant independently of the level of constraint. However, information from parafoveal vision can be utilized more effectively in the high constraint condition because the threshold for identifying a parafoveal word is lower than in the low constraint condition [p. 654]." Ehrlich (1983) noted, however, that the generality of this specific parafoveal processing hypothesis might be quite limited. Specifically, she noted that "the referent of the target word had been established for the subject earlier in the text. It is possible that this repetitive structure is required to produce the fixation location and strong fixation duration effects that were found [p. 200]."

More importantly, the flexibility in readers' strategies that was so important to Shebilske and Fisher (1981, 1983) is probably related to the contextual issues raised by Rayner and Ehrlich but may have been overlooked by Just and Carpenter because of the coarseness of the "gaze" duration measure. Combining fixations into gazes is quite likely a limitation of the recording system rather than a characteristic of the oculomotor system and, as Carrithers and Bever (1984) suggested, may cover up underlying processes and evidence for flexibility. Excluding peripheral and parafoveal complements to the reading proceses makes it more difficult to explain differences in flexibility during reading. The present results and those of Shebilske and Fisher (1983a) suggest a more parsimonious resolution in that it is likely that parafoveal and peripheral complements are fundamental components of flexible reading.

References

Carrithers, C. & Bever, T. G. (1984) Eye-fixation patterns during reading confirm theories of language comprehension. Cognitive Science, 8, 157-172.

Carpenter, P. A. & Just, M. A. (1977) Reading comprehension as eyes see it. In M. A. Just and P. A. Carpenter (Eds.), Cognitive Processes in Comprehension. New York: Wiley.

Carpenter, P. A. & Just, M. A. (1983) What your eyes do while your mind is reading. In Rayner, K., Eye Movements in Reading: Perceptual and Language Processes. New York: Academic Press.

Ehrlich, S. F. & Rayner, K. (1981) Contextual effects on word perception and eye movements during reading. Journal of Verbal Learning and Verbal Behavior, 20, 641-655.

Ehrlich, S. F. (1983) Contextual influences on eye movements in reading. In Rayner, K., Eye Movements in Reading: Perceptual and Language Processes. New York: Academic Press.

Fisher, D. F. (1975) Reading and visual search. Memory and Cognition, 3, 197-209.

Fisher, D. F. (1979) Understanding the reading process through the use of transformed typography: PSG, CSG and automaticity. In Kolers, P. A., Wrolstad, M. E. & Bouma, H., Processing of Visible Language I. New York: Plenum Press.

Fisher, D. F. & Lefton, L. A. (1976) Peripheral information extraction: A developmental examination of the reading process. Journal of Experimental Child Psychology, 21, 77-93.

Hochberg, J. (1970) Components of Literacy: Speculations and exploratory research. In H. Levin and J. Williams (Eds.), Basic Studies on Reading. New York: Basic Books.

Hogaboam, T. W. & McConkie, G. W. The rocky road from eye fixations to comprehension (Technical Report No. 207). Urbana: University of Illinois, Center for the Study of Reading, May, 1981.

Judd, C. H. & Buswell, G. T. (1922) Silent Reading: A study of various types. Supplemental Education Monographs, (23). Chicago: University of Chicago Press.

Just, M. A. & Carpenter, P. A. (1980) A theory of reading: From eye fixations to comprehension. Psychological Review, 87, 329-354.

Karsh, R. & Breitenbach, F. W. (1983) Looking at looking: The amorphous fixation measure. In Groner, R., Menz, C., Fisher, D. F. & Monty, R. A., Eye Movements and Psychological Functions: International Views. Hillsdale, New Jersey: Lawrence Erlbaum Assoc.

Kliegl, R., Olson, R. K. & Davidson, B. J. (1983) On problems of unconfounding perceptual and language processes. In Rayner, K., Eye Movements in Reading: Perceptual and Language Processes. New York: Academic Press

McConkie, G. (1983) Eye movements and perception during reading. In Rayner, K., Eye Movements in Reading: Perceptual and Language Processes. New York: Academic Press.

O'Regan, J. K. (1983) Elementary perceptual and eye movement control process in reading. In Rayner, K., Eye Movements in Reading: Perceptual and Language Processes.. New York: Academic Press.

O'Regan, K. (1981) The "Convenient Viewing Position" hypothesis. In D. F. Fisher, R. A. Monty & J. W. Senders (Eds.), Eye Movements: Cognition and Visual Perception. Hillsdale, New Jersey: Lawrence Erlbaum Assoc.

Rayner, K. (1983) The perceptual span and eye movement control during reading. In Rayner, K., Eye Movements in Reading: Perceptual and Language Processes. New York: Academic Press.

Shebilske, W. L. (1975) Reading eye movements from an information-processing point of view. In D. Massaro (Ed.), Understanding Language. New York: Academic Press.

Shebilske, W. L. & Fisher, D. F. (1981) Eye movements reveal components of flexible reading strategies. In M. L. Kamil (Ed.), Directions in Reading: Research and Instruction. 30th Yearbook of the National Reading Conference.

Shebilske, W. L. & Fisher,D. F. (1983a) Eye movement and context effects during reading extended discourse. In Rayner, K., Eye Movements in Reading: Perceptual and Language Processes. New York: Academic Press

Shebilske, W. L. & Fisher,D. F. (1983b) Understanding extended discourse through the eyes: How and why. In Groner, R., Menz, C., Fisher, D. F. & Monty, R. A., Eye Movements and Psychological Functions: International Views. Hillsdale, New Jersey: Lawrence Erlbaum Assoc.

Slowiaczek, M. L. (1983) What does the mind do while the eyes are gazing? In Rayner, K., Eye Movements in Reading: Perceptual and Language Processes. New York: Academic Press.

Thibadeau, R., Just, M. A. & Carpenter, P. A. (1982) A model of the time course and content of human reading. Cognitive Science, 6, 101-155.

Eye Movements and Human Information Processing
R. Groner, G.W. McConkie and C. Menz (eds.)

EYE POSITION AND WORD IDENTIFICATION DURING READING

George W. McConkie & Thomas W. Hogaboam

Center for the Study of Reading
University of Illinois at Urbana-Champaign
U.S.A.

College students read text displayed by computer as their eyes were being monitored. On occasional fixations or saccades the text was removed and the subject reported the last word that had been read and tried to guess the next word. Distributions of the location of the last read word with respect to the last fixated word give an indication of what words are being read during a fixation. The data do not support an anticipation model of reading nor the acquisition of peripheral cues concerning upcoming words.

One way to study the on-going mental processes taking place during reading is to interrupt reading at certain times and to have the readers introspect on some aspect of their mental state. This can be done using eye movement technology by programming the computer to detect when the eyes have reached a particular place in the text or have executed a certain movement pattern and then to remove the text from the display screen. This serves as a signal for readers to report their introspections. We will refer to this as the Disappearing Text technique.

The authors conducted a series of pilot studies with themselves and others, causing the disappearance of the text at random times during reading and attempting to see what aspects of processing could be reported. These studies indicated that the dominant experience which the reader has when the text disappears is that certain words are being read. One of the authors (GWM) spent ten hours reading a novel with the text being removed at random times averaging about every tenth line of text, and attempting to introspect on some aspect of the syntactic processing taking place. He was unable to introspectively grasp any aspect of syntactic processing and, as was found previously, the overwhelming experience was that of reading certain words. Attempts to introspect about hypotheses or predictions of upcoming words were equally unsuccessful. While it was possible to predict what words would occur next, this required a special effort and a shift of perspective rather than being a natural part of the ongoing reading process.

For these reasons, the initial studies performed using the Disappearing Text technique, as reported in this paper, investigated the relationship between the location of the words being read and the location of the eyes in the text. This was done by occasionally removing the text during reading and having the reader report the last word which had been read. Distributions of the locations of the last word read, in relation to the location of the last word on which the eyes were centered prior to the text's disappearance, served as data and were compared for different conditions.

The first study reported here compared these distributions when the text disappeared during vs. following a fixation and when the text was simply blanked out vs. being replaced by a masking pattern. The second study manipulated the time during the fixation at which the text disappeared. The third study replicated results from the earlier studies.

EXPERIMENT I

Method

Design

In this experiment, two variables were manipulated, each with two levels. The first variable was Text Replacement Type; when the text disappeared it was replaced either by an unbroken line of upper-case X's or by a blank screen. The second variable was Replacement Time; the text disappeared either 120 msec following the beginning of a fixation, or after the fixation was complete (that is, during the following saccade). These two variables were combined into a 2X2 factorial design, with each of the four conditions occurring four times for each subject during the reading of a single passage. In addition, the text disappeared twice during regressive saccades, but insufficient data were obtained in this condition and it will not be discussed further.

Passage

The passage was 720 words in length and discussed supposed characteristics of gnomes. It was formatted with a maximum line length of 73 character positions, yielding 54 lines of text. This passage was then divided into 18 segments, each being one to five lines in length. The last line of each segment was that on which the text disappeared. The reader had no indication as to when the disappearance would occur. The experimental conditions were assigned to text segments randomly, with the restriction that all four conditions must occur before any of them could be repeated.

Subjects

Eleven undergraduate students were paid to participate in the study. All had been subjects in at least one previous eye movement study and were familiar with the equipment and general procedures.

Procedures

The text was displayed one line at a time on a cathode-ray tube, refreshed every 3 msec, as the reader's eyes were being monitored. After completing one line, the reader pressed a button to cause the next line to appear. Readers were instructed to read and try to comprehend the passage. They were also told that at unpredictable times during reading the text would disappear from the screen, sometimes being replaced by X's and sometimes just being blanked out. When this occurred, they were to immediately report the last word they had read before the text disappeared. In addition, they were asked to guess what the next word was beyond the last word they remembered reading. After recording this report, the experimenter would cause the line of text to reappear and they could continue reading the passage. In this way, the readers could check the accuracy of their reports and guesses. The computer program removed or replaced the text either during or after the fixation which followed the fourth forward saccade on a critical line.

Prior to reading each segment, the reader performed a calibration task by looking directly at a dot and pressing a button, as it moved to each of five locations along the line where text would appear.

The entire session required 20 to 40 minutes, and the time between text segments, during which readers gave their reports, typically ranged from 20 to 60 seconds. Longer intervals occurred when people had difficulty generating a guess about the next word. The time elapsing between the disappearance of the text and the report of the last word read was typically less than 5 sec.

Equipment

Eye movements were monitored using a Biometrics Model SG limbus reflection eye movement monitor, with the eye position being sampled every msec. A bite bar was used to stabilize head position. Text was displayed on a cathode-ray tube with fast-decay phosphor and was refreshed every 3 msec. A description of the equipment and programs used in creating the eye-movement contingent display manipulations and in reducing the data is presented elsewhere (McConkie, Zola, Wolverton, & Burns, 1978).

Results

Data for 27% of the trials were discarded for the following reasons: occurrence of blinks, 11%; fewer than four forward saccades on the line, 8%; equipment failure, 5%; and eye movement patterns that rendered the data uninterpretable, 5%.

For each remaining trial, the last correctly reported word was identified, as well as the first word indicated as being a guess. Subjects frequently reported a three or four word sequence, often a complete or partial phrase, rather than reporting a single word, even though asked to report just the last word read. In earlier pilot work, subjects showed this same tendency; this seemed easier for them to do than to report a single last word read. Sometimes in guessing the next word, a word sequence was also given. In these cases, the last word of the reportedly read sequence, and the first word of the guessed sequence were used as data.

Subjects had little trouble with the task of reporting what they had read. The words reported as having been read occurred on the line of text 88% of the time. Errors were of two types: reporting words not present on the line, and reporting punctuation marks that were not present. The most common error was reporting commas where none occurred. Under 6% of the instances were erroneous word reports.

In contrast to this, subjects' guesses about the following word were correct only 31% of the time. The words "the" and "and" accounted for 36% of the correct guesses, while nouns, verbs and adjectives together accounted for only 32%. Most of the remaining correct guesses were short words such as "in," "of" and "by." Only 9.9% of all guesses were correct content words.

For each correct trial, the distance was computed between the last read word and the word which was fixated during the last fixation on which text was present. This distance was measured in terms of words, regardless of their length. If the last word reported was also the last word fixated, this distance was 0. If the last word reported was the word prior to the last fixated word, this distance was -1. Figure 1 presents the relative frequency distributions for this distance.

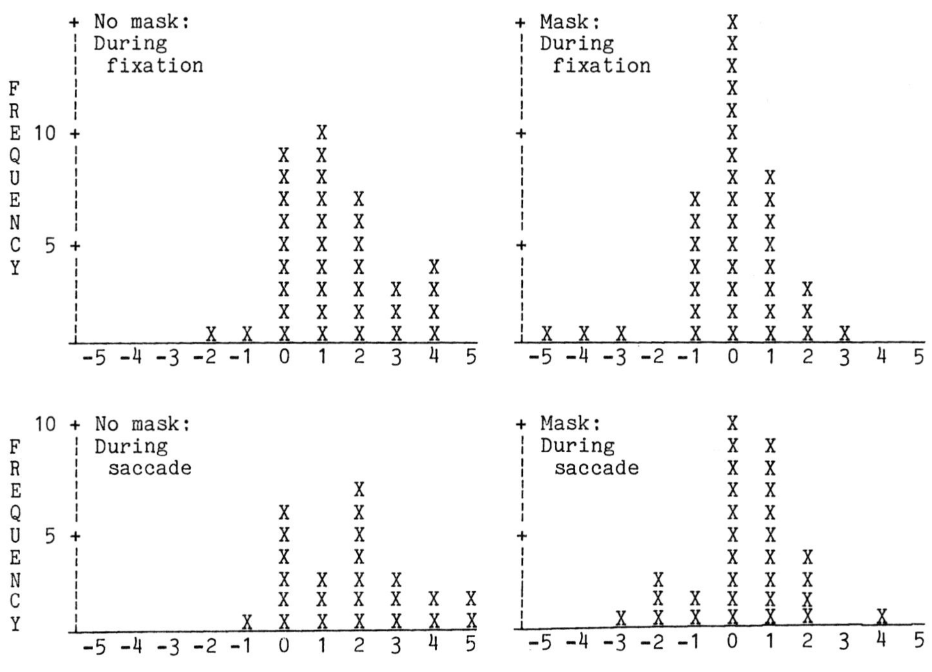

Figure 1: Frequency distributions of the location of the last read word with respect to the location of the last fixation on which text was present. Distance is measured in word units, without regard for word length.

As Figure 1 indicates, the distributions are quite different when the text was masked than when it was simply blanked out. When masked, the median word reported was that which was directly fixated; when blanked, the median word reported was one or two to the right of the fixated word. The data for each condition were grouped according to whether the last read word was the fixated word, a word lying to the left of it, or a word lying to the right. These frequencies were collapsed across the text removal time conditions, and the mask vs. no-mask conditions were compared using a Chi-square test. This yielded a Chi-square value of 14.30 which, with 2 degrees of freedom, is significant at the .001 level. It is clear that the mask interferes with processing that continues in the absence of the mask.

When the text was removed during a saccade, the computer recorded where the following fixation was located, even though the text was not present on that fixation. This makes it possible to ask where the last reported word was located with respect to the location of the word to which the eyes were being sent for the next fixation. A distribution of these data indicates the relationship between the location of the last word read during one fixation, and where the eyes were sent for the next fixation. These distributions are presented in Figure 2.

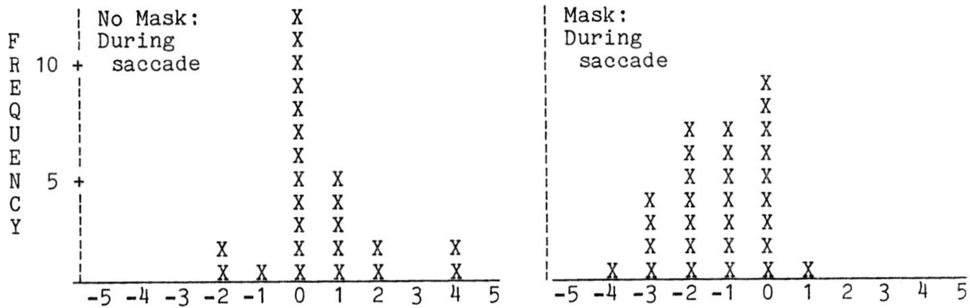

Figure 2: Frequency distributions of the location of the last read word with respect to the location of the fixation following the last fixation on which the text was present. Distance is measured in word units, without regard for word length.

As Figure 2 indicates, in 66% of the cases in which the text was masked the saccade was taking the eyes to a word beyond the last word that could be reported; in all but one of the remaining cases the eyes were going to the last reported word. However, the pattern is quite different when the text was simply blanked out during the saccade. Here, on half the instances the eyes were centered on the last reported word, and on all but three of the remaining instances, the last reported word lay to the right of the fixated word. Grouping the data according to whether the last read word was on, to the left of, or to the right of the word to which the eyes were sent, and comparing these data for the mask and no-mask conditions yields a Chi-square of 18.15 which, with 2 degrees of freedom, is significant at the .001 level.

The time at which the text was removed had very little effect. A Chi-square test on the data collapsed across text replacement type yielded a Chi-square value of 0.73.

Discussion

This study demonstrates that adult subjects are quite able to perform the task of reporting the last word or words read when they are interrupted during reading, and it provides initial data concerning the location of this word with respect to the location of the eyes during the last fixation on which text was present, and to the location of the following fixation.

There was a clear distinction between the accuracy of the last word reported as having been read, and the guess concerning what the next word was. The last read word was highly accurate; the guess was not. Subjects' reactions to the two tasks were also quite different. The last word read was reported with great confidence, whereas subjects felt they had no information about the immediately following word and were making a pure guess. These facts suggest that there was a clear dichotomy between the last word read, which could be reported, and the immediately following word, about which the reader had little or no information beyond that provided by language constraints. It seems likely that the subjects were being accurate in indicating the last word that had been identified, and that the words beyond it simply had not been dealt with; little or no information had been obtained about them that would substantially constrain their identity. The other option, of course, is that whatever information had been obtained from these latter words was quickly forgotten and not available to assist in forming the guess. A more carefully designed study is needed to determine whether the guessing rate for these words might be elevated somewhat as a result of peripherally-obtained information, but with a guessing rate of 31% such influences must be small.

At the end of a fixation, the distance between the last word read and the word being fixated showed a considerable amount of variability. However, it is important to note that the nature of the distribution was strongly influenced by the type of replacement stimulus used when the text disappeared. Apparently, when the text is simply blanked out sufficient visual information is maintained to permit some continued processing of the text. Replacing the text with a mask corrupts this information or otherwise interferes with processing so the last read word does not lie as far to the right. In contrast, studies of letter and word perception do not find effects of masking following presentations of 100 msec or longer (Taylor & Taylor, 1983, p. 175). The masking which occurs during reading may result from the greater complexity of the stimulus pattern presented by a full line of text, or from the possibility that the utilization of the visual information may not take place as early in the exposure period during fixations in reading (Blanchard, McConkie, Zola, & Wolverton, 1984) as it does in word-identification tasks.

Haber & Hershenson (1980, p. 152) suggest, on the basis of research by Breitmeyer & Ganz (1976), that the suppression associated with the making of a saccade serves to isolate individual fixations from the effects of masking from prior and following fixations. The present results do not support that conclusion, since the distribution of locations of the last read word were quite different when a mask occurred on the following fixation than when the screen was simply blanked out. Replacing the text with a mask during a saccade shifted the distribution of the last word read to the left as compared to the blanking condition. Apparently the presence of the mask on the following fixation either corrupted lingering visual information from the prior fixation or interfered with its processing in some way.

In reading, the normal case is to have text present on each fixation, with the potential for the pattern present on each new fixation to reduce the amount that could have been read from the last. Therefore, it is concluded that the results obtained when the text is masked during a saccade give the most accurate indication of what words are being read during a fixation while reading a passage. However, as will be discussed later, even this condition may overestimate what is normally read.

The distribution for the last read word for the condition in which the text was masked during a saccade, presented in Figure 1, indicates that in a majority of cases the last read word was the word on which the eyes were centered during that fixation or the word immediately to the right of it. This agrees with prior research which indicates that the visual region within which letter information is used during a fixation is relatively small and is asymmetric to the right (McConkie, 1983; Rayner, 1983). Instances in which the last read word lay to the left of the fixated word could include cases in which identification of the fixated word had failed and another fixation on it would normally be required, and cases in which the fixated word was simply not attended for some reason. Instances in which the last read word lay further to the right could include cases where the lengths of the words concerned were very short and where the eyes were centered near the end of the fixated word.

Finally, the results indicated that the time at which the text was removed had little effect on the distribution of the last read word. Experiment II was performed to further explore the effects of masking the text at different times during the fixation.

EXPERIMENT II

Method

This study was conducted in the same manner as Experiment I, using the same text and with subjects obtained in the same manner. Four conditions were used in the study, consisting of four different times during the fixation at which the text was removed and replaced by a line of X's. These times were 60, 120 or 180 msec following the onset of the fourth fixation on the line, or during the saccade following the fixation. Each subject received each of these conditions four times according to the same design as was used in Experiment I. Again, subjects were asked to report the last word read and to guess what the next word would be.

Results

As before, subjects' reports were frequently in the form of word sequences, often phrases. The last read word was actually on the line being read 92% of the time, but the following word was guessed correctly only 31% of the time.

Figure 3 presents the distributions of the location of the last read word. The top three distributions present this location with respect to the location of the last fixated word for conditions in which the text was removed during the fixation, either 60, 120 or 180 msec following its onset. The bottom two distributions present data for the condition in which the text was removed during the saccade. In the left distribution, the data are plotted with respect to the location of the last fixated word. This will be referred to as the Fixation N distribution. In the right distribution, these same data are plotted with respect to the location of the following fixation, after the saccade during which the text was removed. This will be referred to as the Fixation N+1 distribution.

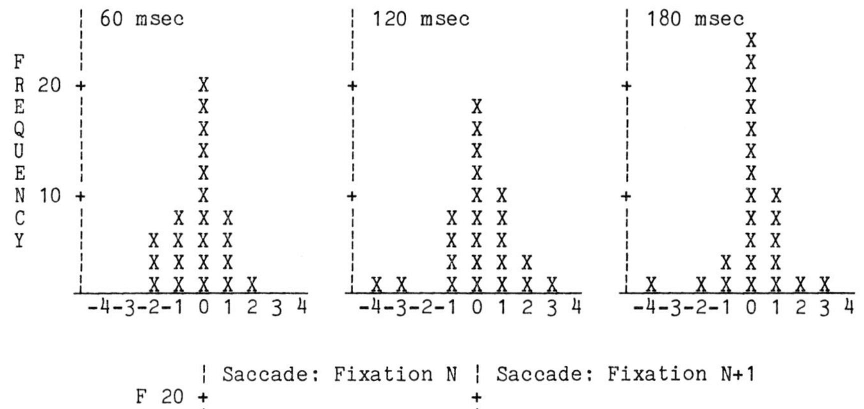

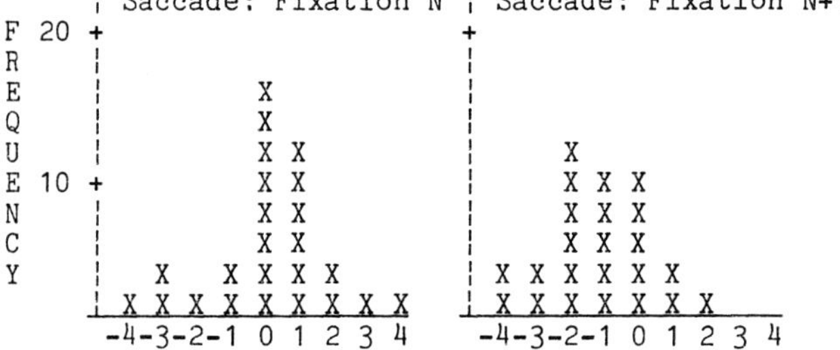

Location of the Last Read Word

Figure 3: Frequency distributions of the location of the last read word with respect to the location of the last fixation on which text was present (Fixation N) or the fixation following (Fixation N+1). The text was removed either 60, 120 or 180 msec following the onset of Fixation N, or during the saccade following Fixation N.

Each distribution was partitioned into three categories: instances in which the last read word was the word fixated, a word to the left of it, or a word to the right of it. A series of Chi-square tests indicated that all the distributions plotted with respect to the last fixated word did not differ from each other, but all did differ significantly ($p<.001$) from the Fixation N+1 distribution. The means of these distributions were as follows: 60 msec, -0.21; 120 msec, 0.08; 180 msec, 0.08; Fixation N, 0.18; Fixation N+1, -1.26.

Discussion

The Fixation N+1 distribution can be taken as indicating the situation that exists at the beginning of a fixation, prior to receiving any visual information. In this distribution, the location of the last read word is plotted with respect to the fixation following the removal of the text, so no information about the text was obtained on that fixation. The Fixation N distribution indicates the situation that exists after a fixation. Here the data are plotted with respect to the location of the last fixation on which the text was seen, and the text was present for the full period of that fixation. Thus, a comparison of these two distributions indicates the degree of advancement through the text that results from a single fixation in reading. The means of these two distributions differ by 1.44, indicating an average advancement of 1½ words as a result of a fixation.

The three top distributions in Figure 3 indicate the situation as a result of having visual information available for three intermediate periods. Thus, we might expect them to show a gradual transition between the two distributions just considered. The difference between the mean for the Fixation N+1 distribution and the 60 msec distribution is 1.05, or about 3/4 of the advancement that occurs during a fixation. The remaining ¼ occurs with additional visual exposure to the text.

These results indicate that the visual system is capable of registering most of the information needed to support reading during the first 60 msec of a fixation in a form little influenced by a visual mask. Providing additional exposure time allowed some further advancement but the added benefit was relatively small compared to the amount of time involved. This finding agrees with the findings of Rayner, Inhoff, Morrison, Slowiaczek & Bertera (1981) who reported that relatively normal reading is possible when the text is present for only the first 50 msec of each fixation.

From the fact that most of the visual information needed for reading can be registered within the first 50 msec of a fixation, Rayner, et al. (1981) argued that this must be the period of word identification, and that the remainder of the fixation is then spent in further processing and determining where the eyes are to be sent next. However, a more recent study (Blanchard, McConkie, Zola, & Wolverton, 1984) suggests that a distinction must be made between the registration and the utilization of the visual information. Blanchard, et al. provide evidence that the utilization of the information in the text can actually take place at any time throughout the fixation. In many instances, readers showed no awareness of a word which was present during the first part of a fixation, and reported having seen only a word that was present during the latter part. Thus, while the nature of the visual system is such that the stimulus pattern present at the beginning of a fixation is registered and can be used for reading, it appears that the normal utilization of that information does not necessarily take place during that early period. In fact, when transmission delays in the visual system are taken into account, it seems unlikely that words are ever identified during the initial 50 msec of a fixation (McConkie, Underwood, Zola, & Wolverton, 1985).

The Fixation N+1 distribution in Figure 3 provides information about eye movement control during reading. It indicates that in the majority of instances when a forward saccade is made the eyes are being sent beyond the last read word. In only about 25% of the instances were the eyes sent to the last read word and seldom were they sent short of it.

EXPERIMENT III

In order to replicate some of the findings of Experiment II, a third experiment was conducted. This study repeated the mask condition of Experiment I, with the text always being removed during a saccade.

Method

The equipment and procedures used were identical to those of Experiment I. Ten subjects participated who were drawn from the same subject pool as in the earlier studies. A new 47-line passage was used, which gave information about backpacking. It was broken into 18 segments, varying in length from 1 to 5 lines. As the subjects read the last line of each segment, the text was replaced with a line of X's during the third forward saccade. When that occurred, the task was to report the last word read and to guess what the next word would be. There was the possibility of 18 data points per subject.

Results

Again subjects were accurate in their reporting of the last read word, in that it appeared on the target line 95% of the time. Guesses of the word following that word were correct 24% of the time, with function words accounting for 70% of the correct guesses. Twenty-six percent of the trials were lost for various reasons. In order to increase the sample size, the data from the Experiment I condition in which the text was masked during a saccade were added to the sample.

When the location of the last read word was plotted with respect to Fixation N (the last fixation on which the text was present), the last read word was the fixated word in 40% of the instances, the word to the left of it in 22%, and the word to the right in 38%. When the location of the last read word was plotted with respect to Fixation N+1 (the fixation following the saccade on which the text was removed), the last read word was the word fixated 25% of the time, it lay to the left 69% of the time, and to the right 5% of the time. It lay one word to the left 22% of the time, and two to the left 24% of the time. Thus, as in Experiment II, the likelihood of sending the eyes to the last read word, or one or two words beyond it, were all approximately equal, and subjects seldom sent their eyes short of it.

The means of the two distributions are -1.50 for Fixation N+1 and 0.07 for Fixation N, again showing an advancement of about 1½ words as a result of making a fixation.

The results from this study are very consistent with those found in Experiment II, in terms of the amount of advancement resulting from making a fixation, and the means and shapes of the distributions.

GENERAL DISCUSSION

The Disappearing Text technique was used in three studies to investigate the relation between the location of the last word that could be reported when the text disappeared and the location of the last fixation on which the text was seen. The results showed both variability and consistency in this relationship. On the one hand, the last word reported as having been read was most commonly the word fixated during the last fixation, or the word to the right of it, in agreement with earlier studies indicating a rightward assymmetry in the perceptual span during reading (McConkie & Rayner, 1976; Pollatsek, Bolozky, Well, & Rayner, 1981). On the other hand, the responses were not restricted to these two word locations. On about one-third of the trials, words from other locations were reported. Most of these were words lying to the left of the fixated word, with the fixated word not being reported. The current data do not permit a conclusion as to whether the fixated word was not reported because it had not been identified on that fixation (either because of inattention to it, having obtained insufficient visual information on that fixation to identify it, or because the reader was not yet ready to utilize that word in the on-going reading and hence did not use the visual information which had been available), or because it had been identified but quickly forgotten. Subjects in the experiment did not report the experience of having known what a word was only to be unable to report it as might be expected if forgetting were the primary reason for this phenomenon.

An argument against the forgetting explanation is the striking difference between the readers' ability to accurately report the last word read, and their poor performance on guessing the next word. If words were frequently being identified and then forgotten, we might expect that some information about the forgotten word would still be available and could raise the guessing probability for the word. However, the guessing rates observed, 24% to 31%, were in the range that would be expected as a result of guessing from context alone, without the aid of perceived information from the word itself. While these observations do not rule out a forgetting explanation, they do provide some evidence against it.

It may be that in some instances in which the last read word lay 2 or more words to the left of the last fixated word, the reader was not attending to the visual information available during the fixation. In normal reading it may have been necessary to later regress to these words in order to read them. The interruption produced by the disappearance of the text prohibited us from observing such regressions, if they would have occurred. It is also possible that readers sometimes ignore portions of the text as they read, but from the parts of the text to which they do attend they are able to satisfactorally comprehend the message. Other studies will be required to investigate these possibilities more specifically.

The distributions obtained in the studies conducted would appear to indicate the distribution of the location of words identified during a fixation while reading. It is important to note, however, that these results may not generalize to normal reading quite that completely. In reading, the fixation studied would have been followed by another fixation on which reading would have continued. In the Disappearing Text task reading is terminated during or after the last fixation, and the reader is then free to focus attention on any cues from the visual display which remain in memory and to use them to try to identify an additional word. It is quite possible that some words reported in the Disappearing Text task would normally not have been identified until the following fixation. Thus, this task may overestimate the frequency with which the fixated word or words to the right of it are identified during a fixation in reading.

However, the fact that the results are quite harmonious with previous studies estimating the size of the perceptual span during reading suggests that any such overestimate is not great.

It has often been suggested that skilled readers form hypotheses and anticipations of upcoming text, and that these facilitate perception of the words (Goodman, 1976). Peripherally obtained information is assumed to facilitate this process by reducing the number of alternatives, thereby leaving relatively little further perceptual work to do when a word is brought into the fovea (Haber & Haber, 1981). If this were the nature of perceptual processing during skilled reading, we might have expected the readers in the studies reported here to make accurate guesses of upcoming words based on the peripherally obtained information, and to make such guesses quite readily when reading was terminated. However, the subjects showed a reluctance to try to guess, felt very unsure of their guesses, and in fact were usually incorrect. These observations do not seem harmonious with a model in which peripheral information about upcoming words is accumulated and anticipations are formulated to facilitate perception. Furthermore, in most cases the word being guessed was the word immediately to the right of the fixated word, or the word just beyond that. In other cases, it was actually the word being directly fixated or a word to the left of it. In only about 3% of the cases did the word to be guessed lie more than 2 word positions to the right of the directly fixated word. Thus, this word was typically within a region in which visual information about it could be obtained from the fovea or near periphery; at least such information as the word length, word shape and extreme letters. Haber, Haber & Furlin (1983) have demonstrated that when readers are given cues to the length and shape of words, their guesses of those words from context rise dramatically. The low guessing rates of the subjects in the present studies indicate that either they had not obtained this type of information from the words not yet read, or, if they had, they were not using it in their guesses. Thus, the data do not support this type of anticipation model of reading.

The results from these studies suggest a model of perception in reading in which there are neither anticipations nor extensive use of peripheral vision for acquiring cues from upcoming words. Rather, words are attended and identified within a small visual area, and the reader has little or no information about words that are not attended and identified, even when they lie within the fovea itself. It is not necessarily the case that a directly fixated word is identified; rather the identification depends on whether it is attended on that fixation. This strong link between attention and identification would account for the variability in the location of the last read word as obtained in these studies. Finally, there is a possibility that where the eyes are sent for the next fixation is related to the location of the last read word, with the eyes sometimes going to that word but more commonly going one or two words beyond it. A mechanism of this sort has the virtue of simplicity; there is no need for complex machinery to preview peripheral stimuli or to form anticipations or eliminate possible words based on certain visual characteristics. Rather, the focus of mental activity can be on language processing with words being attended and identified as needed to support this activity.

The Disappearing Text technique is quite similar to a method used to study the eye-voice span during reading. Although some studies of the eye-voice span have simultaneously recorded eye position and voice (Buswell, 1920;

Fairbanks, 1937), others have obscured the text at particular times and recorded how far the voice continued in the absence of the text (Gray, 1917; Levin & Addis, 1979; Quantz, 1897). This presumably indicates how far the eyes were ahead of the voice at the time the text was obscured. Buswell (1920) noted that the eye-voice spans obtained with this latter technique tended to be larger than the distance typically obtained with actual monitoring of the eyes and voice. This leads to the suspicion that words are sometimes identified beyond the location of the eyes, a suspicion that is confirmed by the present study.

The Disappearing Text technique is similar to that used in the eye-voice span studies, but is used to investigate a somewhat different relationship: how far along the line of text processing proceeds using visual information available from the current fixation. This might be termed the eye-mind span. As with the eye-voice span, the eye-mind span raises both temporal and spatial issues. The current studies have not dealt with temporal delays between fixating and identifying a word. They have focused only on the spatial issue, identifying the distribution of distances of the last read word from the word being fixated.

References

Blanchard, H. E., McConkie, G. W., Zola, D., & Wolverton, G. S. (1984). The time course of visual information utilization during fixations in reading. Journal of Experimental Psychology: Human Perception and Performance, 10(1), 75-89.

Breitmeyer, B. G., & Ganz, L. (1976). Implications of sustained and transient channels for theories of visual pattern masking, saccadic suppression, and information processing. Psychological Review, 83, 1-36.

Buswell, G. T. (1920). An experimental study of the eye-voice span in reading. Supplementary Educational Monographs, 17.

Fairbanks, G. (1937). The relation between eye movements and voice in the oral reading of good and poor silent readers. Psychological Monographs, 48(3), 78-107.

Goodman, K. S. (1976). Behind the eye: What happens in reading. In H. Singer & R. B. Ruddell (Eds.), Theoretical models and processes of reading. Newark, DE: International Reading Association.

Gray, C. T. (1917). Types of reading ability as exhibited through tests and laboratory experiments. Supplementary Educational Monographs, 1(5).

Haber, L. R., & Haber, R. N. (1981). Perceptual processes in reading: An analysis-by-synthesis model. In F. I. Pirozzolo & M. C. Wittrock (Eds.), Neuropsychological and cognitive processes in reading (pp. 167-200). New York: Academic Press.

Haber, L. R., Haber, R. N., & Furlin, K. R. (1983). Word length and word shape as sources of information in reading. Reading Research Quarterly, 18, 165-189.

Haber, R. N., & Hershenson, M. (1980). The psychology of visual perception (2nd edition). New York: Holt, Rinehart & Winston.

Levin, H., & Addis, A. B. (1979). The eye-voice span. Cambridge, MA: MIT Press.

McConkie, G. W. (1983). Eye movements and perception during reading. In K. Rayner (Ed.), Eye movements in reading: Perceptual and language processes (pp. 65-96). New York: Academic Press.

McConkie, G. W., & Rayner, K. (1976). Asymmetry of the perceptual span in reading. Bulletin of the Psychonomic Society, 8, 365-368.

McConkie, G. W., Underwood, N. R., Zola, D., & Wolverton, G. S. (1985). Some temporal characteristics of processing during reading. Journal of Experimental Psychology: Human Perception and Performance, 11 (in press).

McConkie, G. W., Zola, D., Wolverton, G. S., & Burns, D. D. (1978). Eye movement contingent display control in studying reading. Behavior Research Methods and Instrumentation, 10, 154-166.

Pollatsek, A., Bolozky, S., Well, A. D., & Rayner, K. (1981). Asymmetries in the perceptual span for Israeli readers. Brain and Language, 14, 174-180.

Quantz, J. O. (1897). Problems in the psychology of reading. Psychological Monographs, 2.

Rayner, K. (1983). The perceptual span and eye movement control during reading. In K. Rayner (Ed.), Eye movements in reading: Perceptual and language processes (pp. 97-120). New York: Academic Press.

Rayner, K., Inhoff, A. W., Morrison, R. E., Slowiaczek, M. L., & Bertera, J. H. (1981). Masking of foveal and parafoveal vision during eye fixations in reading. Journal of Experimental Psychology: Human Perception and Performance, 7, 167-179.

Taylor, I., & Taylor, M. M. (1983). The psychology of reading. New York: Academic Press.

Eye Movements and Human Information Processing
R. Groner, G.W. McConkie and C. Menz (eds.)

EYE MOVEMENT PARAMETERS IN READING: EFFECTS OF LETTER SIZE AND LETTER SPACING

Dieter Heller[1] & Annelies Heinisch[2]
1) Institut für Psychologie, University of Basel
2) Institut für Pädagogik II, University of Würzburg

In the present experiment, the effects of size of print and letter distance are examined in children who are starting to learn to read as well as in poor readers between 8 and 11 years of age. The texts were presented in three sizes of print (3.5, 6, 8.5 mm) and with three distances between letters (1, 3, 5 mm). Eye movements were registered electrooculographically. The results show a clear effect of letter size and distance on eye movement parameters such as number of fixations, duration of fixation and size of saccades in terms of letter positions. Further it has been shown that fixation duration and number of fixations correlate positively in the group of subjects investigated.

INTRODUCTION

The question of the effect of typographic characteristics on the readability of texts is as old as experimental reading research itself. It remains, however, unanswered in many respects. At present, this question is particularly interesting in the context of the typographic layout of screen text.

Recently, BOUMA (1982), O'REGAN (1981), O'REGAN, LEVY-SCHOEN, and JACOBS (1983), as well as GRONER and MENZ (1984) have been concerned with typographic text characteristics.

The effects found in these studies were rather weak and partly inconsistent. It could be argued that this is due to the flexibility of the reading process which has been demonstrated , for instance, by LEVY-SCHOEN (1980). With respect to the typographic characteristics of texts, flexibility would mean that the skilled reader is able to adapt to less than optimal conditions, at least temporarily.

Therefore, the present study investigated the question of the effect of typographic characteristics on the reading process with children who were beginning readers or had considerable reading difficulties, the rationale being that their reading processes are less flexible so that variations of the layout should produce stronger effects.

Thus our question was: What are the effects of the variation of letter size and letter spacing on the reading process, as reflected in eye movement parameters? Based on present knowledge, the following hypotheses can be stated:

1. Smaller letters should result in longer fixation durations because of their reduced discriminability.

2. Saccade amplitude, measured in letter positions, should not vary as a function of letter size and letter spacing, because the "visual span", according to the model of O'REGAN, is not the determining factor for saccade size in reading.

3. According to McCONKIE and RAYNER (e. g. 1975), it could be expected that fixation duration decreases as letter spacing increases, because less letters would be accessible at a given fixation position.

4. Concerning the effect of letter spacing, one could expect, according to McCONKIE and RAYNER (e. g. 1975), that saccade size, measured in letter positions, decreases, because as the letter spacing gets wider less characters could be preprocessed in peripheral vision.

SUBJECTS AND MATERIALS

18 children participated as subjects; their age ranged from 7;4 to 10;0 corresponding to the first up to the fourth grades. 14 of these children showed varying degrees of reading impairments and therefore attended our remedial reading courses. In order to increase the number of comparatively good readers, we included another four children who did not participate in these courses. At the time of the investigation, the poorest readers were just able to identify words which had been practised frequently; their reading was an effortful process proceeding letter by letter. About one third of the children had overcome their reading difficulties to some degree and could now read quite fluently. The other third were able to read texts appropriate to their age levels without making mistakes.

The reading materials used were hand-written (hand-drawn) texts with the letter size varying from 9 mm to 3 mm; this corresponds to the range of variation found in the text books commonly used for the first and second grades.

In order to make the texts equally difficult, we selected meaningful nouns of a length of four to five letters which had been frequently practised by the children; these words were arranged in random order and embedded in a meaningful context, as shown in the following example:

Rudi is reading all new words to his grandmother: trousers, people, moon, fish, aunt, nail, wine, child, tub, roof, bed, cloth. Granny is proud of him.

Each of the texts produced in this way used one of the nine

combinations of three levels of letter size and letter spacing. The three levels of letter spacing (measured from the end of a given letter to the beginning of the next one) were 1 mm, 3 mm, and 5 mm; the three levels of letter size (measured as the size of upper case characters) were 3.5 mm, 6.0 mm, and 8.5 mm. The following table (table 1) summarizes the typographic characteristics of the 9 texts presented in our experiment.

Table 1: Typographic characteristics of the texts used. The cell entries are the average distances from the middle of one character to the middle of the next one in degrees of visual angle (given an eye-text distance of 31 cm).

		letter spacing		
		1 mm	3 mm	5 mm
letter size	8.5 mm	1.16°	1.65°	1.90°
	6.0 mm	0.91°	1.37°	1.66°
	3.5 mm	0.65°	1.05°	1.39°

The children read each of the nine texts, in a half-loud voice, and were instructed to read for their own understanding. While reading, their eye movements were recorded by means of an EOG-system (see HELLER, 1983, for details of the system). All subjects had been familiarized with the experimental set-up in several preexperimental sessions.

RESULTS

The following table (table 2) gives an impression of the reading skills of our children. The values presented are the overall means over all subjects (the data were collected only from the lines with the random ordered meaningful nouns).

Table 2: Eye movement parameters (overall means and standard deviations)

	number of fixations per word	fixation duration msec	number of progressions per word	amplitude of progressions in degree	number of regressions per word	amplitude of regressions in degree	number progressions plus regressions per word	amplitude of progressions plus regressions in degree
$\bar{X}$	3.86	415.3	2.69	3.02	.90	- 1.75	3.59	2.73
s	2.25	226.9	1.86	3.92	1.28	1.67	2.66	2.35

As can be seen from table 2, in order to read one word the subjects needed approximately four fixations of an average duration of 415 msec. The mean saccade amplitude was 2.73 degrees, i. e. on average a single saccade bridged two letter positions.

It is interesting to compare these data with those obtained from adults. The data of MÜLLER (1982) allow a direct comparison, for he had used the same recording system and analysis programs as well as zero order approximations of 3- to 4-letter words. Table 3 provides a comparison between our results and the data obtained by MÜLLER.

Table 3: Eye movement parameters: Comparison between children and adult readers

	fixation duration per word msec	number of fixations	total reading time msec
children, 4 to 5 letter words	415	3.86	1603
adults, 3 to 4 letter words	274	1.08	296

A striking feature of our data is the wide range of variation, reflecting the large variability in the reading skills of our subjects: The number of fixations per word varies between 1.83 and 6.98, the fixation duration varies from 309 msec to 495 msec, and the saccade amplitude varies between 4.76 degrees and 1.56 degrees.

Looking at the interrelations between the eye movement parameters and reading errors, there is a striking pattern of correlations. This pattern is presented in the following diagram.

Concerning the correlation between the number of fixations and fixation duration, the positive covariation is unusually high and not in accordance with the normal expectation. On the basis of the present data, however, it is not possible to decide wether the sign and magnitude of this correlation is a result of the text material used or whether it is a characteristic of the children tested. A reanalysis of HELLER's (1976) data (recorded with children who were somewhat older and comparatively better readers) also revealed a positive correlation between the number of fixations and fixation duration, both for the meaningful texts and for the zero order approximations (three-letter words).

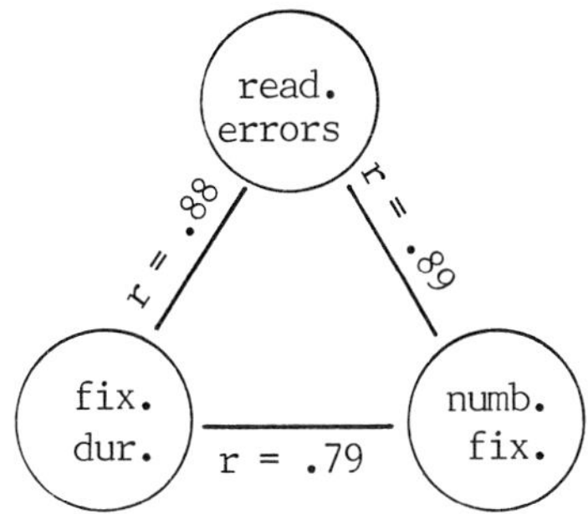

Figure 1: Correlation between reading errors, fixation duration, and number of fixations

Another correlation for adult readers can be calculated from the data of LEVY-SCHOEN. This correlation turns out to be negative, i. e. consistent with the expectation. The three correlations are summarized in the following table (table 4).

Table 4: Correlations between the number of fixations and fixation duration: Comparison between subjects of differing reading skills, 1 = poor readers, 3 = good readers.

1	Heller & Heinisch	r = .79
2	Heller (1976)	r = .39
3	Levy-Schoen (1980)	r = -.92

The following hypothesis can be derived from the correlations presented in table 4: As the reading skills increase, the correlation between the number of fixations and fixation duration develops from a positive into a negative relationship. This change in sign can be conceived of as reflecting the decreased identification demands encountered at a given fixation position.

Turning to the effects of the varying typographic characteristics, the differences between the texts were tested in an ANOVA with the subject means as cell entries.

In this analysis, there were two within-subjects factors, letter spacing and letter size, each consisting of three levels. In addition, there was one between-subjects factor, reading performance. The resulting ANOVA comprised the factors "reading skills" (2 levels), "letter spacing", and "letter size" (3 levels each). The dependent variables were "fixation duration" and "saccade size" measured in letter positions (subject means).

This ANOVA revealed the following significant effects ($p<0.01$)

which are illustrated in the subsequent figures:

Firstly, a main effect of "letter size" (figure 2). This effect is in accordance with the prediction that smaller characters result in longer fixation durations. However, this increase in fixation duration with decreasing letter size should be interpreted in a conservative way, i. e. it should be taken into account that the individual durations show a variability of about 50 %.

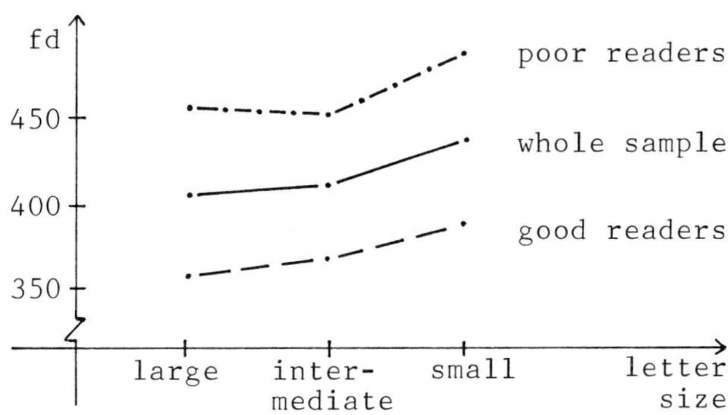

Figure 2: Main effect of "letter size" on "fixation duration" (msec)

The ANOVA did not yield a significant effect of letter spacing on fixation duration, contrary to hypothesis 3 stated above.

"Saccade size" is much more affected by the experimental variation than "fixation duration". It varies both with "letter size" and "letter spacing", as shown in the following two figures (figures 3 and 4).

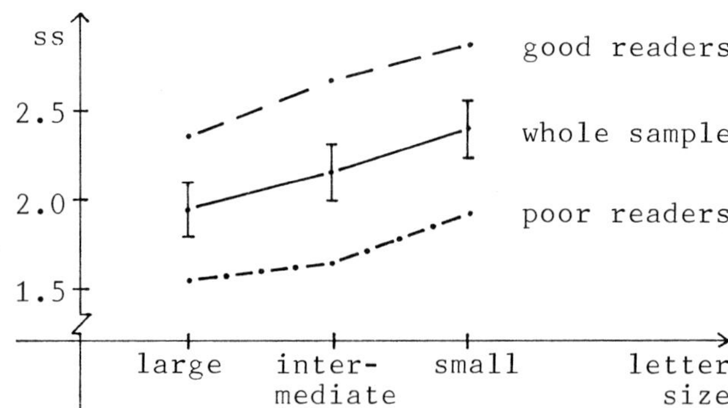

Figure 3: Main effect of "letter size" on "saccade size" (measured in letter positions)

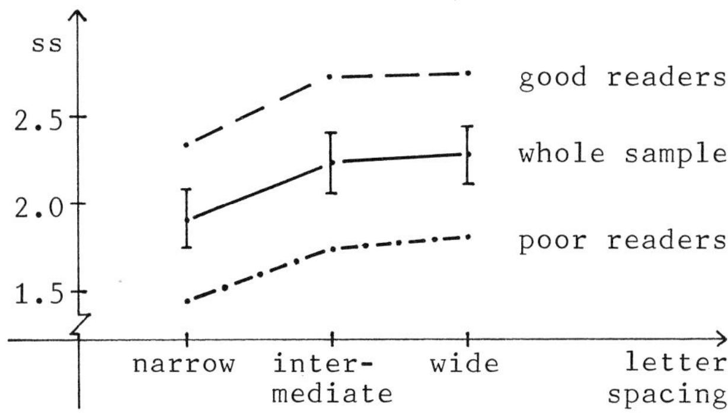

Figure 4: Main effect of "letter spacing" on "saccade size" (measured in letter positions)

In contrast to the expectation, the saccade amplitudes increase with increasing letter spacing and decreasing letter size, i.e. the subjects bridge more letter positions in a single saccade.

However, there is an additional interaction between "letter size" and "letter spacing", as shown in figures 5 and 6.

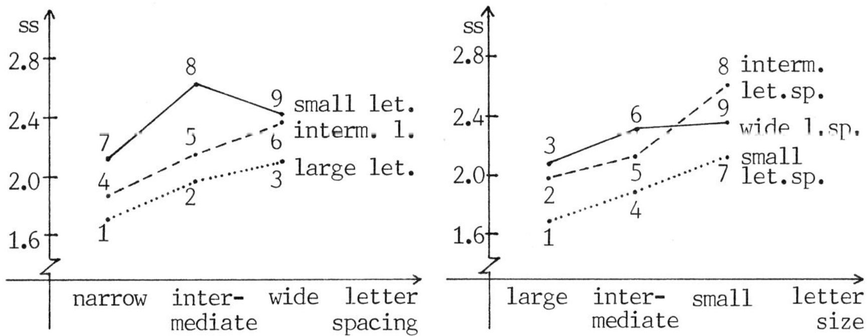

Figures 5 and 6: Interaction between "letter size" and "letter spacing" on saccade size (measured in letter positions). The digits represent the numbers of the texts presented.

As is evident from these figures, the interaction results from a positional change of the texts 8 and 9.

Looking at the mean saccade amplitudes and their rank order which is illustrated in table 5, it can be seen that (within the range of variation investigated) the data fit an additive model of the factors "letter size" and "letter spacing".

Table 5: Mean saccade size per text (in letter positions) and rank order of the mean values

letter size	letter spacing: narrow No. text	$\bar{X}$	rank	intermediate No. text	$\bar{X}$	rank	wide No. text	$\bar{X}$	rank
large	1	1.70	9	2	1.97	7	3	2.07	6
inter-mediate	4	1.89	8	5	2.11	4	6	2.33	3
small	7	2.10	5	8	2.61	1	9	2.38	2

Assuming the following rank order for the effects of both factors:

	3	2	1
3			
2			
1			

by adding up, the following matrix results:

	3	2	1
3	6	5	4
2	5	4	3
1	4	3	2

The following figure (figure 7) illustrates the relationship between the rank order of the texts expected on the basis of the additive model and the rank order actually obtained for the saccade amplitudes.

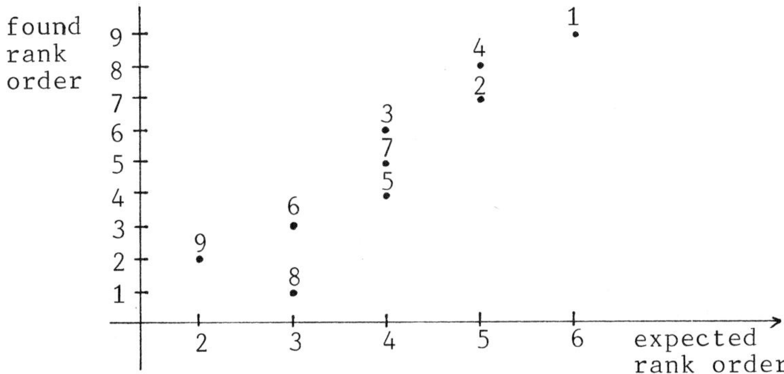

Figure 7: Relationship between the rank order of the texts expected and the rank order actually found for the saccade amplitudes. The digits represent the numbers of the texts.

With respect to the change in rank between the texts 8 and 9 (the original size of which is shown in the following cut-outs), it is suggestive that the facilitatory effect of "letter spacing" ceases at the letter-to-letter distance of text 9 (in relation to the letter size, the distance between the letters is highest for text 9) and the words start to "fall apart".

text 8 H o s e   L e u t e   M o n d

text 9 F o t o   A m s e l   S e i f e

With respect to the hypotheses of McCONKIE and RAYNER and O'REGAN concerning saccade amplitude (hypotheses 2 and 4), it can be stated that the present data are at variance with the predictions for all texts (see table 5): For all letter sizes, more letter positions are bridged in a given saccade as the letter spacing increases, i. e. increasing the letter spacing, within the range chosen, has a facilitatory effect on the reading performance of our subjects. This result, however, questions neither the notions of McCONKIE and RAYNER nor the grain model of O'REGAN; our data indicate only that these ideas are not applicable to the reading processes of children. The results presented lead to the suggestion that, depending on the reading skills, there is an optimum number of characters to be presented per fixation.

REFERENCES:

[1] Bouma, H., Legein, Ch. P., Mêlotte, H. E. M. and Zabel, L., Is large print easy to read?, in: Institute for Perception Research, IPO Annual Progress Report, 17 (1982).

[2] Groner, R. and Menz, C., Orientierung im Text und Augenbewegungsparameter beim Lesen, Vortrag auf der 26. Tagung exp. arb. Psychologen (April 1984).

[3] Heller, D., Über das Elektrookulogramm beim Lesen, Ph. D. Thesis, Universität Erlangen (1976).

[4] Heller, D., Problems of on-line processing of EOG-data in reading, in: Groner, R., Menz, C., Fisher, D. F., and Monty, R. A. (eds.), Eye Movements and Psychological Functions (Lawrence Erlbaum Ass., Hillsdale, N.Y., 1983).

[5] Lévy-Schoen, A., La flexibilité des saccades et des fixations au cours de la lecture, L'Année Psychologique, 80 (1980) 121-136.

[6] McConkie, G. W. and K. Rayner, The span of the effective stimulus during a fixation in reading, Perception and Psychophysics, 17 (1975) 578-586.

[7] Müller, H., Die Steuerung der Augenbewegungen beim Lesen, Dipl.-Arbeit (Würzburg, 1982).

[8] O'Regan, K., Elementary perceptual and eye movement control processes in reading, Sloan Conference on Eye Movements, Amherst (June, 10-13, 1981).

[9] O'Regan, J. K., Lêvy-Schoen, A., and Jacobs, A. M., The effect of visibility on eye movement parameters in reading, Perception & Psychophysics, 34 (1983) 457-464.

Eye Movements and Human Information Processing
R. Groner, G.W. McConkie and C. Menz (eds.)

EXPERIMENTS ON VISUAL ORIENTATION IN READING: EFFECTS OF LINING, LETTER SPACING AND INSERTED ELEMENTS

Christine Menz and Rudolf Groner

Department of Psychology
University of Bern
Bern
Switzerland

The effects of spatial organization of printed text on eye movement dynamics was examined. Twelve experienced readers were presented with a text divided in six paragraphs of equal length. The layout conditions of these paragraphs varied according to spacing of letters and lining. Letter spacing was either single, double or each letter was flanked by a dash, interword spaces being filled with three dashes. Letters were positioned on a line or displaced in the vertical direction by a random amount not exceeding one letter height. The results show that experienced readers rely very much on the physical attributes of printed text. Word shape and word boundaries are important cues for word identification, for structuring and orientation in text and for reading speed. Comprehension was not impaired by the most perturbing layout conditions.

INTRODUCTION

Much recent work in reading research has been centered around the question of spatial arrangement of printed text and reading performance. Tinker (1963) emphasized the importance of word shape information which is especially yielded in lowercase print. Word shape can be manipulated by changing the size, case and spacing of characters or by filling interword spaces. In the present experiment the major focus is on changes in eye movement dynamics due to typographic manipulations of word shape by letter spacing, bumpy lining and insertion of elements. Unfortunately the work done so far in this area is at most concerned with two of these variables.

Among studies varying case and size of typeface, two different views are held. On one hand Smith, Lott and Cornell (1969) used six different variations of print (upper- and lowercase with and without size alternation, alternation of size and case). The subjects had to search for target words in prose passages. Thereby word identification was significantly impaired if both size and case for upper- and lowercase characters were altered. Performance was better if case was not altered throughout the words. Case alternations had no influence on performance if size was held constant. So they concluded that word identification is based upon letter integration and not upon a shape-dependent perception. McConkie and Zola (1979) supported a similar view. They presented text in alternating case while eye movements were recorded. In between fixations visual features of individual letters were changed which did not affect reading performance. They concluded that such kind of information is not integrated across fixations. And they argued that the abstraction of a canonical representation of the letter string, rendering variations irrelevant, is the physical signal for the reader.

On the other hand Coltheart and Freeman (1974) criticized the experimental paradigms of Smith (1969) and Smith et al. (1969) for insensitivity. Instead of a reading aloud or searching task they tachistoscopically presented eight-letter words with constant character size but varying case (upper-, lowercase, case alternation). Dependent variable was the number of correctly recognized words. As opposed to Smith and Smith et al. they found an impairment of word identification in the alternating case conditions independent of character size. These results support a view about analyzing print which takes account of the manifold physical attributes of the visual configuration.

The inconsistence of the results reported so far might be an artifact since task requirements and methods of measuring reading performance differ a lot. Rudnicky and Kolers (1984) examined the effect of size and case alternations in various reading tasks. Their data support the results of Smith (1969) and of Coltheart and Freeman (1974). Both size and case alternations affected reading. The size effect was stronger, but in the reading aloud condition the difference was submerged during the eye-voice span. They found that any disturbance in the typographic integrity impairs reading. They conclude that through years of practice readers seem to acquire skills for analyzing shape.

Furthermore they tested whether these analytical operations are transferable from upper- to lowercase print and vice versa. The results confirm that such skills do exist and that they are well applicable to lowercase print. It is a support of what Tinker found. Word shape seems to be a very useful source of information if lowercase print is used. But it is of minor importance with uppercase print.

In another series of experiments the major focus is on eye guidance in reading text with case alternation and blurred word boundaries. Pollatsek and Rayner (1982) have investigated the functions of interword spaces. They had either all spaces to the right of a fixation filled or all but the first or just the first space filled. The onset of a space-filler was delayed (0-150 msec) compared to the onset of a fixation. The space-fillers were either random letters, digits or a kind of grating. If the space-fillers appeared with a delay more than 50 msec they had no effect in the first-space-preserved condition. There was little effect of the various space-fillers. Reading impairment was observed for the other conditions independent of the delay time. They concluded that filled spaces in the parafovea impair eye guidance while the filling of spaces in the fovea disrupts the identification of the momentarily fixated word. Letters as space-fillers had a stronger interfering effect on reading than digits or gratings. This supports the findings of Malt and Seamon (1978). Through practice experienced readers learned not a generalized strategy for processing interword space-fillers but they learned the nonmeaningfulness of a specific stimulus. So the degree of interference depends on the physical cues of the fillers.

Various studies (Fisher, 1975; Fisher & Lefton, 1976; Spragins, Lefton & Fisher, 1976) were conducted to examine whether peripheral cue accessibility is related to development. The text material was printed in normal or alternating letters with spacing between words normal, filled or absent. The data confirm that reliance upon peripheral cues increase with increasing reading experience. In the most perturbed conditions performance was reduced to a letter-by-letter processing. An experienced reader seems to rely more on spatial cues than an unexperienced one. Cues of word shape and word boundaries were found to be interdependent, a result that supports the Hochberg (1970) model.

An important factor that should be taken into account with spatial arrangement of print is visibility. Studies on visibility in relation with eye movements were conducted in order to find optimal display conditions for reading (Paterson & Tinker, 1947; Tinker & Paterson, 1955). Heller (chapter 12 in this volume) found evidence that optimal spatial relations between letter size and letter spacing affect reading performance even of beginning readers. O'Regan, Levy-Schoen and Jacobs (1983) investigated visibility accentuating more the question why the conditions mentioned were optimal. The results show that under visibility changes (viewing distance and character spacing) saccade sizes were affected by factors probably related to word length and word boundaries or to linguistic processing and not to the visual span. Fixation durations appeared to be affected by the closeness of the letters to the reader's acuity threshold.

Manipulations of word shape by using alternating size and case of characters yielded not consistent results about the role of word shape in reading. Interword spaces proved to be an important cue for a selective direction of eye movements. Furthermore saccade size seems to be affected by word length and word boundaries and not by visual span, i.e. "the size of the region around the eye's fixation point in which letters can be recognized with a given accuracy" (O'Regan, Levy-Schoen & Jacobs (1983), p. 457) if letter spacing is varied. Foveal processing as well as peripheral processing may be disturbed by manipulations of word shape, word boundaries and letter spacing. All these three aspects are somehow interdependent. And the present experiment which takes into account all three aspects was conceptualized in order to find a more specific description of this relationship. Word shape was manipulated not by size and case alternations of single letters but by randomly varying the letter position in the vertical direction up to a certain amount. This new paradigm has the advantage that possible effects of word shape manipulations are not confounded with variations in the constituent letters. So the discussion will not deviate from the main point to less relevant questions such as whether size or case has a more interfering effect on reading lowercase print.

Assuming now that spatial manipulations of word shape, word boundaries and letter spacing are relevant cues specially for the peripheral search guidance and for the structuring and orientation in the text, they would become manifest in eye movement dynamics. They would be indicated by an increase in the reading time, a decrease in the perceptual span because of some kind of tunnel-effect and a change in the fixation pattern (Spragins et al., 1976).

EXPERIMENT

Method

Subjects

Twelve adults from the Universities of Bern and Basel served as subjects in the experiment. All subjects were practiced with the eye movement recording equipment used. The subjects were naive concerning the purpose of the experiment. They all had normal or corrected to normal vision.

Apparatus and Material

Eye movements were recorded with an infrared system, the ASL Remote Eye View Monitor and TV Pupillometer System, Model 1994-SB. It was interfaced with a NOVA 3/12 computer equipped with a Megatek graphical system. Eye movements from the left eye were sampled with a frequency of 50 Hz. The computer stored a complete record of the eye movement pattern under all conditions.

The material was displayed on a CRT Hewlett-Packard 1321A . Letters appeared white on a black background. As text material we used an outline about the ecological situation of owls in Germany and Austria.

The text was divided into segments of six lines. Line length was maximum 65 character spaces. By pressing a button the subject could display such a segment on the CRT. The subject was sitting in a distance of about 1 m to the CRT. So a display segment subtended a visual angle of 20.5 deg in the horizontal and 15.5 deg in the vertical axis.

Figure 1 shows the experimental variations introduced by this experiment.

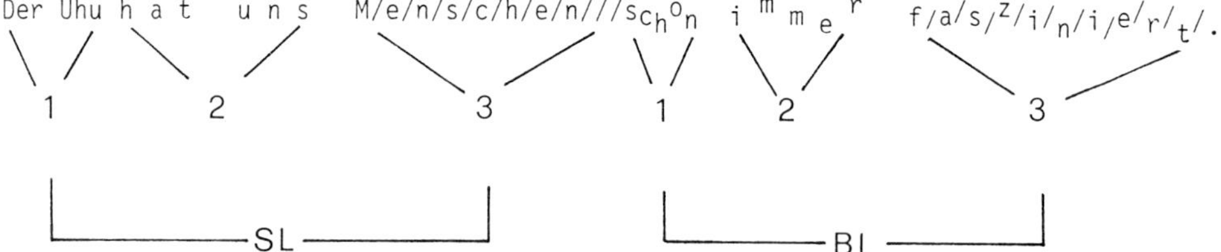

Figure 1: Examples of the six layout conditions used in the experiment. Varied was letter spacing (single(=1), double(=2) and insertion of dashes(=3)) and lining (straight(=SL) and bumpy(=BL)).

The letters could be positioned either the usual way all on one straight line (=straight lining) or displaced in the vertical direction for a random amount not exceeding a letter height (= bumpy lining). In addition interletter and interword spacing could either correspond to the standards of the graphic system (=single spacing), or each letter could be flanked by a blank comparable to double spacing or each character could be flanked by a dash while interword spaces were filled with three dashes (=filled with dashes). A complete crossing of the factors Lining and Spacing resulted in six display conditions that were tested (Fig. 1). Therefore the text was divided into six paragraphs of equal length. Excluding the warming-up trials, 50 segments were presented. For each lining condition five segments were presented in standard spacing and ten segments in double spacing respectively in the inserted dash condition.

Procedure

When a subject arrived for the experiment she or he was seated in a dentist chair. The head was supported at the back and on the forehead to avoid head movements during the experiment. The eye movement recording system was calibrated by first linearizing the system and checking whether all data are acceptable within the range of the CRT. In a second step fine calibration followed. Together with an accoustic signal squares appeared in succession on random positions with three random digits successively displayed in the square. The subject had to report these numbers. During the fixation of the digits eye movements were recorded. On the basis of these data the fixation positions were computer-interactively calibrated. By calculating the regression parameters eye movement data could be related to the CRT positions (Menz, Groner & Bischof, 1984). After the calibration the subject was given a written instruction about the experimental task. The instruction was displayed on the CRT serving at the same time as warming-up. It contained examples of all six conditions involved in the following experiment. Luminance of the CRT was adjusted to a comfortable level for the subject and held constant throughout the experiment. The subject had to read the text silently. A button had to be pushed to display the successive text segments. Before a new segment was displayed a fixation square appeared at the beginning of the first line. The calibration was redone after the warming-up and then the subject started reading. The 2 x 3 factorial design yielded six display conditions which were counterbalanced for all subjects. The subject started either with the bumpy lining condition or with straight lining. After a short break in the middle of the text the lining condition changed. At the end of the experiment comprehension was tested. Therefore 60 words in the text were replaced by numbers and the subject had to choose the corresponding word out of three alternatives. The whole session lasted about 1.5 hrs.

Results

Reading performance was assessed by the overall measure, the reading time per text segment, by saccade size, i.e. regression and progression size, by fixation duration and number of fixations. All these data were calculated from the eye movement recordings and will be described successively. The five performance measures were submitted to analyses of variance, mixed model with repeated measurements with lining (straight or bumpy) and spacing (single, double or filled with dashes) as between factors and subject as within factor.

Mean reading times across the three layout conditions are shown in Figure 2. The data give an overall impression of the effects the various conditions had on both perceptual and cognitive components of the reading process. The ANOVA yielded highly significant differences between straight and bumpy lining, $F(1,11) = 34.33$, $p < 0,001$; and between the three spacing conditions, $F(2,22) = 58.14$, $p < 0.001$; indicating that in both lining conditions the dash condition is the most time consuming while the time difference between single and double spacing is much smaller. The interaction of Lining by Spacing was also statistically significant, $F(2,22) = 13.48$, $p < 0.001$; and there were notable difference among subjects.

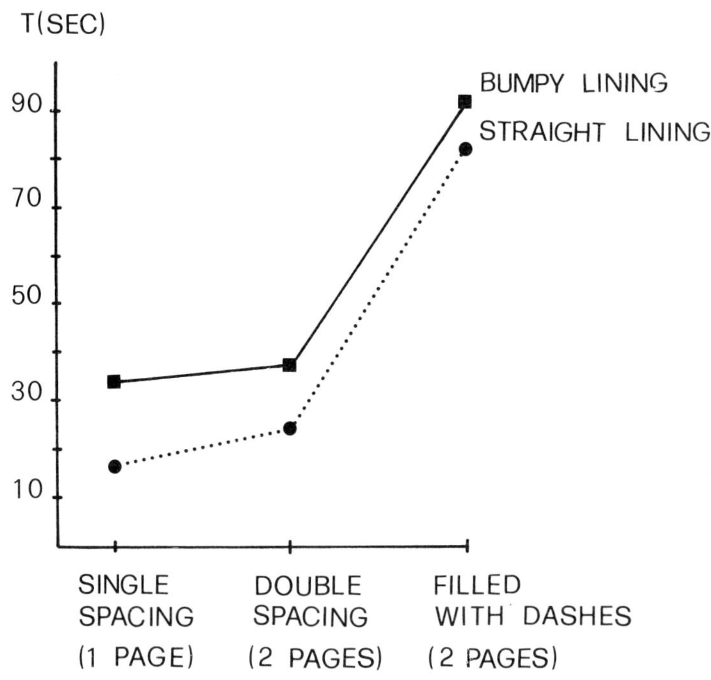

Figure 2: Mean reading times for equal text amount (i.e., one text segment (=page) in the single spaced condition corresponds to two text segments in the double spaced and filled with dashes conditions.

The influence of the various layout conditions on the perceptual span is represented with the parameters relative progression size and relative regression size. Here the dependent variable is the mean number of effective letters subtended by one saccade. Figure 3 plots the data for the relative progression size. The ANOVA yielded again highly significant differences among spacing, $F(2,22) = 52.35$, $p < 0.001$; and lining, $F(1,11) = 15.23$, $p < 0.001$. Furthermore the interaction Lining by Spacing was significant, $F(2,22) = 4.44$, $p < 0.025$; indicating that progression size is systematically longer for straight lining compared to bumpy lining, but the difference between the lining conditions is getting smaller as spacing is doubled and dashes are filled in.

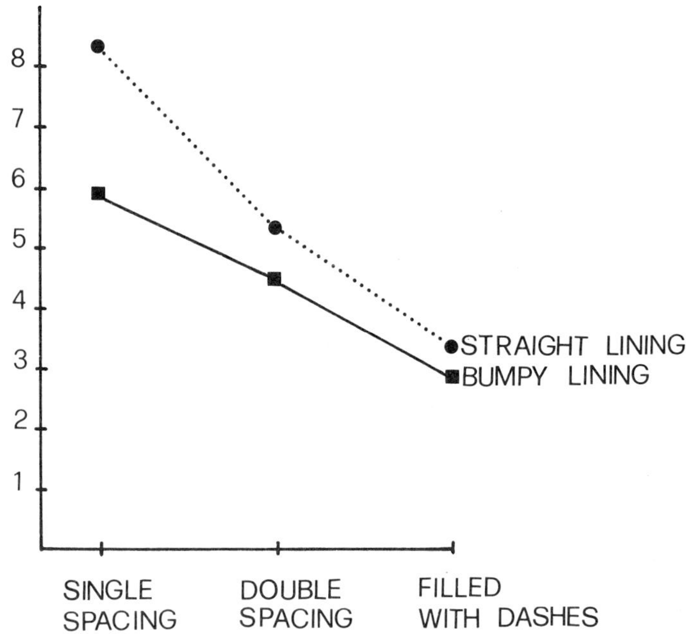

Figure 3: Mean progression size, in number of effective letters skipped, as a function of letter spacing.

The analysis of the relative regression size showed a significant main effect of spacing, $F(2,22) = 8.5$, $p < 0.002$; and a significant interaction of Lining by Spacing, $F(2,22) = 5.93$, $p < 0.01$ (see Fig. 4). The most drastic decrease of regression size under the straight lining condition can be stated between double spacing and the condition with inserted dashes. Under the bumpy lining condition regression size is most drastically decreasing when spacing is doubled.

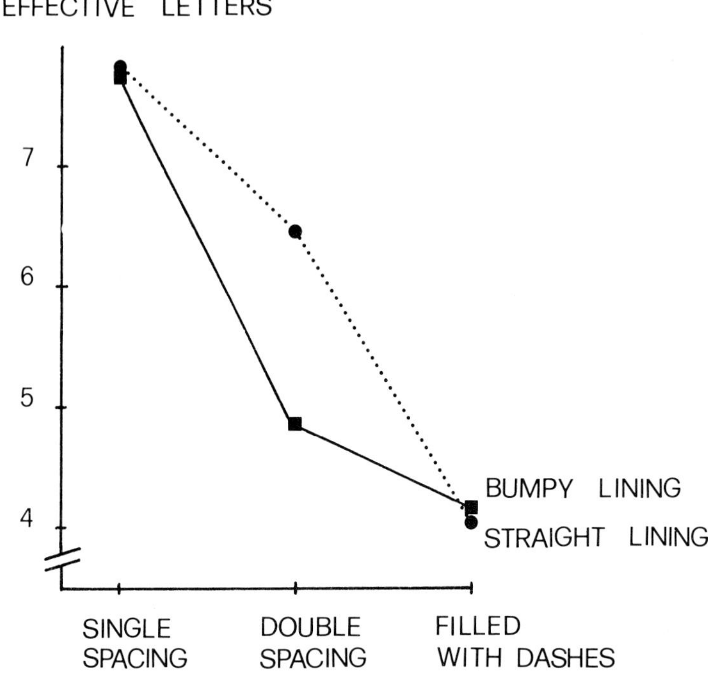

Figure 4: Mean regression size, in number of effective letters skipped, as a function of letter spacing.

Effects of the various layout conditions on fixation duration and number of fixations are illustrated in Figure 5 and Figure 6. The analysis of the mean fixation durations showed significant main effects of spacing, $F(2,22) = 30.4$, $p < 0.001$; and lining, $F(1,11) = 31.35$, $p < 0.001$. In addition, a Spacing by Lining interaction, $F(2,22) = 8.59$, $p < 0.002$ was significant, indicating that the bumpy lining condition yielded systematically longer fixation durations and that there is a common trend in the lining factor to show the shortest fixation durations in the double space condition and the longest in the dash condition. The greatest disparity between the two curves is stated for the single spacing condition.

Figure 6 plots the data for the number of fixations. Again we found highly significant differences between the lining conditions, $F(1,11) = 33.56$, $p < 0.0$ and between the three spacing conditions, $F(2,22) = 37.21$, $p < 0.001$. The increase of the number of fixations induced by the bumpy lining condition is larger for single and double spacing than for the text with inserted dashes, indicated by the significant interaction of Lining by Spacing, $F(2,22) = 5.54$, $p < 0.02$.

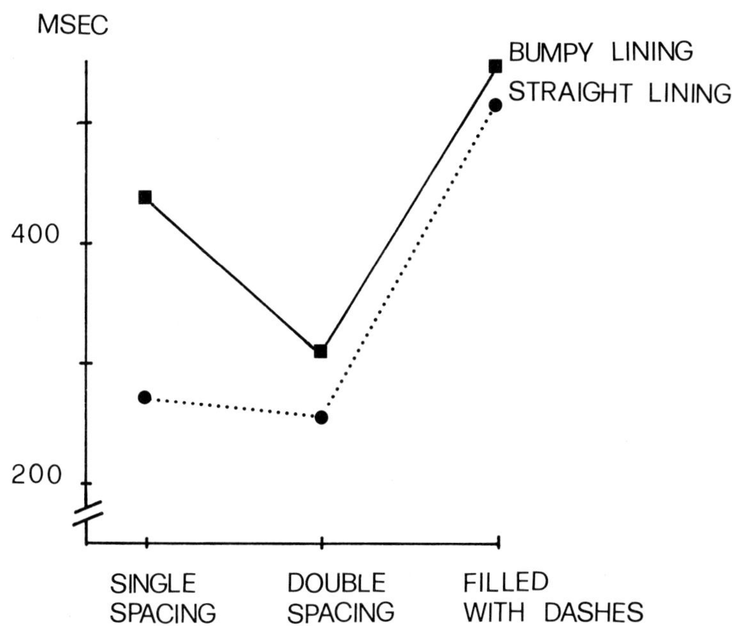

Figure 5: Mean fixation duration as a function of letter spacing.

Fixation durations and number of fixations were integrated in one plot (Fig. 7) to examine more specifically their relations under the various experimental conditions . The rectangles visualize the product of fixation duration and number of fixations which equals net reading time, i.e. omitting the time spent on saccades. Overall an increase or decrease of fixation duration is just partly compensated by an increasing or decreasing number of fixations. The compensation is quite good for the straight, single spaced condition. If the fixation duration increases in the inserted dashes condition or decreases with double spacing, it is less compensated in the number of fixations. For the bumpy lining condition the compensation is steadily decreasing.

In the analysis of the comprehension test the number of correctly recognized words were counted. As reported above, mean reading times differed significantly for the six layout conditions. That means that more processing time is spent on the identification of words. It was tested whether these long processing times affect remembering. Therefore correlations between the number of correctly recognized words in the corresponding passages and the reading times were calculated. A statistically significant correlation, t(22) = 2.11, p = 0.05, was found for the most perturbed condition with inserted elements independent of lining. All other correlations were not significant.

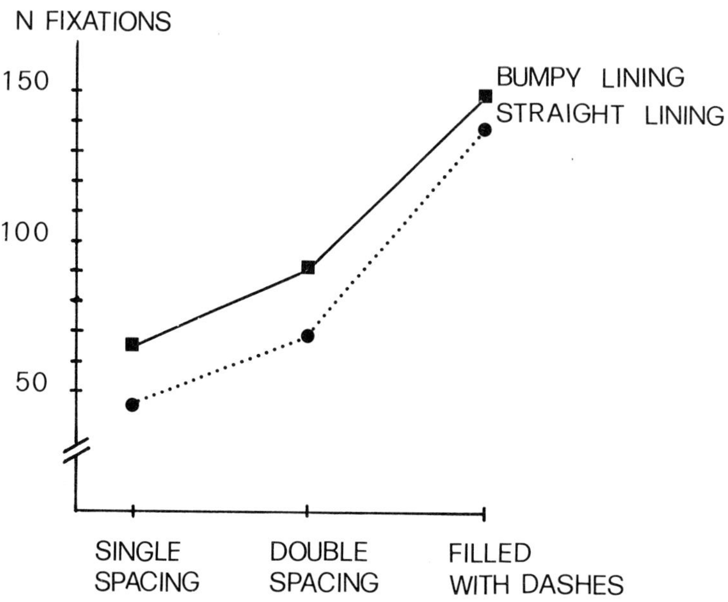

Figure 6: Number of fixations for equal text amount (i.e., one text segment in single spacing corresponds to two in double spacing and in the condition with inserted dashes) as a function of letter spacing.

As learning measures the data were submitted to an analysis of variance, mixed model with repeated measurements with lining and spacing as between factors and subject as within factor. Main effects and interaction failed to reach significance while there were notable differences among subjects.

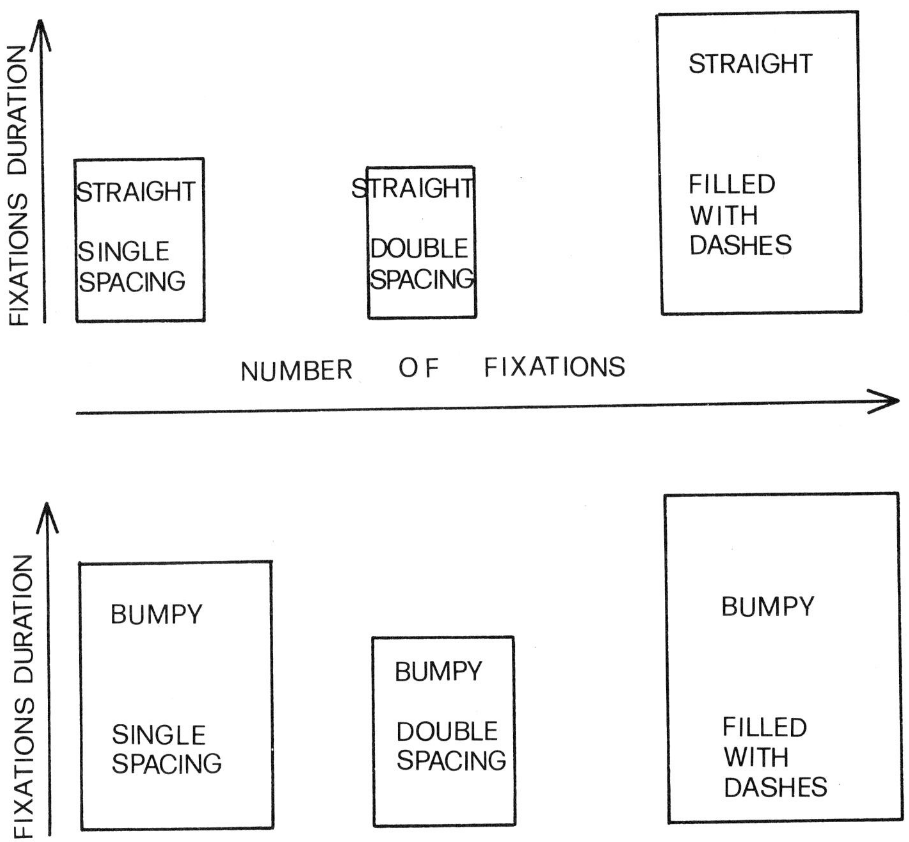

Figure 7: Relations between mean fixaton durations and number of fixations under the various layout conditions with the number of fixations on the abscissa and the mean fixation durations on the ordinate.

DISCUSSION

We varied a number of physical attributes of typography in order to investigate their contribution to reading performance. The results show evidently that sophisticated and efficient reading strategies of adults are easily disturbable by manipulations of the text layout. This finding is consistent with results of Spragins et al. (1976), saying that the role of spatial information such as word shape is even more important for the experienced reader than the unexperienced one.

Adams (1979), Rayner (1983) and McConkie and Zola (1979), among others, claim that information conveyed by word shape is provided by the constituent letters. In the present experiment word shape was manipulated independently of case and size of letters. The results show that the bumpy lining condition is affecting word identification, indicated by longer and more fixations, by shorter saccades and longer reading times compared to straight lining. This holds to a view which Rudnicky and Kolers (1984), among others, affirm. They write (p. 245), "....the physical signal is part and parcel of the processing and of the mental representation of the words conveyed, an active participant in the processing."

The manipulation of visibility by changing character spacing affected the way the eye scans the text. The size of progressions and regressions is decreasing indepenent of the factor lining. The number of fixations increases while for both lining conditions the fixation durations are shorter compared to the single spacing condition.

It is evident that fixation durations are proportional to the amount of information processed at each fixation. Reading time, on the other hand, is hardly prolonged with double spacing. This indicates that this kind of visibility change affects mainly the saccade control strategies (see O'Regan et al., 1983) of the readers. The strategy change, however, does not affect the reading speed.

Peripheral cues such as word length and word boundaries (McConkie & Rayner, 1976; Rayner & McConkie, 1976) were missing in the most perturbing conditions with dashes filled in between letters and words. In addition to the lack of peripheral cues a new, not letter-like stimulus (i.e., the dash) is imposed for processing. This kind of manipulations resulted in a severe impairment of the reading process indicated in all eye-movement parameters measured. Progression size was reduced to 4-5 letters, regression size to 4 letters. Fixation durations increased while the number of fixations was three times higher than in the single spacing condition, independent of lining. These results show that the dashes between letters interfere with word identification, indicated by longer fixation durations and more fixations, and with orientation in text, indicated by a decrement of saccade size. Comprehension processes are severely delayed. These findings partly replicate and extend the work of Fisher (1975), Fisher and Lefton (1976), Spragins et al. (1976) and Pollatsek and Rayner (1982). The bumpiness of lining is hardly affecting saccade size. The reading process is never reduced to a letter-by-letter processing, as Spragins et al. (1976) found, and the decrement of saccade size is not combined with constant fixation durations and number of fixations. The finding of Malt and Seamon (1978), that the disruptive effects of the interword filler is reduced with practice, could not be replicated. Our subjects did not develop strategies allowing them to treat the single, nonletter filler dash as not meaningful. Two reasons might be responsible for this inconsistence. The practice times might have been too short and in addition to the filling of interword spaces, fillers were inserted between letters.

All the spatial manipulations used in the present experiment had no effect on the comprehension of the text. Eye guidance, however, seems to be very sensitive to orientation cues in the text such as word length and word boundaries and to word shape information. This shows that efficient readers take account of the manifold physical attributes of print that affect reading speed. Thus optimal conditions should be defined where the visual system has to rely most parsimoniously on the typographic display. As the visual system is flexible and reacts task-dependently (see Rudnicky & Kolers, 1984) it is important to further investigate specific models, taking into account reading material and task requirements.

REFERENCES

Adams, M.J. Models of word recognition. Cognitive Psychology, 1979, 11, 133-176.

Coltheart, M., & Freeman, R. Case alternation impairs word identification. Bulletin of the Psychonomic Society, 1974, 3, 102-104.

Fisher, D.F. Reading and visual search. Memory & Cognition, 1975, 3, 188-196.

Fisher, D.F., & Lefton, L.A. Peripheral information extraction: a developmental examination of reading processes. Journal of Experimental Child Psychology, 1976, 21, 77-93.

Hochberg, J. Components of literacy: speculation and exploratory research. In H. Levin and J.P. Williams (Eds.), Basic studies on reading (pp. 74-89). New York: Basic Books, 1970.

Malt, B.C., & Seamon, J.G. Peripheral and cognitive components of eye guidance in filled-space reading. Perception & Psychophysics, 1978, 23, 399-402.

McConkie, G.W., & Rayner, K. Identifying the span of the effective stimulus in reading: literature review and theories of reading. In H. Singer & R.B. Ruddell (Eds.), Theoretical models and processes of reading. Delaware: International Reading Association, 1976.

McConkie, G.W., & Zola, D. Is visual information integrated across successive fixations in reading? Perception & Psychophysics, 1979, 25, 221-224.

Menz, Ch., Groner, R., & Bischof, W.F. Optimierte Eich- und Auswertungsverfahren bei der Cornea-Reflexionsmethode. Vortrag an der 26. Tagung experimentell arbeitender Psychologen, Erlangen-Nürnberg, 1984.

O'Regan, K.J., Levy-Schoen, A., & Jacobs, A.M. The effect of visibility on eye-movement parameters in reading. Perception & Psychophysics, 1983, 34, 457-464.

Paterson, D.G., & Tinker, M.A. The effect of typography upon the perceptual span in reading. American Journal of Psychology, 1947, 60, 388-396.

Pollatsek, A., & Rayner, K. Eye movement control in reading: the role of word boundaries. Journal of Experimental Psychology: Human Perception & Performance, 1982, 8, 817-833.

Rayner, K. The perceptual span and eye movement control during reading. In K. Rayner (Ed.), Eye movements in reading (pp. 97-120). New York: Academic Press, 1983.

Rayner, K., & McConkie, G.W. What guides a reader's eye movements? Vision Research, 1976, 16, 829-837.

Rudnicky, A.I., & Kolers, P.A. Size and case of type as stimulus in reading. Journal of Experimental Psychology: Human Perception & Performance, 1984, 10, 231-249.

Smith, F. Familiarity of configuration vs. discriminability of features in the visual identification of words. Psychonomic Science, 1969, 14, 261-263.

Smith, F., Lott, D., & Cornell, B. The effect of type size and case alternation on word identification. American Journal of Psychology, 1969, 82, 248-253.

Spragins, A.B., Lefton, L.A., & Fisher, D.F. Eye movements while reading and searching spatially transformed text: a developmental examination. Memory & Cognition, 1976, 4, 36-42.

Tinker, M.A. Legibility of print. Ames: Iowa State University, 1963.

Tinker, M.A., & Paterson, D.G. The effect of typographical variations upon eye movements in reading. Journal of Educational Research, 1955, 49, 171-184.

Eye Movements and Human Information Processing
R. Groner, G.W. McConkie and C. Menz (eds.)

COMPARABLE PRIMING EFFECTS OBTAINED IN LEXICAL DECISION, NAMING AND READING TASKS

John S. Kerr and Geoffrey Underwood

Department of Psychology
University of Nottingham
Nottingham NG7 2RD
England.
Tel. (0602) 506101 ext. 3126

ABSTRACT

This study used three different experiments to investigate whether lexical priming occurs during reading. Materials consisted of sets of three words: a pair of high-associate synonyms, one of which was chosen as the target word, the other as the priming word, and a control word. Lexical decision and naming tasks established the presence of a priming effect with these materials. In the third experiment subjects' eye movements were recorded as they read sets of three sentences which included the materials used in the single word studies. It was found that subjects fixated the target word for less time if they had just read the priming word as compared to the control word. The conclusion is that lexical priming occurs during reading.

INTRODUCTION

Does lexical priming facilitate reading during sentence comprehension? The present experiments were intended as an attempt to replicate and extend Kennedy (1978), an experiment which used eye movement data to suggest that lexical relationships influence fixation patterns. Kennedy recorded the eye movements of subjects while they read sets of three individually presented sentences from a CRT screen. These sentences formed a natural narrative or descriptive sequence. In the experimental condition there was a "strong semantic relationship" between a word in the first sentence of the set and a word in the last sentence, i.e. a priming relationship between two high-associate synonyms. This relationship was not present in the control condition, although the congruity of the sequence was maintained. For example:

> It is unwise to wander on a MOUNTAIN. (TRACK)
> People can get lost there.
> A HILL is not always easy to climb.

Kennedy found that in the priming condition subjects "reached the critical word earlier and in general spent longer looking at it" than in the control condition where there was no priming.

In his explanation of this effect, Kennedy used the process of anaphoric reference: he argued from Sanford & Garrod's (1977, 1981) position that, in reading sequences of sentences, readers engage "in part in a search for cross-reference". Thus the "primed" word engages attention earlier and is fixated for a longer duration, indicating the presence of a reference process.

There are two problems with this account. Firstly the claim that anaphoric reference is involved in the Kennedy experiment is not justified. There is no reason to expect readers to undertake referential processing merely on the basis that two words are associated, indeed Sanford & Garrod (1977) found it necessary to disconfirm a priming explanation of different reading times in their experiments on the effect of conjoint frequency on the time taken for reference resolution. Secondly, priming is a different process from reference, the essential feature of which is a reduction in response time for a primed word, be it lexical decision, naming, or fixation time.

Unfortunately, Kennedy gives only one example of the materials used in his experiment (see above). In this example it is possible to make an anaphoric reference, that is, compute that "It is unwise to wander on a hill", though since "hill" suggests a different entity from "mountain" it is not a good reference. If all of Kennedy's materials were like this, the result would be longer fixations on the critical words due to the presence of referential processing. Any priming process would affect fixation time in the opposite direction.

We intend to consider both Kennedy's and the present experiment from the standpoint of an explanation in terms of lexical priming. It is of some interest that Kennedy's primed words are fixated earlier than unprimed words - the implication being that the primed word is already available to the reader before it is encountered, its presence in peripheral vision being sufficient to attract the eye. It has been established with single-fixation tachistoscope studies that the meanings of parafoveal words can influence the processing of fixated words (e.g. Balota & Rayner, 1983; Bradshaw, 1974; Underwood, 1981; Underwood & Thwaites, 1982). These studies establish the plausibility of the notion of parafoveal information controlling future eye movements, but Kennedy's experiment establishes the case during free-reading for sentence comprehension. Kennedy's longer fixation times for primed words presents a problem for the priming explanation, however, since the essence of priming is that it reduces the time required for processing. For this reason a replication of Kennedy's experiment is necessary: the predictions of the priming model would be that primed words would be fixated earlier and for less time than those words unprimed. Weight would be added to the argument if it were also shown that the chosen materials produced a reliable priming effect in the more "traditional" paradigms of lexical decision and naming tasks. For this reason three experiments were performed using the same targets, primes, and controls in lexical decision, naming and reading studies.

Experiment 1: Lexical Decision

METHOD

Subjects

Two volunteer groups of 12 Open University students attending summer school at Nottingham University participated in the experiment.

Materials and Design

19 sets of 3 words were prepared. These consisted of a pair of high-

associate synonyms (Postman & Keppel, 1970) e.g. look-see, and a control word which was less related or unrelated to the target (see Appendix 1). The choice of words was limited by whether a congruous set of sentences could be constructed around them for the purposes of the reading task. The number of sets (19) was also due to the limitations of experiment 3. One of the synonyms was chosen as the target word: on a primed trial this was preceded by its associate; on an unprimed trial it was preceded by the control word from that set. These materials were randomised once (whilst maintaining priming/control relationships) with 34 non-words (English words with one letter altered, of varying length 3-6 letters) and with 9 words of a similar type to the targets, chosen at random.

The experiment was divided into two sections: those targets primed for one group of subjects were unprimed for the other group, and vice-versa. Each subject therefore saw 81 letter strings, of which 19 were targets, and performed under both primed and non-primed conditions.

Apparatus

Stimuli were prepared using a Kroy lettering machine with a lower case Century Schoolbook 8pt. typeface. These were mounted on slides and presented using a Kodak carousel slide projector modified for tachistoscopic presentation with a Forth Instruments FI 272 pulse generator set at a presentation time of 500 milliseconds. This was connected to a digital timer which was stopped by the subject pressing one of two buttons labelled "yes/word" or "no/non-word". Stimuli were back-projected onto a white screen positioned approximately 1 metre in front of the subject. All equipment was situated in a dimly-lit, soundproof laboratory.

Procedure

The subject was seated 1 metre in front of the projection screen and instructed that he/she was to decide whether the letter string presented was a word or not and press the appropriate button as quickly as possible. Subjects were told that the first 12 trials were for practice and that the experimenter would say "ready" before each trial. Stimuli were then presented serially for 500 milliseconds each, with an inter-stimulus interval of approximately 1.5 seconds, during which the experimenter noted the subject's reaction time for that trial. When they had completed the experiment subjects were debriefed.

Results and Discussion

Primed	Unprimed
558 (54)	588 (52)

Table 1. Mean lexical decision times (milliseconds), for the words used in Experiment 1, with standard deviations in parentheses

The results are shown in Table 1. Only those words which appeared in both sections of the experiment (targets) were used in the analysis. The non-word data were ignored. Means for each subject in each condition were calculated and an analysis of variance was carried out on these data treating subjects as a random factor. A similar analysis was carried out using the means for each set of materials, with materials treated as random factor: minF' was then calculated. Trials where the subject made an incorrect response were excluded from the analyses (the error rate was less than 1%). It took significantly less time to decide that a primed word was a word, than the same word unprimed, F1 $(1,23) = 10.21$, $p < 0.005$; F2 $(1,17) = 11.19$, $p < 0.005$; minF' $(1,37) = 5.34$, $p < 0.05$.

Meyer & Schvaneveldt (1971), Anderson (1983), and others explain this effect as being due to a process of spreading activation in semantic memory: when an element in semantic memory is activated, this activation spreads to related elements, e.g. reading "doctor" will activate elements like "nurse", "operation" and "stethoscope". If one of these related elements is subsequently encountered, less stimulus information will be required for that word to be accessed. Thus, in a lexical decision task, reaction time will be reduced for a word if it is preceded by an associated word.

Experiment 2: Naming

Subjects

Two groups of 11 subjects from the same population as experiment 1 were used. No subject had participated in the previous experiment.

Materials and Design

The sets of priming pairs and controls used in the lexical decision task were added to 41 words of similar type to the targets for practice and fillers. The design used in experiment 1 was repeated here. Subjects therefore had to name 79 stimulus words of which 19 were targets.

Apparatus and Procedure

The procedure was the same as that of experiment 1 except that subjects were required to name the word presented as quickly as possible. Naming times were measured by means of a timer started by the pulse which operated the projector, and stopped by the subject's response through a voice key.

Results and Discussion

Primed	Unprimed
575 (79)	594 (89)

Table 2. Mean naming times (milliseconds), from Experiment 2 with standard deviations in parentheses.

Trials where the subject made an incorrect response were not included in the analysis; these were again less than 1%. Analyses were carried out as for experiment 1. These showed that it took significantly less time (19 milliseconds) to name a primed word, than the same word unprimed, F1 $(1,21) = 8.44$, $p < 0.01$; F2 $(1,17) = 2.06$, $p = 0.17$; minF' = N.S.

It can be seen from the results that a priming effect of a similar order (19 as compared to 30 milliseconds) to the lexical decision task was obtained with the same materials, using a naming task. The implication is that the effect is due to input (lexical priming)and not due to output processes.

Experiment 3: Reading

METHOD

Subjects

Two groups of 8 volunteer undergraduates at the University of Nottingham participated in the experiment.

Materials and Design

19 sets of sentences were prepared. Each set consisted of 3 short sentences connected in a thematic way. The last sentence contained the target word. In the primed condition, the first sentence of the set contained a high associate synonym of the target; in the unprimed condition this was replaced by a less associated or unassociated word which was congruous with the context of that set. For example:

Bill went to the ruins to have a look. (/walk.)
It was enjoyable.
There was a lot to see.

The priming relationship in this case is between look-see. The control word is walk.

The position of the target in the third sentence was varied between sets, it was either at the end, as in the example above, or at the beginning. Between each set of three slides a calibration slide was placed: this consisted of two two-digit numbers, one of which was in the same position as the target which occurred on the immediately preceding slide. Subjects were instructed merely to look at the two numbers.

The experiment was divided into two sections: those targets primed for one group of subjects were unprimed for the second group, and vice versa. Each subject therefore saw 19 sets of sentences, half (10 or 9) of which contained a priming relationship between words in the first and third sentences.

Five dependent measures were taken: the time spent on the first fixation of the target; the total time fixating the target, that is the first fixation plus any regressive fixations; the reading time for the target sentence; and the number of regressive saccades to the target. Finally, the time elapsing between the appearance of the third (target) sentence on the screen and the subject's fixation of the target word.

Apparatus

Horizontal movements of the left eye were recorded using a device which monitors the position of the iris-sclera border by means of reflected infra-red radiation (Wilkinson, 1976). The device consists of emitters, a simple optical arrangement for focus, and detectors all mounted on an adjustable band placed on the subject's head. A chin rest and frame was used to restrict head movements. Output from the eye movement detector operated a Watanable WTR 211 pen recorder running at 10 millimetres per second. Overall accuracy is approximately +/-20' of arc in a range of 60 degrees (Wilkinson, 1976).

Stimuli were mounted on slides and presented on a Bell and Howell Auto-Focus back projector modified so that the key operated by the subject to advance the projector also sent a pulse to the pen recorder, thus indicating the time each slide was on the screen. All the apparatus was situated in a sound-proof cubicle.

Procedure

Subjects were seated 40 centimetres in front of the projector with the chin rest adjusted to a height such that subjects had to look slightly upwards to see the middle of the screen, where the sentences appeared. Calibration was achieved by having subjects fixate letters in the middle line of a letter grid which extended across the screen. Calibration slides were placed throughout the materials (after each target sentence) to aid in the analysis of the eye movement recordings. After calibration subjects were instructed that they were to read, silently and as naturally as possible, sets of three related sentences. This was followed by a calibration slide, which consisted of two numbers which they simply had to look at. They were told to go at their own pace, pressing the key for the next slide as soon as they were ready. The end of the experiment was signalled by a marker slide. Subjects were then debriefed.

Results and Discussion

1 Duration of First Fixation: Priming x Target Position (milliseconds)

		PRIMED	UNPRIMED
Target Position	BEGINNING	276 (73)	315 (67)
	END	359 (85)	398 (151)

2 Total time on Target (milliseconds)

PRIMED	UNPRIMED
345 (70)	405 (119)

3 Sentence Reading Time (milliseconds)

PRIMED	UNPRIMED
2663 (397)	2679 (404)

4 Number of Regressive Saccades to Target (means per subject)

PRIMED	UNPRIMED
1.8 (1.4)	1.6 (1.3)

5 Time Elapsed to First Fixation of Target (milliseconds)

PRIMED	UNPRIMED
1796 (369)	1840 (285)

Table 3. Mean values and standard deviations for each dependent variable recorded in the reading task, Experiment 3.

Analyses of variance were performed on the data from each of the dependent measures, the means of which are shown in Table 3. Only the first two measures, first fixation and inspection durations, produced F values greater than 1. On the first fixation subjects spent 39 milliseconds longer looking at the target, regardless of its position, when that target was unprimed than when it was primed $F1\ (1,15) = 6.35$, $p < 0.05$; $F2\ (1,18) = 4.95$, $p < 0.05$. Including regressive fixations (total time on target) the difference increased to 60 ms: $F1\ (1,15) = 9.91$, $p < 0.01$; $F2\ (1,18) = 5.58$, $p < 0.05$.

These results show a clear effect of reduction in fixation time on a word when a high associate synonym of that word had recently been read, implying that lexical priming occurs during reading. No significant reduction in sentence reading time was found, nor was there any difference in the speed with which the subject fixated the target word. The number of regressive fixations was small throughout the target sentences, and not different across the two conditions. A large increase was observed between fixation times for targets at the beginning and end of the sentences; this is accounted for by integrative processing which Just & Carpenter (1980) call sentence wrap-up.

General Discussion

The results of the three experiments reported above demonstrate a reduction in reaction/reading time (differences of 30, 19, and 39 milliseconds) for a word when a high associate synonym of that word has previously been processed. Although the three experiments required different responses, they are otherwise comparable: similar sets of primes and controls constituted the materials in each case, and each task required the target to be retrieved. It does not necessarily follow that the same process produced the priming effect in each task, but it does seem likely.

Priming in naming and lexical decision tasks has been regularly demonstrated (for example, Meyer & Schvaneveldt, 1971; Forster, 1981; Stanovich & West, 1983). The most widely accepted explanation of this effect is the spreading activation model. This theory (Anderson, 1983 provides a recent version) requires that for an element in semantic memory to be retrieved, the activation associated with that element must reach a threshold value. Elements may receive input from various sources. stimulus information, context and memory. When an element is accessed, activation spreads throughout the network of which that element is a part, causing related elements to be activated to an extent correlated with their degree of association with the original element.

The spreading activation model of priming accounts adequately for the data described above, including the presence of a priming effect in the reading task. However there are possible alternatives.

Forster (1981) offered an explanation of priming in which context has effect after the word has been accessed. Context may modify the process of deciding that the correct entry has been located by providing information other than stimulus features; "the candidate entry can also be checked for compatibility with the context" (Forster, 1981, p467). Forster does not apply this context-checking explanation to the results from his single word priming studies, rather he uses it to account for sentence context effects, implying that lexical and sentence context effects have different mechanisms. A further alternative advanced by Forster is that context modifies decision processes after lexical access has been accomplished, in which case the context effect may be dismissed as a methodological artifact. For Forster the important feature of these two accounts is that they locate the effect temporally posterior to presentation of the target and so, in the case of a sentence context, do not disconfirm the theory of autonomy of levels of processing which he wishes to advance.

Pre-access explanations of the context effect, such as spreading activation, have received a great deal of support from single word studies, and so it is parsimonious to accept this as an adequate account of the mechanisms involved in producing the priming found in experiments 1 and 2 above; further there is no reason to reject this as an explanation of the presence of priming in the reading task, experiment 3. It should be said that post-access, context checking may not be totally rejected; however the load put on the processor by a checking procedure would seem likely to interfere with the reading process, also there is no reason why this should be performed if a reader is not explicitly searching for related words.

The present results fail to replicate those of Kennedy (1978). Kennedy, in a reading task similar to experiment 3 above, found an effect in the opposite direction . primed words were fixated for longer than the same words unprimed. There are two possible reasons for this. Firstly, in the materials used by Kennedy the ratio of experimental trials (sets of 3 sentences which contained associated words in the first and third sentences) to control trials (no priming relationship) was unbalanced in favour of the experimental sets, that is, the majority of trials contained synonyms. This may have caused the subjects to engage in a search for synonyms and process them explicitly as targets. This would explain the longer fixation time for "primed" trials, and also Kennedy's other main finding that, when primed, targets were fixated sooner, the subject being aware of the presence of the synonym through the processing of items in peripheral vision (Jennings & Underwood, 1983).

If lexical priming occurs during the reading of text, and it seems likely from the foregoing that it does, of what use would this be to the reader? It may be the case that lexical priming is in fact of little help to the reader, being merely a result of the way lexical items are stored and accessed. Alternatively lexical priming would be of use to a processor which used schemata as a basis for comprehension in the way suggested by Kleiman (1980) in a model of sentence processing in which schemata (e.g. Rumelhart, 1980; Anderson, 1983) are seen as connected to a semantic network (Collins & Loftus, 1975). By asking subjects to make a lexical decision about sentence completions, Kleiman found that not only were best completions of the sentences facilitated in terms of reaction time, but also normative associates to the best completions, even when this resulted in an unlikely completion.

Kleiman explained this in terms of his hybrid model in which, on reading a sentence, a suitable schema is accessed and some of the slots in the schema are filled by information in the sentence. Unfilled slots cause activation of the default values for those slots and association spreads through the semantic network to associates of those values.

Auble & Franks (1983) proposed an extension of Kleiman's model in which sentence comprehension is seen as "a process of retrieving schemata which fit the meaning of the sentence. This retrieval is achieved through spreading activation in a semantic network" (Auble & Franks, 1983, p399). Thus when a sentence is read, activation spreads from the words in the sentence to related concept nodes resulting in retrieval of the schema which receives the most activation.

Auble & Franks tested an hypothesis from this theory: normative associates of words in a sentence will be activated even when unrelated to the meaning of the sentence as a whole. Using auditory presentation of targets masked by white noise they failed to find facilitation of associates to words in the sentence, except when the associate was related to the meaning of the whole sentence and the sentence was understood.

The present sentence reading experiment would appear to contradict this, since the target words, primed or not, always bore the same relationship to the meaning of the whole set of sentences, being only slightly changed by the replacement of the priming words by the controls (see Method of Experiment 3). However comparing Auble & Franks' task with the present one is unjustified since they are so different.

In conclusion, the explanation of sentence comprehension utilising schemata in combination with a semantic network remains viable and is supported by the present experiment which shows a lexical priming effect, manifested by a reduction in fixation time on targets, during the comprehension of sentences.

References

Anderson, J.R. A spreading activation theory of memory. Journal of Verbal Learning and Verbal Behaviour, 1983, 22, 261-295.

Auble, P. & Franks, J.J. Sentence comprehension processes. Journal of Verbal Learning and Verbal Behaviour, 1983, 22, 395-405.

Balota, D.A. & Rayner, K. Parafoveal visual information and semantic contextual constraints. Journal of Experimental Psychology: Human Perception and Performance, 1983, 9, 726-738.

Bradshaw, J.L. Peripherally presented and unreported words may bias the perceived meaning of a centrally fixated homograph. Journal of Experimental Psychology, 1974, 103, 1200-1202.

Collins, A.M. & Loftus, E.F. A spreading activation theory of semantic processing. Psychological Review, 1975, 82, 407-428.

Forster, K.I. Priming and the effects of sentence and lexical contexts on naming time: Evidence for autonomous lexical processing. Quarterly Journal of Experimental Psychology, 1981, 33A, 465-495.

Jennings, G.D.J. & Underwood, G. The influence of parafoveal information in a simple reading task. Paper presented to the Second European Conference on Eye Movements, Nottingham, 1983.

Just, M.A. & Carpenter, P.A.A. A theory of reading: From eye fixations to comprehension. Psychological Review, 1980, 87, 329-354.

Kennedy, A. Reading sentences: Some observations on the control of eye movements. In G. Underwood (ed.) Strategies of information processing. London: Academic Press, 1978.

Kerr, J.S. & Underwood, G. Fixation time on anaphoric pronouns decreases with congruity of reference. Paper presented to the Second European Conference on Eye Movements, Nottingham, 1983.

Kleiman, G.M. Sentence frame contexts and lexical decisions: Sentence acceptability and word relatedness effects. Memory and Cognition, 1980, 8, 336-344.

Meyer, D.E. & Schvaneveldt, R.W. Facilitation in recognizing pairs of words: Evidence of a dependence between retrieval operations. Journal of Experimental Psychology, 1971, 90, 227-234.

Morton, J. Interaction of information in word recognition. Psychological Review, 1969, 76, 165-178.

Postman, L. & Keppel, G. (eds.) Norms of word association. New York: Academic Press, 1970.

Rumelhart, D.E. Schemata: The building blocks of cognition. In R.J. Spiro, B.C. Bruce & W.F. Brewer (eds.), Theoretical issues in reading comprehension: Perspectives from cognitive psychology, linguistics, artificial intelligence and education. Hillsdale, N.J.: Erlbaum, 1980.

Sanford, A.J. & Garrod, S.C. Understanding written language. New York: Wiley & Sons, 1981

Stanovich, K.E. & West, R.F. On priming by a sentence context. Journal of Experimental Psychology: General, 1983, 112, 1-36.

Underwood, G. Lexical recognition of embedded unattended words: Some implications for reading processes. Acta Psychologica, 1981, 47, 267-283.

Underwood, G. & Thwaites, S. Automatic phonological coding of unattended printed words. Memory and Cognition, 1982, 10, 434-442.

Wilkinson, H.P. Wide range eye and head movement monitor. Quarterly Journal of Experimental Psychology, 1976, 28, 123-124.

Acknowledgements

This work was supported by a research studentship to the first author from the Social Science Research Council, and Project Grant No. GRC/02259 to the second author from the Science and Engineering Research Council. We are grateful to C.I. Howarth, E.A. Maylor and two anonymous reviewers for their comments on this work, and to H.P. Wilkinson for his technical expertise.

Eye Movements and Human Information Processing
R. Groner, G.W. McConkie and C. Menz (eds.)

ON THE PURPOSE OF READING AND THE IMMEDIACY OF PROCESSING PRONOUNS

Wietske Vonk

Max-Planck-Institut für Psycholinguistik
and
University of Nijmegen
Nijmegen, The Netherlands

This study deals with the immediacy of processing pronouns in relation to the purpose of reading as induced by the task. Subjects had to read sentences such as *Harry won the money from Albert because he was a skillful player*. The gender of the pronoun and of the antecedents was varied to create conditions with and without a gender cue on the basis of which the pronoun could unambiguously be assigned. The verb phrase of the subordinate clause was congruent or incongruent with the causality implicit in the main verb. Reading times and eye movements were recorded. The results give evidence for the immediacy of processing being controlled by a strategy of selection of information dependent on the reading task.

A central topic in research on sentence processing is the question of what linguistic cues are used in interpreting the sentence and when that information is used in the time course. One particular position is formulated as the *immediacy assumption* (Just & Carpenter, 1980). According to this assumption, the reader tries to interpret the words as soon as he/she encounters them. The words are interpreted as soon as possible, even at the risk of making erroneous interpretations. Related to the immediacy assumption is the *eye-mind assumption* that posits that the eye remains fixated on a word as long as it is being processed. According to these assumptions, the processing of the information is not delayed and the information is processed as completely as possible. These assumptions do not claim that *buffering* the information and delaying the interpretation never occurs. In fact, the restriction "as soon as possible" and "as completely as possible" is a built-in qualification of the immediacy of processing.

It is indeed an empirical question whether information is processed immediately or whether the processing is delayed. There may be several reasons why information is not processed immediately. Sometimes the interpretation is postponed and information is buffered because additional information is necessary for a complete interpretation. There may be, however, another reason why particular information is not processed immediately. In many sentences there are several cues that can be used for a particular interpretation. The question is then whether all these cues will be used immediately. If not, which ones are used and how is the selection made of the cues that are used? It is conceivable, for instance, that a particular interpretation can be based on lexical information, to be derived from a particular word, as well as on contextual information to be derived from the integration of larger units. An example is the sentence *Mary won the money from Albert because she was a skillful player*. The antecedent for *she* in this sentence can be found on the basis of the gender information of the pronoun itself, as well as on the basis of the relation between *won* and *skillful player*. An interesting suggestion with respect to this issue is that, if buffering takes place, the advantage of buffering lexical information may be smaller than the advantage of buffering contextual information and that higher integrative processes may benefit from a processing delay (Dee-Lucas, Just, Carpenter, & Daneman, 1982).

This paper deals with the situation in which several cues can be used as the basis for a particular interpretation. Assuming that not all cues are used immediately, the question is which cues are used and when, how the cues are selected, and to what extent the selection depends on the task of the reader. The assumption in this paper is that the immediacy of processing is determined not only by properties of the text, but also by the interaction between the reader and the text. The purpose of the reader, the task the reader sets himself or herself, and the knowledge of the reader may determine under what conditions the linguistic cues in the text are used and how immediately they are used.

In this paper, the understanding of pronouns will be studied in relation to the purpose of the reader as induced by the task. The sentences are such that there are two different linguistic cues that can be used to assign the antecedent to the pronoun: A lexical factor and a contextual factor. Table 1 illustrates the sentences the readers had to process and the factors under consideration.

Table 1.
Example sentences illustrating the factors Congruency (1a vs. 1b and 2a vs. 2b) and Gender Cue (1a vs. 1c and 1b vs. 1d) for NP1-biasing (1 a-d) and NP2-biasing (2 a-b) verbs.

(1a) Harry won the money from Albert because he was a skillful player.
(1b) Harry won the money from Albert because he was a careless player.
(1c) Mary won the money from Albert because she was a skillful player.
(1d) Mary won the money from Albert because he was a careless player.
(2a) Harry didn't trust Albert because he was so secretive.
(2b) Harry didn't trust Albert because he was so suspicious.

The first factor is the gender information of the pronoun. In contrast to sentence (1a) of Table 1, sentence (1c) contains gender information on the basis of which one can unambiguously assign the antecedent of the pronoun.

The contextual factor can best be explained in relation to the verb of the main clause. Caramazza, Grober, Garvey, and Yates (1977) claim that a property of the main verb in sentences such as (1a) and (2a) influences the assignment of the pronoun in the subordinate clause (cf. Brown & Fish, 1983). They term this property the *implicit causality* of the verb. The main verb creates a context for the subordinate clause in which one particular assignment of the pronoun is preferred. The presence of *won* leads the reader to the initial assumption that the pronoun in the *because* clause is anaphoric with the subject of the main clause. The verb phrase *didn't trust* induces the initial assumption that the pronoun is anaphoric with the surface object of the main clause. This preference in assigning was demonstrated in a sentence completion task in which sentence fragments up to the conjunction were presented. The completions of sentence fragments with main verbs like *win, confess, sell,* and *lie*, indicated that the pronoun is anaphoric with the subject nounphrase (NP1) of the main clause; those of sentence fragments with main verbs as *trust, punish,* and *fear,* showed that the pronoun is anaphoric with the surface object noun phrase (NP2) of the main clause. The verbs of the first type will be called NP1-biasing verbs, those of the second type NP2-biasing verbs.

These biases do not completely determine the interpretation. They can be contradicted without the sentence becoming unacceptable or unnatural. The pronoun in (1b) does not refer to the subject, but to the object of the main clause, thus conflicting with the NP1 bias of the main verb. The information of the second clause is thus *incongruent* with the bias of the main verb. The same is true for sentence (2b). In this sentence the information in the subordinate clause is incongruent with the NP2 bias of the main verb.

Caramazza et al. (1977) found both a congruency effect and a gender cue effect in the pronoun assignment. The time it took to assign the pronoun was shorter when the subordinate clause was congruent with the bias of the main verb than when it was incongruent. So, congruency is one factor that readers may use in interpreting pronouns. Readers also use the gender information: Sentences in which the gender of the pronoun unambiguously determined the antecedent were processed faster than sentences without such a cue. It is interesting to note that the congruency of the subordinate clause still had an effect when the pronoun could be assigned on the basis of the gender alone.

These effects were found in a task in which the subject had to read the sentence in order to *explicitly* identify the referent for the pronoun: For each sentence the subject had to name the antecedent of the pronoun as quickly as possible. What was measured was the vocalization latency, which includes the time for naming the answer.

This experiment demonstrates that somewhere in executing the task two distinct types of information are used. But the central issue is when exactly in the process these types of information are used. It is quite plausible that the naming task consists of two separate subprocesses, the processing of the sentence and, subsequently, the execution of the answer.

Pronoun assignment

A verification task was used in which subjects were asked to read a sentence and afterwards had to verify a statement with respect to that sentence. This allows for a separation of reading time (time for reading the sentence) and verification time (time for executing the answer). Eye movements were recorded while subjects read the sentences, because this method is more sensitive to on-line processes than reading time registration.

Examples of experimental sentences are shown in Table 1. Eight NP1-biasing and eight NP2-biasing main verbs were selected on the basis of a sentence completion task. For each verb, one sentence with a continuation congruent with the verb and one sentence with a continuation incongruent with the verb were constructed. In a preliminary experiment the *naturalness* of the sentences was checked. The incongruent sentences did not differ from the congruent ones in the naturalness judgements of the subjects. The sentences were presented in two conditions: A condition with a gender cue (the names in the main clause are of different gender) and a condition without a gender cue (the names are of the same gender).

In order to prevent readers from using a strategy of focussing on the assignment of pronouns, filler sentences with the conjunctions *before* and *after*, not containing pronouns, were added to the set of experimental sentences. Moreover, several kinds of verification statements were used, only some of them requiring the assignment of the pronoun.

The experimental verification statements required the integration of the two clauses of the experimental sentences, e.g., for sentence (1a), *Harry was a skillful player*. Filler verification statements were simple verifications that did not require the integration of the two clauses, like, for sentence (1a), *Harry won the money*, and statements about the filler sentences. For filler sentences, like *Mary had finished the soup before Anna came to the table*, verification statements were, for instance, *Anna had finished the soup*, and *Anna was eating first*.

Subjects had to read the sentence, press a button in order to get the verification statement on the screen, and press a *yes* or a *no* button to give the verification answer. Before a sentence was displayed, a fixation point was presented at the point where the first word of the sentence would appear. The sentence appeared when the subject pushed a button. The eye movements were measured while subjects read the sentences on the display until they pressed the button for the verification sentence to appear.

The data were obtained with a corneal-reflectance eye tracking system (Gulf & Western), with a sample frequency of 50 Hz. Subjects read with two eyes, but eye movements were recorded from the left eye only. The sentences were written in lower and upper case. Three characters equalled about 1.5

degree of visual angle. The reading time was the time from the onset of the sentence to the moment the subject pressed the button. The verification latency was measured from the onset of the verification statement to the moment the subject pressed the *yes* or *no* button. There were ten subjects.

Verification and reading times. The verification latencies showed an effect of both the congruency factor and the gender cue factor (the probability of the *min F'* statistic being less than 5%), and no interaction between these factors. The verification latencies were on the average 150 msec shorter for the congruent sentences than for the incongruent ones; they were also on the average 150 msec shorter for sentences which had a gender cue than for sentences without such a cue. The results are comparable to the results of Caramazza in his naming task.

It is interesting that the reading times for the sentences did not give the same pattern. The congruent sentences were on the average a significant 200 msec shorter than the incongruent ones, but there was no effect of the gender cue. The question now is what is going on during reading.

Eye fixations. The eye fixations on the verb phrase of the second clause will be discussed first. If the main verb biases the reader towards an interpretation of the verb phrase of the subordinate clause that is congruent with the main verb bias, then the congruency effect is expected to show up immediately during the fixation of that verb phrase.

The data that have been analysed are fixations in the first pass of reading the sentence; regressions were not included. Because the verb phrases in the sentences were not of completely equal length, the statistical analysis is based upon the fixation duration per character.

The average fixation duration per character on the verb phrase of the second clause was a significant 2.8 msec longer in the incongruent sentences than in the congruent ones. This corresponds to a difference of 80 msec on the average for the whole verb phrase. So, the reader utilizes the biasing information in the main verb: The immediate longer fixation duration on the verb phrases that are not congruent with the expectancy created by the main verb testify to that.

No effect of the gender cue was found in the fixation duration on this part of the second clause, nor was there an interaction between the two factors, testifying that, during the reading of the verb phrase, the gender information apparently plays no role although it could have already been fully used.

What about the fixations on the pronoun? Could the gender information already have been used during the reading of the pronoun? Before answering this question, a study will be briefly presented in which the same kind of sentences were used in a *naming* task (Vonk, 1984). In that study only congruent sentences were used, but with different conjunctions in the subordinate clause (cf. Ehrlich, 1980). The interesting result in this study concerns the question of how early the gender cue information is used. The eye movement data showed a difference in eye fixations on the pronoun. The fixation duration on the pronoun in the first pass through the sentence was a significant 50 msec *longer* when there was a gender cue. Besides the longer fixation duration in case the pronoun was fixated, the pronoun was more often fixated when there was a gender cue. So, when the pronoun is informative, it is fixated more often and longer. The duration of the first fixation after the pronoun was not effected by the gender cue, testifying to the immediacy of the use of the gender information.

Does the same effect occur in eye fixations in the present *verification* experiment? There appears to be no effect of the gender cue factor at all: The average fixation duration on the pronoun when there is a gender cue is 178 msec, and when there is not it is 187 msec.

There was also no effect of the congruency factor. A main effect of congruency cannot really occur; at this point in the reading process the congruent or incongruent information is simply not yet available. But there is some ground to expect an interaction of congruency and gender cue: If the reader is already biased by the main verb to a plausible antecedent, then the reader will notice when the gender of the pronoun is incongruent with that plausible antecedent, and this then will lead to a longer fixation duration in the incongruent condition with a gender cue. But no such effect was observed.

With respect to the first fixation after the pronoun there was again no effect of the gender cue factor, nor was there an effect of the congruency factor.

Conclusion

The data can be interpreted in terms of a *rational selection of information* principle. This implies the following: The purpose of reading, in this case induced by the task, determines what information is relevant. The information that is relevant is immediately processed as soon as it is encountered. A closer examination of the tasks is appropriate.

In the naming task the attention of the reader is very much addressed to the pronoun. The reader has to name aloud the antecedent of the pronoun. It is clear from the eye movement data of the naming experiment that when a pronoun is informative, the fixation duration on the pronoun increases immediately.

The task in the verification experiment focusses the reader much less on the pronoun. In only one fourth of the items, the task asks for the resolution of the pronoun, the task being to verify what a particular person *had done or felt*. The relevant information for the verification is primarily the content of the verb phrase. Accordingly, an effect was found in the total fixation duration on the verb phrase of the second clause in the first pass of reading: Incongruency of the second verb phrase is noticed immediately and requires more time. Corresponding with this result no effect is found on the pronoun.

In conclusion, the reader is able to very quickly establish what the relevant information is, and this information is processed immediately. What the relevant information is, is at least in part determined by the requirements of the reading task. From the fact that the gender cue is not used when the pronoun is first encountered in the verification experiment, one can conclude that not all the information that could have been used is used immediately. One may conclude that the immediacy is controlled by a strategy of rational selection of information.

Acknowledgements

L. Damen conducted the experiments, and L.G.M. Noordman gave many comments and suggestions on an earlier draft of the paper. Their contributions are gratefully acknowledged.

REFERENCES

Brown, R., & Fish, D. (1983). The psychological causality implicit in language. *Cognition, 14*, 237-273.

Caramazza, A., Grober, E., Garvey, C., & Yates, J. (1977). Comprehension of anaphoric pronouns. *Journal of Verbal Learning and Verbal Behavior, 16*, 601-609.

Dee-Lucas, D., Just, M.A., Carpenter, P.A., & Daneman, M. (1982). What eye fixations tell us about the time course of text integration. In R. Groner and P. Fraisse (Eds.), *Cognition and Eye Movements*. Amsterdam: North-Holland Publishing Company.

Ehrlich, K. (1980). Comprehension of pronouns. *Quarterly Journal of Experimental Psychology, 32*, 247-255.

Just, M.A., & Carpenter, P.A. (1980). A theory of reading: From eye fixations to comprehension. *Psychological Review, 87*, 329-354.

Vonk, W. (1984). Pronoun comprehension. In A.G. Gale and F. Johnson (Eds.), *Theoretical and Applied Aspects of Eye Movement Research*. Amsterdam: Elsevier Science Publishers B.V. (North-Holland).

B. Visual Search and Problem Solving

Eye Movements and Human Information Processing
R. Groner, G.W. McConkie and C. Menz (eds.)

VISUAL SEARCH AND PROBLEM SOLVING

Introduction

In this part, a broad variety of articles are presented ranging from simple visual scanning to complex problem solving. The common perspective is the view that the eye movements and fixations provide the means of studying visual information processing in considerable detail and close to the basic operations of visual intake.

The central aim of the paper by Ellis and Smith is a thorough test of the statistical properties of consecutive fixations (= dependencies, in contrast to random movements). Their subjects judged future relative positions of air-crafts on dynamic displays. Based on a large sample of more than 100'000 fixations they observed statistical dependencies which could not simply be attributed to spatial regularities on the display. The authors conclude that these regularities reflect the information seeking strategies used by the subjects.

Groner and Menz pursue this issue further by studying the influence of the stimulus, task and subject on scanning patterns. A complete factorial design makes it possible to assess the contribution of each variable separately as well as their mutual interaction. The authors demonstrate two different kinds of dependencies, local scanpaths (= patterns of consecutive fixations) and global scanpaths (= differences in the distribution of fixations in different parts of the inspection period).

The next paper by Gonzalez and Kolers approaches one of the most central questions underlying eye movement research, in which way the location of a fixation is related to the processing of the material fixated. The authors distinguish between two different aspects: salience (=importance of a region as a potential source of information), and subsequent interpretation made about the information obtained there. An immediately following question resulting from this distinction would be whether the two processes are serial or (at least partly) parallel, in which latter case fixation durations could not directly be used as an indicatior of the amount of cognitive processing spent at the respective location. An experiment which appears in several ways as a continuation of the last one is the next one by R. Hansell, P. Kolers and P. Sousan on taxonomic judgements. The process of classification is analyzed by relating eye movements to subjective scaling weights of different features and their similarity. It is shown that the process of efficient classification requires a minimum number of fixations which falls into two parts: a primary process of peripheral vision where information is Gestalt-like organized, followed by a secondary central vision process which is under cognitive control.

In her paper L.C. Hall fully exploits the potential of eye movement research for investigating the perceptual, cognitive and linguistic development of different groups of children, comparing learning disabled and deaf with normal children. It is amazing how, even for the young and handicapped children language served a directive function which still improved with age. In this way it is possible to assess inobtrusively the role of second language systems in the regulation of visual search and possibly extend these findings to other settings.

G. Lüer, R. Hübner and U. Lass start their experiment in complex problem solving on the assumption that, if this skill depends on the subject's capacity to build up an internal representation of the problem environment, eye movement research might provide the means of tracking that process. In their task of running a factory, the subjects have to search the necessary information from a display where details were given randomly dispersed on a 5 x 5 matrix. The scanpaths were decomposed by spectral-analytic methods which led the authors to the conclusion that systematic and balanced explorative behaviour is the decisive difference for distinguishing between successful and unsuccessful problem solvers.

The final paper by G. Deffner attempts to put into relation strategies derived from a theoretical task analysis with empirical scanpaths. This is done by identifying small basic units of gaze fixation sequences and assembling them to correlates of the proposed strategies. Although an empirical validation of this approach seems difficult at the moment, it still provides an interesting example of a model-directed analysis of gaze sequences.

Some chapters in this part provide a good example for the two approaches: exploratory research and model-directed analysis. Since it appears that still essentials of the fundamental processes are yet unknown, more research should be directed towards methodological studies (like the one by Gonzalez and Kolers) which deal with basic implications of this kind of research.

Eye Movements and Human Information Processing
R. Groner, G.W. McConkie and C. Menz (eds.)

Patterns of Statistical Dependency in Visual Scanning

Stephen R. Ellis and James Darrell Smith

Department of Physiological Optics
University of California
Berkeley, California 94720 USA
and
NASA Ames Research Center
Moffett Field, California 94035 USA

A method to identify statistical dependencies in the positions of visual fixations was applied to eye movement data from subjects who viewed dynamic displays of air traffic and judged future relative position of aircraft. Analysis of these data has identified statistical dependencies in scanning that were independent of the physical placement of the points of interest. Identification of these dependencies is inconsistent with random-sampling based theories used to model visual search and information-seeking[1].

1. INTRODUCTION

The distribution of visual fixations on stimuli in the visual field is usually not uniform and the time spent viewing each of their component features is usually not equal (Buswell, 1935; Yarbus, 1967; Monty, Senders, 1976; Senders, Fisher, & Monty, 1978; Fisher, Monty & Senders, 1981). Certain features are often more "popular" than others. The resulting distribution of fixations, may be expressed as a zero order probability vector where each element is the probability of viewing a particular feature. When the scanning among the features is otherwise random, this vector constrains the transition pattern. One aspect of this constraint is that transitions between features, with high probability of viewing occur with corresponding high frequency (Senders, *et. al*, 1966). Thus, a high frequency of transition itself is not a necessary indication of a statistical association of fixations on pairs of features (Carpenter and Just, 1978).

Somewhat surprisingly, oculomotor information seeking during a variety of tasks such as visual search, (Krendel & Wodinsky, 1960; Engel, 1977; Inditsky & Bodmann, 1980; Kraiss & Knaeuper, 1983) instrument monitoring, (Senders, *et. al.*, 1966; Weir and Klein, 1970; Hofmann, *et. al.*, 1973; Papin, *et. al.*; Wewerinke, 1981). computer-menu scanning (Card, 1983) and during solution of seriation problems (Groner and Groner, 1982) may be modeled as random or stratified random sampling with replacement. This apparent randomness in visual scanning is especially surprising in view of evidence from more controlled experiments which shows that subsequent fixations may be directed by information acquired at the current fixation (Rayner and Pollatsek, 1978; Kapoula, 1983) If the underlying cognitive processes directing eye movements during information-seeking can be made periodic and statistically stationary, evidence of that direction ought to be evident as statistical dependencies in the observers' scanning during free viewing.

The following experiments were designed to exhibit these dependencies in an information seeking task. Periodicity and stationarity of the processing of visual information in this task was encouraged by periodicity in presentation and training of the subjects. We endeavored to measure to what extent our subjects' scanning eye movements could be described as random and thereby to infer the extent to which their control may be autonomous from presumptively repetitive ongoing cognitive processing. If the decision where to fixate next were controlled by open-loop repetitive information gathering strategies (Kolers, 1976; Bouma & de Voogd, 1974), i.e. left-right scan as in reading, or by closed-loop strategies in which the decision is based on information gathered in the previous fixation (Rayner & Pollatsek, 1981), scanning ought not to be random.

EXPERIMENT 1

2. METHODS

2.1. Display Conditions

A series of 48 track-up, moving map air traffic displays was generated on a calligraphic computer graphics system (Evans and Sutherland PS 1) and videotaped for presentation. (See Palmer *et. al.* 1980,1981 for similar displays). Each display depicted an encounter between two aircraft at the same altitude, the pilot's own ship and an intruder. An example of a specific encounter is in Figure 1.[2]

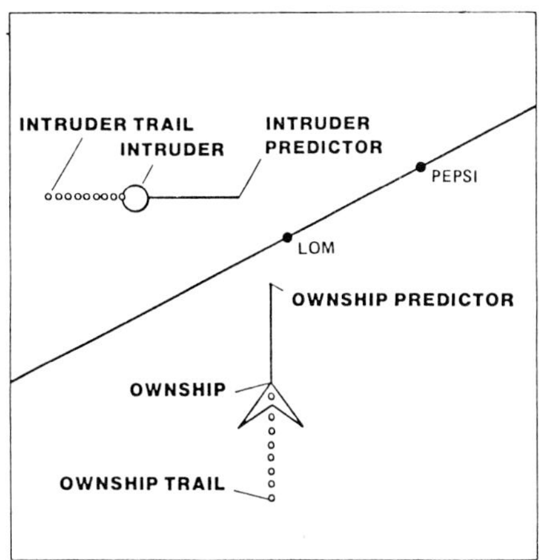

Figure 1. Representative encounter between ownship and an intruder approaching from left. Map range is 10 nautical miles from ownship to top of the display. The boldface labels did not appear on the display when viewed by the subjects.

All aircraft had 32 seconds of previously tracked positions displayed as 8 dots of trail, one for each update, and had a 32 second predictor which indicated its future position if it did not maneuver[3]. Equal numbers of intruders were randomly determined to pass in front and behind ownship. All trajectories crossed near LOM, one of two geographical locations shown. Each encounter consisted of seven 4-second updates; two updates before the intruder appeared, and five updates afterwards. In order to avoid the mixing of different scan strategies, analysis was restricted to the final five updates during which the intruder was visible.

The encounters represented both straight and turning (1.5 deg./sec) horizontal encounter geometries. Intruders approached randomly but equally often from the left and right of ownship. There were four different types of encounters producing different target movements on the display: neither aircraft turning, intruder only turning, ownship only turning, and both aircraft turning. Variation of the encounter geometry of each type of encounter was accomplished by varying the position of point of minimum separation. and intruder heading difference Details of these encounters have been described elsewhere (Ellis and Stark, 1982). Significantly, the turning of ownship caused the other parts of the map to rotate around it.

The resulting set of encounters provided a wide variety of encounter geometries in terms of display coordinates. This variety would prevent stereotyped scanning such as a left-to-right reading pattern from masking a scanning strategy based on information present on the display. The variety can help ensure that any scanning strategies are not a consequence of the particular placement or movement of the aircraft and ground symbols on the display. Subjects signaled the in front and behind judgements with a toggle switch.

Direction of gaze data were recorded with a Gulf and Western 1994 pupilometer-based television eye monitor which was calibrated by fixations at reference points in a 5 X 5 array, 14 degrees/side, centered in the subjects forward field of view. The eye monitor performed within specification providing at least 1 degree overall accuracy in measuring eye position. The eye monitor output (x,y direction of gaze and pupil diameter), the subjects signals, and the time markers from the videotape were all digitally recorded at 30 hz.

2.2. Subjects

Eight airline pilots were subjects in the experiment. All were familiar with the display and the front/behind judgement from at least 3 hrs previous testing.

During an orientation before the experiment, the subject's attention was diverted from the recording of their eye movements. They were told that the purpose of the experiment was to determine if pupilary changes could be used to predict their in front/behind judgements. The meaning of all parts of the symbology was reviewed and each subject was given about 20 minutes practice making in front/behind judgements. This training and the selection of experienced subjects resulted in asymptotic, near perfect performance of the task which provided stable behavior for analysis.

After the experiment, the data were transferred to a PDP-11/70 computer where they were linearized and reduced to fixations at least 90 msec. long in a manner similar to Karsh and Breitenbach (1984).

After identifying the positions, duration, and onset time of all fixations, the data were correlated with records of the positions of all points of interest as a function of time after the beginning of each encounter. Each fixation was assigned to one of eight possible points of interest: the end of ownship's trail (OST), ownship present position (OS), the end of ownship's predictor (OSP), the end of intruder's trail (IT), intruder's current position (I), the end of the intruder's predictor (IP), location PEPSI (PEP), and location LOM (LOM). All fixations not within 1 degree of any of the above points of interest were assigned to a category call BIN. The data were then tabulated to determine overall distribution of fixation duration as well as separate distributions for each point of interest. Per cent of time spent at each point of interest was determined.

3. RESULTS

3.1. Distribution of Fixations

The individual distributions of fixation durations had the usual positive skew, 1.84 to 2.64, a range of means somewhat longer than that usually found for scanning of graphical stimuli, 341 to 554 msec., and standard deviations ranging from 282 to 498 msec. The pilots distributed their fixations across the eight points of interest in a stereotyped manner as indicated in Figure 2.

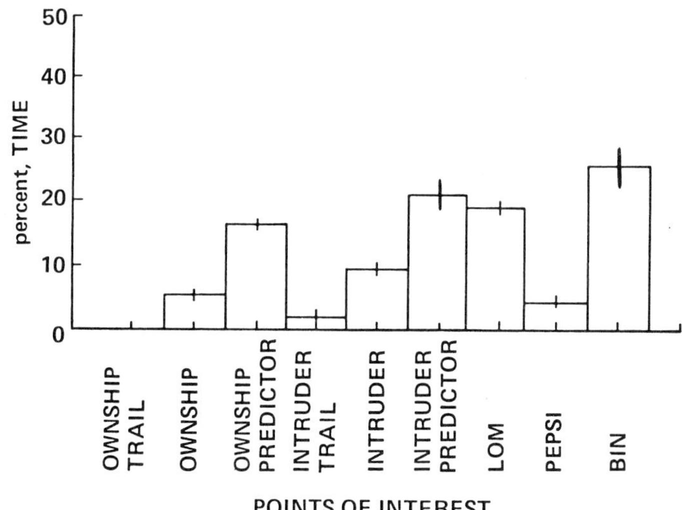

Figure 2. Pilots' distribution of fixational attention shown by across subjects means of per cent of time each pilot spent viewing each point of interest. Error bars represent +/- 1 standard error.

Their distributions of fixation reflect the differential usefulness of the spatial information at each point of interest for the in front/behind judgement that they made (Palmer, *et. al.*, *1980)*. The higher proportion of viewing time on the location LOM probably occurred because it was close to the point of intersection of the flight paths for all the encounters. With the exception of LOM, the per cent of time viewing each point of interest was approximately constant, +/- 8%, during the course of the encounter. The time spent viewing LOM increased about 40% as a function of time after the appearance of the intruder, i.e. as a function of each 4 second update period ($F = 15.02$, $df = 1,7$ $p < .01$). This increase in viewing of LOM corresponded to a decrease in of about 30% in unclassified fixations which were generally at points intermediate between the ends of the predictors on the aircraft.

3.2. Analysis of Transition Frequencies

We have examined the possibility that each subject's probability of viewing each point of interest can predict the frequency of transitions among them. To do so we calculate expected frequencies of transitions, as described in the appendix, and compare them with observed transition frequencies. This comparison was made on a subject by subject basis with a chi-square goodness of fit test on the entire distribution of observed and expected transitions.

The method of analysis is illustrated in Table 1 with the data from one subject. The table contains a of matrix of his observed and expected 1st order observed transition frequencies.

A Singles Subject's First Order Transition Frequencies Between 8 Points of Interest

From	To: OST	OS	OSP	IT	I	IP	LOM	PEP
Ownship trail (OSP)	- -	1 (0)	0 (0)	0 (0)	0 (0)	0 (0)	0 (0)	0 (0)
Ownship (OS)	0 (0)	- -	11 (4)	1 (0)	3 (4)	6 (8)	6 (6)	5 (1)
Ownship predictor (OSP)	0 (0)	12 (4)	- -	0 (2)	8 (16)	14 (30)	30 (21)	5 (3)
Intruder trail (IT)	0 (0)	0 (0)	0 (2)	- -	6 (2)	1 (3)	2 (2).	0 (0)
Intruder (I)	0 (0)	2 (4)	9 (16)	6 (2)	- -	**47** **(29)**	12 (23)	2 (3)
Intruder predictor (IP)	0 (0)	4 (8)	21 (30)	0 (3)	**54** **(30)**	- -	40 (43)	4 (6)
Waypoint LOM (LOM)	0 (0)	2 (6)	10 (24)	0 (2)	23 (23)	47 (43)	- -	5 (5)
Waypoint PEPSI (PEP)	0 (0)	5 (1)	7 (3)	1 (0)	3 (3)	7 (6)	7 (5)	- -

Total number of transitions = 429
Chi-square = 82.1, df=47, $p<.005$

Table 1. This table compares one pilot's observed pattern of transitions between points of interest on the CDTI display with the pattern of transitions, parenthesized numbers, that would have been observed had he only been taking a stratified random sample of the information at the points. were collapsed. The bold-face font indicates which of the observed transitions were identified as sufficiently different from the expected values to be considered evidence for statistical dependency in the scanning. The main diagonal is undefined, since we are unable to observe a transition from a point of interest to itself.

As shown by the chi-square statistic at the bottom of Table 1 [4], there is statistically significant deviation between the overall observed and expected transition patterns and, thus, there is evidence for something other than stratified random sampling during the scanning. As seen in Table 2, the chi-square tests for seven of the eight subjects show a highly reliable difference between the observed and expected transition frequencies. For no subject, can the chi-square test alone measure the magnitude of the deviations from stratified random sampling.

Accordingly, in order to assess the extent of the deviation, each subject's expected transition frequencies were regressed against his corresponding observed frequencies (Tukey, 1977). In such a regression a perfect prediction corresponds to a linear regression with a slope of 1.0 and correlation of 1.0. As is clear from Figure 3, the slope of the regressions for each subject are quite close to 1.0 (dashed line) and there is a strong linear relation between the observed and expected frequencies.

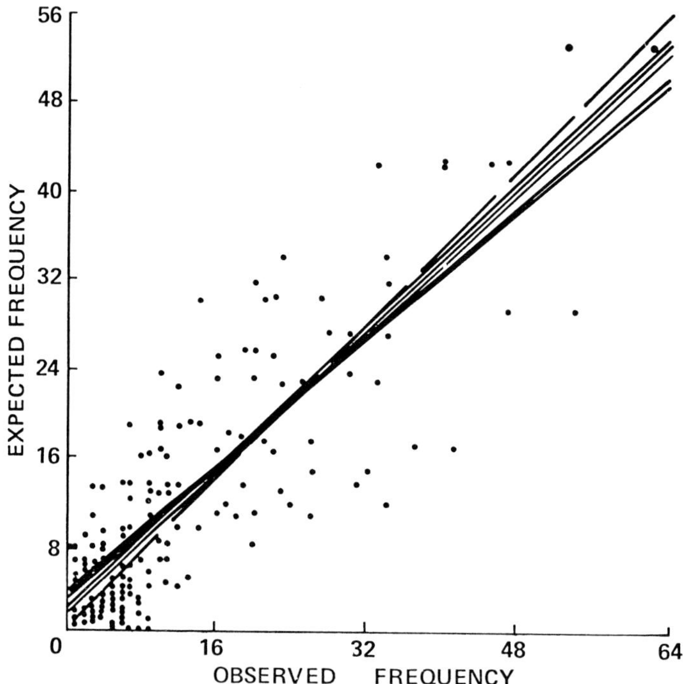

Figure 3. Scatter plot of observed transition frequency versus that expected based on assumption of stratified random sampling and the observed 0-order sampling probabilities. The plot collapses across all subjects. Regression were calculated separately for each subject and drawn through the plot. The dashed line represents the equation that would be seen if stratified random sampling completely described the scanning.

The strength of this relationship is measured by two correlations between observed and expected frequencies which are shown for each subject in Table 2. The first is the Pearson correlation corresponding to the regression shown in Figure 4. The second is a Pearson correlation based on log transforms of both expected and observed frequencies which to some extent corrects for the skew in the marginal distributions. As seen from Tables 1 and 2, though the stratified random sampling model used to calculate the expected frequencies provides an approximation of the actual 1st order transition pattern, there is noticeable deviation from them (see Figure 3).

Subjects	X-sqr(df)	X-sqr statistical significance	Number of transitions	Corr	Corr(df) log
1	35.3(47)	------	154	.97	.84(39)
2	152.5(47)	p<.001	417	.96	.79(51)
3	134.8(47)	p<.001	409	.94	.71(43)
4	97.3(47)	p<.001	348	.95	.75(49)
5	82.1(47)	p<.005	270	.93	.79(43)
6	84.5(47)	p<.005	431	.97	.84(57)
7	178.8(47)	p<.001	429	.96	.82(48)
8	78.2(47)	p<.005	275	.94	.72(43)

Table 2. Results of subject by subject analyses of each subject's entire 1st order transition matrix. The chi-square values represent goodness-of-fit tests of stratified random sampling as a model of the scanning data.

3.3. Identification of Statistical Dependencies

In order to isolate terms in the chi-square calculations that contribute to the overall deviation one may treat each term as a separate test with 1 degree of freedom. For example, in Table 1, after the collapsing of the cells with small expected frequencies to a single cell, there remained 21 separate terms for the chi-square calculation. Thus, there are 21 separate tests, 20 of which may be treated as independent. If one adjusts the over all probability of the Type II error to 0.05, the separate terms may be tested. The results of this procedure are shown in Table 1 in which boldface font is used to indicate transitions that reliably contribute to the overall statistical dependency in the scanning.

Similar analyses were carried out on the transition patterns for the other 7 subjects in the experiment and the results from 2 others are summarized in Figure 4. In essence the analysis provides a filter to apply to the transition pattern in order to identify transitions genuinely indicating statistically dependent "linkage" between information presented at a pair of points of interest. As is shown in Figure 4, the transitions exhibiting statistically dependent associations do not necessarily correspond to those with the most frequent transitions.

If the dependencies identified in the scanning were caused by closed-loop control in which information acquired during the current fixation influenced the next fixation, evidence of this interaction could be found in a positive correlation between fixation duration and preceding saccade length. This correlation could be attributed to the peripheral preprocessing that is possible when fixations are made such that subsequent points of interest fall within the functional field of view during preceding fixations (Kapoula, 1983).

PERCENT OF TRANSITIONS

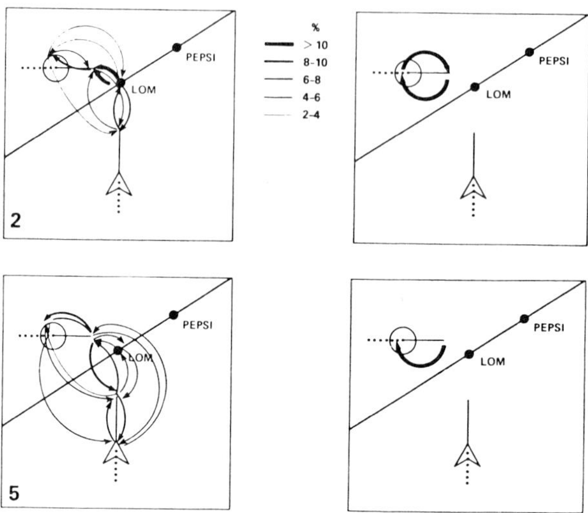

Figure 4. Representative scanning patterns from 2 of 8 pilots. Left-hand panel shows each subject's transition pattern among points of interest on the CDTI display. According to the legend, thickness of the arrows connecting pairs of points on these panels codes the relative frequency of each transition. Corresponding right-hand panels identify only those transitions which exhibit true statistical dependencies for each subject respectively. Thickness of the arrows in right-hand panels has no special significance.

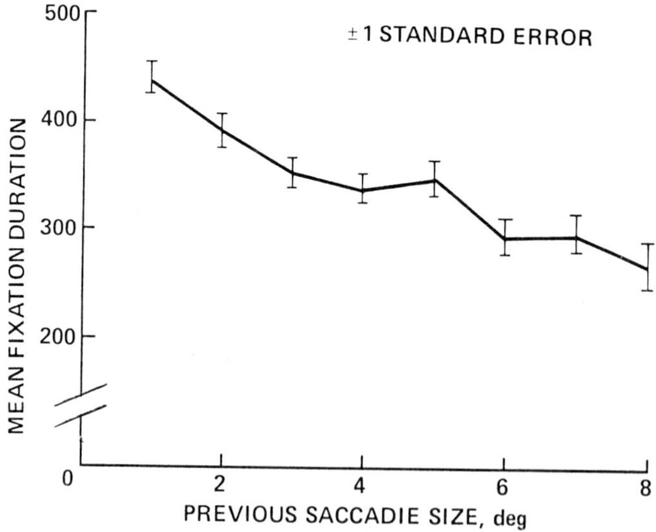

Figure 5. This figure summarizes the decrease in mean fixation duration as a function the size of the preceding saccade.

We examined this aspect of our scanning data subject by subject and found no evidence for this kind of correlation. In fact, in our task there was a slight reverse effect. All of the subjects showed statistically significant negative correlations between previous saccade size and fixation duration. They ranged between -.14 to -.54. Across subject means summarize the results in Figure 5. Inspection of the scatter plots underlying these correlation, indicated that these correlations stand up to correction of the positive skew of fixation duration by log transforms. Breakdown of this analysis by update period to check for changes during the course of an encounter showed the generally linear decrease of fixation as a function of preceding saccade size was present through out the encounter.

4. DISCUSSION

4.1. Causes of Statistical Independence in Scanning

As shown above, a random sampling model can provide an approximation of the actual pattern of transition among points of interest. To the extent this approximation is correct the results are consistent with visual sampling models that assume the search for information is autonomous of subsequent processes that use it. e.g. Smallwood (1967). These types of models would see the eye as a "buffer filler" which is not under the tight control of the higher order information processing that underlies interpretation of visual information[5] (Kolers 1976; Bouma and de Voogd, 1974).

However, the collection of the eye movement data over time and across different display conditions, raises the possibility that the randomness of the data could arise as an artifact of the mixing of a variety of scanning strategies making the transition pattern of nonstationary[6].

To the extent this mixing occurred, the present experiment would be biased against detection of statistically dependent 1st order transition patterns. But the only evidence for this mixing in any case is weak. It is the change in the per cent of time viewing point LOM. This change in viewing probability probably arises as an artifact of LOM being within 1 degree of visual angle of the intersection of the flight paths. As each encounter progressed, the pilots frequent fixations between the ends of the predictors, which were classified in the BIN, moved closed to LOM. Thus, due to inevitable inaccuracy in classification of fixations towards the end of each encounter, the percentage of viewing time assigned to LOM increased and the percentage assigned to BIN decreased.

A more likely alternative cause for the stratified random sampling characteristic of the scanning data in this experiment could be that the measures taken to insure stationarity in the scanning may have had the paradoxical effect of encouraging random sampling. In this view, the efforts to overtrain the pilots to asymptotic, near perfect performance on the in-front/behind discrimination may caused them to develop such efficient decision strategies that the subparts of the strategies were able to be simultaneously active.

Under these conditions, the display serves the pilot as a kind of random access memory allowing immediate acquisition of any fact needed for further analysis without the need for search (Groner and Groner, 1982). This is a situation characteristic of the well trained pilot who is able to simultaneously monitor and control several different aircraft systems. Less well trained pilots have to consciously shift their attention from one display to another and conceively might exhibit considerably more statistical dependency in their scanning eye movements (Tole *et. al*, 1982; Ellis and Stark, 1981).

4.2. Causes of Statistical Dependencies in Scanning

In general two causes of statistical dependencies may be distinguished: closed-loop control and open-loop control. In the first case information acquired during fixation is thought to direct the subsequent saccade. In the second case direction of the next saccade is thought to be due to information processing independent of the current visual information in the visual field. In visual tasks that explicitly benefit from peripheral preprocessing, evidence presented by Kapoula (1983) shows that fixation durations on subsequent points of interest can be determined by their proximity to previous fixations. This kind of evidence clearly suggests that sequences of fixations are influenced by closed-loop control processes[7].

Scanning data also, however, can exhibit statistical dependencies due to open-loop control. The left to right scanning in reading English text is not a consequence of the specific information present in the text, though the specific fixations may be, but only of the habitual lexicographical layout. Such open-loop scanning is not necessarily under the control of ongoing information processes may simply be filling an input buffer. Alternatively, open-loop control of scanning could be based on internal information processing in which the processes themselves drive the subjects sequence of fixations. An example of this could be movements of the eye to answer "visual questions" raised by previous viewing (Hochberg and Brooks, 1978) or scanpaths hypothetically linked to the memory trace for an object (Noton and Stark, 1971).

Our data do not exhibit the same relationship between fixation duration and previous saccade size which was used by Kapoula as evidence for the directing role of peripheral preprocessing, a role that illustrates closed-loop control. Our subjects task, however, was quite different from that used by Kapoula and this difference probably explains the different result.

In her experiment the subjects were required to make a fine visual discrimination requiring high resolution foveal vision. In this task peripheral preprocessing of the target of the next fixation could be reasonably expected to reduce its duration since some aspects of the targets identity would be known before the fixation is made. In our task subjects were required to judge relative position of two targets and would benefit from simultaneous viewing of both. Accordingly, the longer fixation durations we found associated with the shorter preceding saccades could reflect this simultaneous viewing of both targets. When the targets are close together and both can be included in the functional field of view, fixations are longer allowing processing of the positions of both targets. The fixations to the more widely separated parts of the displays would not necessarily allow simultaneous viewing of the current and previously viewed targets. Thus, these fixations would be of shorter duration compared to those preceded by shorter saccades. Accordingly, despite the differences with Kapoula's results, our results are consistent with peripheral information influencing fixation duration . They do not, however, explicitly differentiate whether subsequent fixation position is determined by open or closed loop processes.

In order to differentiate between open or closed loop control one would have to determine the effect of the spatial location of the points of interest on statistical dependencies identified in the scanning. If one could show that the closer points of interest were more likely to be the end points of statistically dependent transitions, one could argue that the dependencies were due to peripheral preprocessing taking place during the preceding fixation. If involvement of a point of interest in a dependent transition were not related to its proximity to another point, the dependency could then be attributed to open-loop control. Since in our experiment, the layout of the points of interest was randomized, the open-loop control could be not be attributed to habitual scanning pattern like a left-right reading raster, but rather to the ongoing processing of the visual information. Unfortunately, the data from the present experiment do not provide sufficient numbers of dependencies for this analysis. The principle conclusion to be drawn from this experiment, then, is that random sampling models of visual information seeking in dynamic visual environments can not completely account for the pattern of information seeking we observed. More deterministic models are required.

EXPERIMENT 2

In order to increase the number of dependencies identified from each subject to assist analysis of the incidence of the dependencies, a second experiment was conducted. In this experiment considerably more scanning was analyzed among a greater number of points of interest. We analyzed about 129,000 fixations made by 23 subjects who viewed a 48 dynamic cockpit traffic displays generated in a manner similar to that of Experiment 1.

5. METHODS

The displays used in this experiment have been described in detail elsewhere (Smith, Ellis, and Lee, 1984). Intruding aircraft and the subjects' own ship were presented on a CRT as chevron shaped symbols associated with data tags showning their speed and altitude. The addition of data tags was the principle change in format as compared to Experiment 1 and provided new points of interest. The intruding aircraft approached the subjects' own ship along straight trajectories with randomly selected heading differences varied in 22.5 degree increments.

The subjects' task was to monitor the impending traffic conflicts to determine which of two intruding aircraft posed the greater collision threat. Subjects were told to select an avoidance maneuver if warranted by the collision threat by pressing an appropriate membrane switch mounted near the display. The task thus required the integration of vertical separation information in the data tag with horizontal separation information shown by symbol position on the map. Details of similar display configurations have been presented elsewhere (Palmer, *et. al.*, 1980, 1981; Smith, Ellis, and Lee, 1984)

The encounters ran for a maximum of 100 sec each., but subjects could choose to discontinue monitoring if no maneuver was needed. Therefore, the amount of data taken from each subject and processed by computer varied somewhat (see Table 2, col 3). The physical conditions of the stimuli, the characteristics of the encounters, and the computer processing of the eye movement data was comparable to that in Experiment 1

Subjects were briefed and then performed several practice runs until they were familiar with the task. After some practice runs and calibration of the eye tracker, the subjects began the first of three sessions of 16 encounters each. Subject's fixations of 90 ms. or longer were resolved by a computer program as in Experiment 1. Subjects fixations were automatically assigned to the closest (within 1 deg.) of eleven possible features on the display : Own ship's data tag, current position, predictor tip; Intruder's data tag, current position, predictor tip; and Pseudointruder's data tag, current position, predictor tip; switch locations for maneuver selections, and numbers signaling danger level features.

5.1. Subjects

Twenty three subjects, fourteen airline pilots and nine nonpilots, participated in this experiment.

6. RESULTS

As in Experiment 1, we identified statistical dependencies in the eye movements between features of the display by using the per cent of time each subject viewed each feature as an estimate of his 0-order viewing probability. The data for every subject showed evidence for statistically significant deviation from statistical independence (p.<.01).

Subject	Number of Transitions Analyzed	Number of Significant Transition Types	Number of Significant Pairs	Probability of Pairs	Expected Number of Pairs
1	1416	18	5	0.0625	1.67
2	4481	19	6	0.0074	1.93
3	1256	12	2	0.1959	0.78
4	2923	14	4	0.0168	1.04
5	1701	15	1	0.3418	1.31
6	2317	13	3	0.0148	0.89
7	794	5	2	0.0027	0.12
8	2551	15	4	0.0256	1.31
9	2351	14	5	0.0045	1.04
10	1027	15	5	0.0085	1.31
11	639	11	3	0.0474	0.66
12	1163	8	2	0.0132	0.37
13	2414	14	6	0.0012	1.04
14	2007	15	4	0.0256	1.31
15	1728	20	9	0.0000	2.02
16	1695	14	4	0.0168	1.04
17	2523	19	5	0.0222	1.93
18	1416	11	4	0.0166	0.66
19	920	8	3	0.0044	0.37
20	2091	14	4	0.0168	1.04
21	2580	17	4	0.0297	1.53
22	1727	11	2	0.1358	0.66
23	1211	3	0	0.9595	0.04

Table 3. This table presents a subject by subject breakdown of the total number of transitions from one feature to another counted for each subject, the number of transition types (i.e. ownship to ownship predictor) that exhibited statistical dependency for each subject, the number of pairs of statistical dependencies found for each subject, the probability that this number of pairs could occur by chance, and the expected number of pairs given the 0-order viewing probability.

As in Experiment 1, the specific transitions contributing to the deviation from statistical independence, cell by cell chi-square tests were calculated for each cell where the expected frequency of transition was greater than 5. Column 3 in Table 3 lists the number of first order transitions from each subject which were determined to exhibit statistical dependency.

Most significantly, the richer pattern of transitions among the larger number of points of interest revealed patterns in the incidence of the dependencies. The dependencies in scanning occur in matched pairs of transition to and from specific pairs of points as shown by the counts of numbers of pairs in Table 3. We call these dyads.

In order to estimate the number of dyadic pairs that could occur in our data by chance we have conducted Monte Carlo simulations for each of the subjects using their 0 order viewing probabilities. These enabled generation of sampling distributions based on 100,000 simulation runs per subject so that the probability of the statistic, "number of paired transitions," in a sample could be determined.[7] All 23 subjects had more paired transitions identified in their individual scanning data than the statistically expected number of pairs as determined by our simulations (sign test $p < .001$). On a subject by subject basis we have determined that the scanning of 19 of 23 subjects had statistically significantly more paired transitions than expected by chance (See Table 3)

We examined the possibility that the frequency of occurrence of a paired-transition could be related to the spatial proximity on the face of the display of the features involved. For those features for which statistical dependencies were identified during the course of the experiment, we first calculated their mean physical separation on the display during the course of the encounters. Then we correlated those distances with the frequencies with which each pair of features exhibited paired dependency. Despite substantial variation in the frequency of paired dependencies and in mean separation distance, both the pearson and spearman correlations between them were quite small ($r^2 < 0.1$), inconsistent, and not statistically reliable[8]. Furthermore, inspection of the scatter plot corresponding to these correlations showed no deviations from linearity that could complicate analysis. Thus, we were unable to relate the occurrence of a pair of statistical dependencies to the distance separating the the features involved.

7. DISCUSSION

The occurrence of matched pairs of statistical dependencies is particularly interesting since it shows that the pattern of scanning deviates in systematic ways from the kind of random sampling which has been used to model visual search and information seeking. Since the random variation in the heading difference of the intruding aircraft positioned it in a variety of locations with respect to ownship and the other fixed parts of the display, the statistical dependencies involving the intruders can not be attributed to spatial regularities in the scanning such as left to right raster scanning. Rather these dependencies, which accounts for about 83% of all identified, may reflect the information seeking strategies used by the subjects to resolve the aircraft separation question. An interesting additional aspect suggesting the generality of paired dependencies is that their occurrence is consistent with anecdotal reports that when repetitive spatial sequences of fixations are observed, the sequences are noted to occur in reverse order (Noton and Stark, 1971; Parker, 1978).

Several explanations for the cause of such statistical dependencies in eye movements have been proposed. Noton and Stark (1971) , for example, suggested that the neural traces of characteristic patterns of eye movements occurring during the recognition of visual material might be part of the substrate for memory encoding processes. They conjectured that repetitive eye movements thus might be triggered during recognition of a previously viewed image. (but see Locher and Nodine, 1974). Alternatively, the dependencies in scanning could be due to internal "cognitive models" developed during the scanning (Stark and Ellis, 1981; Ellis and Stark, 1978; Ellis and Stark, 1979). Another possible mechanism related to the pairing could arise from statistical contingency setup between the information present at the pair of involved features. Such a contingency produces the type of sensory stimulus conditions used in sensory-sensory learning protocols, notably sensory preconditioning, which are used to establish an associative link between pairs of stimuli (Brogden, 1939; Seidel, 1959). Thus, the pairing of the contingencies observed during the problem solving may be involved with the establishment of reciprocal associatives link between the information present at the pair of involved features.

APPENDIX

8. Measurement of Statistical Dependencies in Visual Scanning

In order to understand what is meant by statistical dependency in visual scanning it is helpful to consider three alternative modes of scanning among points of interest. The description of these modes of scanning first requires the distinction of three types of probabilities: 1) p(i), p(j), or p(l), the simple probability of viewing a particular point of interest i, j, or l respectively[9], 2) p(i to j), the probability of a transition between distinct points of interest i and j conditioned only on the assumption that unobserved transitions occur from each point to itself[10], and 3) p(i,j), the conditional probability of viewing point of interest j given previous viewing of point of interest i.[11]

These three probabilities allow the description of the three modes of scanning among points of interest to sample visual information. Visual sampling of points of interest may be completely random, stratified random, or statistically dependent[12]. In the random case, each point is viewed with equal probability, and, as a consequence, all transitions between pairs of points are equal. In the stratified random case, the points of interest are viewed with different probabilities. This distribution may be dependent upon the particular task the viewer must undertake, but now only the transitions to and from particular pairs of points need be equal. Notice that by chance alone there are many transitions between the more probable fixation points of interest. This case may be described alternatively as a 0-order Markov process and thus, the probability of fixating any point of interest is statistically independent of fixation on the preceding point. Accordingly, p(i to j) or p(i,j) are calculable from p(i) and p(j). Only in a statistically dependent case, do some of the transition frequencies illustrate the deviations from statistical independence which indicate statistical dependencies characteristic of at least 1st order Markov processes. In this case p(i to j) or p(i,j) are not calculable from p(i). It is noteworthy, as illustrated in this example, that the illustrated dependencies are not necessarily the most frequent transitions.

In the random case, sampling among the points of interest is completely unconstrained. In the stratified random sampling case, however, a differential probability of viewing the various points of interest leads to a constraint on the scanning sequences which may produce the impression of sequential scanning,. Under these conditions transitions between high probability points of interest are likely simply due to the zero order probability of viewing the respective points. Accordingly, any claim for statistical dependency in the transition patterns among points of interest must first show that the extent of the "sequenciness" exceeds that which could be produced by the zero order probabilities.

In order to detect truly statistically dependent transitions in scanning eye movement data we have adapted an equation cited by Senders *et. al*, (1966) for describing stratified random sampling. They noted that the joint assumption of 1) statistical independence of the transitions and 2) the existence of unobserved transitions from each point of interest to itself provides a means of calculating p(i to j), probability of a transition between any two distinct points of interest, i,j, provided p(i), p(j), the zero order probabilities of the two points are known.

$$p_e(i \text{ to } j)=\frac{p(i)p(j)}{1-\sum_{l=1}^{n}p(l)^2},\ i\neq j \tag{1}$$

The denominator of this expression corresponds to the probability of a all transitions between distinct points of interest. Most importantly, it provides a way to calculate expected transition frequencies f_e(i to j), between points of interest based solely on the expected transition probabilities and the total number of observed transitions, N.

$$f_e(i \text{ to } j)=N p_e(i \text{ to } j) \tag{2}$$

These calculated expected frequencies may then be compared by chi-square tests with the observed transition frequencies

FOOTNOTES

[1] Preliminary reports of the research contained in this paper were presented at the 17th Annual Conference on Manual Control June 16-18, 1981, JPL Publication 81-95 and the 1982 Meeting of the Human Factors Society. The authors are pleased to acknowledge programming assistance provided by James A. Woods, Robert Krones, and Stephen Gonick of Informatics, Inc. and assistance in collection of the data provided by Edward Denz and Bruce Hornstein. Lawrence Stark was partially supported by the NASA cooperative agreement NCC 2-86 from NASA Ames Research Center during the conduct of the reported research.

[2] The videotapes of the encounters were time marked to establish synchrony with the eye movements taken while the subjects made in front/behind judgements. The tapes were played back on a TV monitor so that the display subtended a rectangle of 12 by 10 degrees with average luminance of about 0.3 mL. The outlines of the symbols had a luminance of about 1.0 mL. Complete aircraft symbols on the display subtended a visual angle of 3.5 The monitor was viewed from a distance of 75 cm by the subject who sat in a chair in an experimental room.

[3]The miss distances for all encounters were set at 1846 meters (6000 feet) while the map position of ownship was updated every 0.1 second. The intruder position was updated every 4 seconds.

[4] The number of degrees of freedom in this chi-square test are n(n-2) - 1 if n is the number of points of interest. Two degrees of freedom are lost at each point of interest because we were unable to observe transitions from a point to itself, hence the main diagonal of the transition matrix is empty and the nature of transitions requires that the number of visits to each point of interest equal the number of exits. This latter property was only approximately true of the data because of interruptions in recording of eye position when the eye monitor lost track of the eye.

[5]Models like this could be likened to a real time data acquisition system, such as DEC's RT11, which use a direct memory access device to fill an input buffer.

[6]In a nonstationary process changing genuine statistical dependencies could be obscured by mixing in the overall analysis. Concerned about this possibility, Hofmann, *et. al.* (1973; Clement, Reference Note 1) , examined scanning data collected from pilots making instrument approaches, which exhibit some stratified random sampling characteristics, but concluded that it was "essentially stationary."

[7] We generated these sampling distribution with two different assumptions. One case was simple random sampling without replacement. The second was random sampling without replacement with the proviso that once a transition from a particular feature was selected as a statistically dependent one, no other transition from that feature could be selected as statistically dependent. These two cases are the extremes of a continuum of interpretations concerning the of attribution of statistical dependency to a particular transition. The first case of completely uniform sampling of all possible transitions allows the possibility that that all transitions from a particular feature could be selected as statistically dependent. The second case treats selection of a particular transition as statistically dependent as if it represented a certainty of transition from one feature to another. Thus, in this case it would be impossible for there to be more than one statistical dependency in scanning from a given feature and the number of dependencies cannot exceed the number of features. In general we have found that regardless of the interpretation we give to statistical dependencies in our simulations, our data provide amble evidence that the dependencies occur in pairs more often than expected by chance alone. In reporting the p[illegible]bly of the number of paired dependencies occurring by chance we always use the larger of the two numbers we determined from our Monte Carlo studies.

[8] The pearson correlation was $r = -0.170$, $df=16$, $p > .05$ and the spearman correlation was $r = 0.315$, $df=16$, $p > .05$. The mean of the separation of the features in degrees of visual angle was 5.13, sigma = 3.78, N=18. The mean frequency of paired contingency between pairs of points having any paired contingency associated with them was 4.72, sigma = 3.59, N = 18.

[9] Although this probability may be defined by the number of times a point of interest is visited, in this paper it is defined by the percentage of time spent on each particular point. The conclusions of this paper, however, are insensitive to the choice of definition.

[10] This is sometimes called at "link value."

[11] The latter two probabilities, p(i to j) and p(i,j) may be related to each other by $p(i,j) = [N/n(j)]\ p(i \text{ to } j)$, where N is the total number of transitions among all points of interest and n(j) is the number of exits from a particular point j.

[12] All sampling is assumed to be done with replacement.

REFERENCE NOTES

1) Clement, W. F. personal communication, 1981.

REFERENCES

Bouma, H. & de Voogd, A. H. On the control of eye saccades in reading. *Vision Research*, 1974, *14*, 274-284.

Brogden, W. J. Sensory preconditioning. (1939) *Journal of Experimental Psychology*. *25*, 232-332.

Buswell, G.T., *How people look at pictures*. University of Chicago Press, Chicago, 1935.

Card, Stuart. Visual search of computer command menus. in *Attention and performance X*, Bouma, H., and Bouwhuis, D. eds., Hillsdale N.J., Lawrence Erlbaum Associates, 1983

Carpenter, P., Just, M. Eye fixations during mental rotation. chapter in Fisher, D., and Monty, R. A Senders, J. (eds) *Eye movements and higher psychological functions*. Hillsdale N.J., Lawrence Erlbaum Associates, 1978, 115-133.

Ellis, S.R. & Stark, L., Eye movements during the viewing of necker cubes. *Perception*, 1978, *7*, 575-581.

Ellis, S.R. & Stark, L., Reply to Piggins, *Perception*, 1979, *8*, 721-722.

Ellis, S. R. & Stark, L., Pilot scanning patterns while viewing cockpit displays of traffic information. Proceedings of the 17th Annual Conference on Manual Control, U.C.L.A, June 16-18, 1981, JPL Publication 81-95, pp 517-524.

Ellis, S. R. & Stark, L., Contingency in visual scanning of cockpit traffic displays. Proceedings of the Human Factors Society, 26th annual meeting, (1982) 1005-1009.

Engel, F. L. Visual conspicuity, visual search, and fixation tendencies of the eye. *Vision Research*, 1977, *17*, 95-108.

Findlay, J. M. Local and global influences on saccadic eye movements. chapter in Fisher, D., and Monty, R. A Senders, J. (eds) *Eye movements perception and cognition*. Erlbaum Press, Hillsdale, New Jersey, 1981, 171-180.

Fisher, D. F., Monty, R. F., Senders, J. W. (eds) *Eye movements: cognition and visual perception.* Erlbaum Press, Hillsdale, New Jersey, 1981.

Groner, Rudolf, Marina, Groner. Towards a hypothetico-deductive theory of cognitive activity. chapter in *Cognition and eye movements.* Groner,R. and Fraisse, Paul. (eds) North-Holland, New York, 1982.

Hochberg, J., & Brooks, V. Film editing and visual momentum. chapter in Fisher, D., and Monty, R. A Senders, J. (eds), *Eye movements and the higher psychological proceedings.* Erlbaum Press, Hillsdale, New Jersey, 1978, 293-313.

Hofmann, L.G., Clement, W.F., and Blodgett, R. E. Further examination of pilot instrument scanning data and development of a new link estimator. Proceedings of the 9th Annual Conference on Manual Control, MIT, Cambridge, Mass., May 23-25, 1973.

Inditsky, B., Bodmann, H.W. Quantitative models of Visual Search. *Proceedings of the 19th Symposium of CIE.* Kyoto, Japan, 1979. *CIE Publication N. 50,* 1980,197-201.

Kapoula, Zio. The influence of peripheral preprocessing on oculomotor programming. chapter in *Eye movements and msychological functions: international views.* Erlbaum Press, Hillsdale, New Jersey, 1983.

Karsh, Robert, Breitenbach, Francis W. Looking at looking: the amorphous fixation measure. chapter in Groner, Menz, Fisher, & Monty, R.A.(eds) *Eye movements and psychological functions: international views.* Erlbaum Press, Hillsdale, New Jersey, 1984.

Kolers, P. A. Buswells discoveries. chapter in Monty, R.A. & Senders, J. W. (eds) *Eye movements and psychological processes.* Erlbaum Press, Hillsdale, New Jersey, 1976.

Kraiss, K.F., Knaeuper, A. Using visual lobe area to predict visual search time. *Human Factors*, 1983, *24*, 673-682.

Krendel, E. S., Wodinsky, J. Search in an unstructured visual field. *Journal of the Optical Society of America*, 1960, *50*, 562-568.

Locher, Paul J., Nodine, Calvin F. The role of scanpaths in the recognition of random shapes. *Perception and Psychophysics* 1974, *15*, 308-314.

Noton, D. & Stark, L.: Scanpaths in saccadic eye movements while viewing and recognizing patterns. *Vision Research*, 1971, *11*, 929-942.

Palmer, E.A., Jago, S., Baty, D.L., and O'Connor, S. Perception of Horizontal Aircraft Separation On a Cockpit Display of Traffic Information, *Human Factors*, Oct. 1980, *22*, 605-620.

Palmer, E.A., Jago, S.J. and DuBord, M.: Horizontal Conflict Resolution Maneuvers with a Cockpit Display of Traffic Information. Proceedings of the 17th Annual Conference on Manual Control, UCLA, Los Angles, Calif., June 1981.

Papin, J.P., Naureils, P., Santucci, G. Pickup of visual information by the pilots during a ground control approach in a fighter aircraft simulator. *Aviation, Space, and Environmental Medicine.* May, 1980, 463-469.

Parker, R. E. Picture processing during recognition. *Journal of Experimental Psychology, HPP*, 1978, *4*, 281-293.

Rayner, K. & Pollatsek, A. Eye movement control during reading: evidence for direct control. *Quarterly Journal of Experimental Psychology.* 1981, *33A*, 351-373.

Seidel, R. J. A review of sensory preconditioning. *Psychological Bulletin.* 1959, *56*, 58-73.

Senders, J. W., Grignette, M.C., & Smallwood, R.: An investigation of the visual sampling behavior of human observers. *NASA CR 434*, January 1966.

Smallwood, Richard D. Internal models and the human instrument monitor. *IEEE Transactions on Human Factors in Electronics.* September, 1967, *HFE-8*, No. 3, 181-187.

Smith, J.D., Ellis, Stephen R., Lee, Edward. Perceived threat and avoidance maneuvers in responses to cockpit traffic displays. *Human Factors*, 1984, *26*, 33-48.

Stark, L., Ellis, Stephen R.: Scanpaths revisited. Chapter in Fisher, D., and Monty, R. A Senders, J. (eds) *Eye movements perception and cognition.* Erlbaum Press, Hillsdale, New Jersey, 1981.

Stark, L., Ellis, Stephen R.: Scanpaths revisited. Chapter in Fisher, D., and Monty, R. A Senders, J. (eds) *Eye movements perception and cognition.* (1981) Erlbaum Press, Hillsdale, New Jersey

Tole, John, Stephens, A.T., Vivaudou, M., Harris, R. L. Sr., Ephrath, A. Entropy, instrument scan, and pilot workload. *Proceedings of the International Conference on Cybernetics and Society*, Seattle, 1982, New York, IEEE.

Tukey, J. W. *Exploratory data analysis.* Addison-Westley, Reading, Massachusetts, 1977.

Weir, P. H., Klein, R. H. Measurement and analysis of pilot scanning and control behavior during simulated instrument approaches. *NASA CR 1535*, June 1970.

Wewerinke, P. H. A model of the human observer and decision maker. Proceedings of the 17th Annual Conference on Manual Control, U.C.L.A. June. 16-18, 1981, JPL Publication 81-95, pp 557 - 570.

Yarbus, A. *Eye movements and vision.* Plenum Press, N. Y., 1967, (originally published, Moscow, 1965).

Eye Movements and Human Information Processing
R. Groner, G.W. McConkie and C. Menz (eds.)

THE EFFECT OF STIMULUS CHARACTERISTICS, TASK REQUIREMENTS AND INDIVIDUAL DIFFERENCES ON SCANNING PATTERNS

Rudolf Groner and Christine Menz
Department of Psychology
University of Bern
Switzerland

Using a complete factorial design, this paper investigates the relative contribution of the stimulus, task and subject, and their mutual interactions to the determination of the individual scanpath, that is, the order in which people look at pictures. Twelve adult volunteers served as subjects. The stimuli consisted of matrices of random dot patterns: variation being created by altering the dot densities in selected submatrices, and the tasks consisted of free inspection, of search for a small dot configuration, and of concept identification. - After a report of the effects on saccade amplitudes and fixation durations, the individual scanpaths were analyzed according to two different schemes, viz. local and global scanpath analysis.

INTRODUCTION

When looking at a picture, there are at least three factors which determine the individual scanpath. A lot of research has been done on the influence of stimulus features (e.g. Buswell, 1935; Berlyne, 1958; Yarbus, 1967, Mackworth & Morandi, 1967), and it has repeatedly been demonstrated that the novelty or informativeness of stimulus parts is the decisive factor for predicting the frequency or duration of fixations. There exists also a large body of empirical data on individual differences in eye movement data (e.g. Wagner & Cimiotti, 1975; Snow, 1978; Menz & Groner, 1981; Menz & Groner, 1982; Witruk, 1982) showing quite different scanning patterns for different subgroups of individuals. Finally, a third factor has been much less systematically explored, i.e. the role of different tasks as applied to the same set of stimuli (for a rather sketchy treatment of this question, see Yarbus, 1967; or Reusser & Groner, 1981). It is clear that all three factors mentioned above play an important role in picture perception, and a comprehensive theory of human visual information processing should include their respective contributions as well as their mutual interactions.

The experiments reported here attempt to explore these relationships by means of a factorial experiment where all three factors, stimulus, task, and individual differences, have been varied under all possible combinations.

There is one major obstacle to such an enterprise: if one and the same stimulus is shown repeatedly to the same individual (although under different task conditions), we must expect that some kind of habituation will take place, with the consequence that a reduced amount of visual exploration will be observed. On the other hand, if we want to investigate the role of the stimulus variable, its perceptual properties should remain essentially the same over different replications. There is no easy escape from this dilemma. The way we have chosen is that of a typical laboratory experiment : presenting stimuli which have no previous meaning attached to them and providing the possibility of slight variations without changing the gross features of the global picture. These requirements are satisfied by random dot patterns as they were used in perception research by French (1954), Julesz (1964) and others. The characteristics of these stimuli with respect to high spatial frequencies can be altered by changing the dot densities in some arrays of the stimulus. (For an investigation of the effect of dot density see Barlow, 1978). Figure 1 shows two examples of stimuli as they have been used in our experiments.

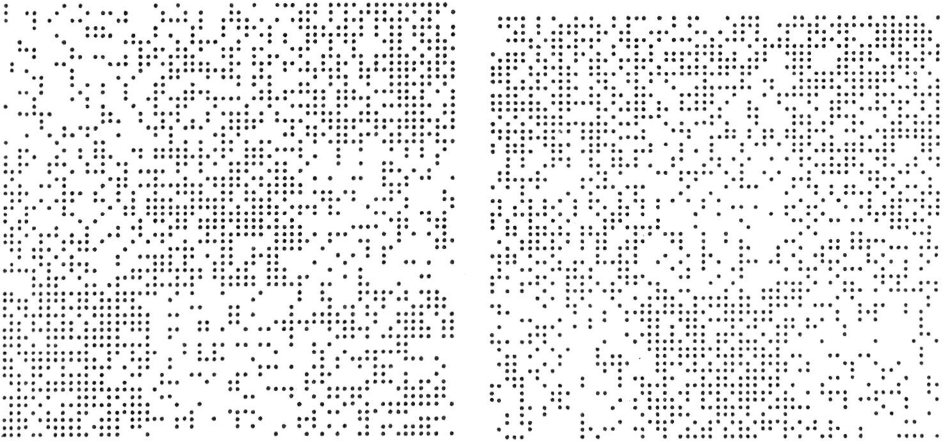

Figure 1 : Two examples of random dot patterns as they were used in our experiments. The relative size of dots compared with the inter-dot spaces was actually smaller. (For details of size and how the stimuli were constructed see below).

After having defined our independent variables, the central question is now: which variables of visual exploratory behavior are affected by the experimental treatment ? In addition to conventional measures like saccadic amplitudes, fixation durations etc, it is of still greater interest to see whether the scanning patterns, defined as the sequential organization of fixations, are also influenced by the stimuli, tasks, subjects, and their interactions.

Such patterns (termed "scanpaths") have been found by, among others, Noton & Stark (1971), Locher and Nodine (1974), Stark & Ellis (1981), and Ellis &

Smith (this volume). Groner, Walder & Groner (1984) extended the concept of scanpaths by distinguishing between "local scanpaths" as consistent patterns of successive fixations and "global scanpaths" as the distribution of fixations on a larger time scale irrespective of their immediate succession. The hypothesis of these authors was that local scanpaths are regulated by the momentary fixation plus peripheral information and operate in a bottom-up control mode, whereas global scanpaths are monitored by the hypothesess (c.f. Groner, 1978; Groner & Groner, 1982, 1983) of the subject operating in a top-down mode. In a facial recognition experiment Groner, Walder & Groner (1984) found not only local and global scanpaths, but also a considerable variability between different subjects with respect to the two types of scanning behavior. Our present experiments are intended to follow up their previous results under somewhat different and more systematic conditions.

METHODS

Subjects Twelve university students and research assistants (four females and eight males, age 18 - 38) served as subjects. All of them had normal vision.

Apparatus All stimuli were presented on a Hewlett Packard 1321A CRT display (P4 phosphor) controlled by a Megatek MG-552 graphics processor from display instructions held in the memory of a Data General Nova 3/12 computer. Eye movement recordings were made with an Applied Science Laboratories corneal reflection system, model 1994, at a sampling rate of 50 Hz. The recordings were digitized and saved with all relevant experimental parameters on the computer which also controlled the timing and sequence of stimulus presentation.

Stimuli All stimuli generated on the screen were random dot squares with a side length of 42 cm thus subtending a visual angle of 26 deg at the viewing distance of 1 m. The dot positions were spaced at 6.95 mm distance yielding a 60 x 60 matrix for the full square; their size was approximately 0.7 mm or 2.5' of visual angle. The dot luminance was 0.3 cd/m2, the background of the screen was less than 0.01 cd/m2, and the general background illumination was approximately 0.6 lm.

The stimuli were computed according to the following algorithm: each square was divided into 9 subsquares of 20 x 20 dots side length, and within each subsquare the presence or absence of a dot at a dot position was computed by a random number generator with constant probability. Two different stimuli were defined by their respective matrices of dot probabilities as shown in Figure 2. This procedure ensured that a large number of stimuli could be generated that were not identical although having the same general shape.

Procedure The subjects were seated on an adjusted dentist chair with two headrests, one supporting the forehead and the other one the occipital part. Some effort was taken to avoid uncomfortable immobilization of the subject, while keeping head movements to a tolerable minimum of $\pm$ 1 cm.
After a computer-assisted calibration of the eye camera lasting 1-2 minutes, four warming-up stimuli were displayed consisting of random dot patterns with densities different from those shown in Figure 2. Immediately following

a first block of 10 trials (5 instances of each stimulus in randomized order) was run under the condition of free inspection, i.e. the subjects were told that they were going to see some stimuli each for 20 seconds but were given no explicit instructions about what to do with them or where to look.

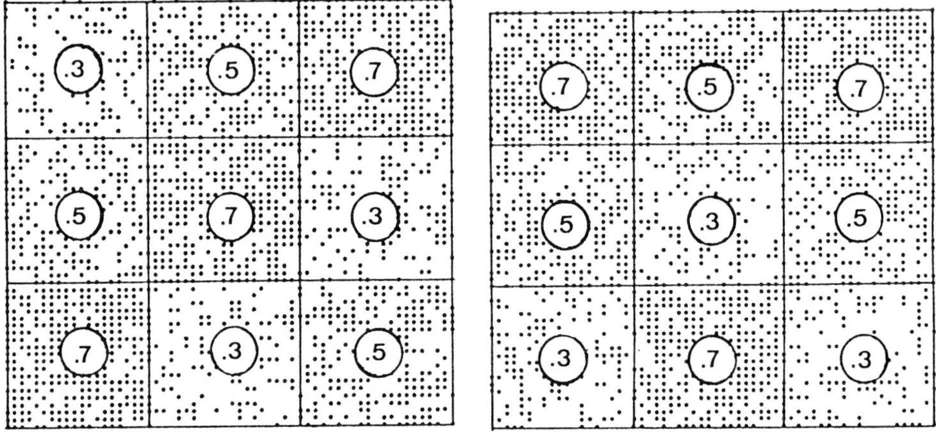

Figure 2 : The design of the two stimuli. It should be noted that although for all instances the probabilities of dots in the subsquares remain constant, the fine-grain structure within the subsquares is always different.

After a short break and recalibration, two more conditions were run with their order randomized over the subjects. One of them was a condition of continuous search where a target consisting of a 3 x 5 dot array (⁝⁝⁝) was to be detected anywhere in the stimulus. Actually, this target was never present, but the subjects were not aware of this fact. Again, 10 trials (5 instances of each stimulus) were presented in a randomized order each lasting for 20 seconds, exactly as in the condition of concept identification. Here the subjects were instructed to guess immediately at the end of each trial whether it had been a "GAM" or a "REF". At the beginning of the experiment these names were meaningless and the subjects had to guess. They received feedback according to the scheme that the stimulus on the left of the Figures 1 and 2 was "GAM" and the one on the right was "REF".
During all stimulus presentations eye movements were recorded and stored together with the calibration parameters for further data processing.

Design Twelve subjects were run under all conditions. This procedure resulted in a full factorial design with repeated measures on the same subjects. Figure 3 summarizes the design of the experiment.

In a first step of data analysis, the recordings were calibrated and processed by a computer program which deleted blinks and artefacts,identified saccades and fixations, and calculated statistics. Finally, the data were further reduced by applying a gaze grid which consisted of the areas of the nine subsquares (Fig. 2), and the dwells and transitions were identified. Three types of data analysis were performed on the data : ANOVAs with repeated measurements for saccadic amplitudes and fixation durations, and loglinear model analysis (Goodman, 1978; Dixon et al., 1981) for the identification of local and global scanpaths (Groner et al., 1984). The details of this method will be explained in the section below prior to the results.

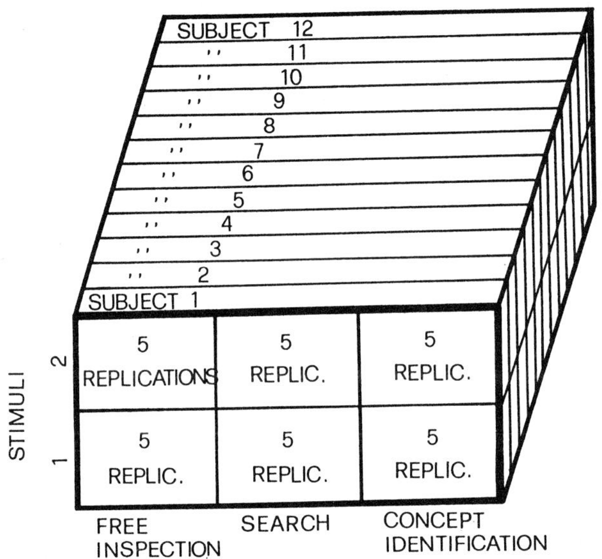

Figure 3 : The complete factorial design of stimulus x task x subject with 5 replications in each cell.

RESULTS AND INTERPRETATIONS

With respect to saccadic amplitude, the ANOVA revealed two significant results: the main effect of individual differences between subjects ($F(11,288) = 33.47$, $p < .001$) and the interaction between subjects and tasks ($F(22,288) = 9.66$, $p < .001$). Figure 4 presents these results. All subjects showed smaller saccades under the search condition, but the difference between free inspection and concept identification was not in the same direction over different subjects. It could be argued that the relatively simple and well defined search task induced a more similar strategy in all subjects compared with the more complex concept identification task or the unconstrained free inspection condition.

Interestingly, with respect to fixation duration there was no result statistically significant due to the large individual differences (Figure 5). The grand mean over all observations amounted to 459 msec with a range of the individual cell means from 350 to 635 msec and an average within-cell mean squares of 163. Both results, the long fixation durations and the large variability are quite surprising. To explain these findings, more experiments are needed, but at the moment it might be concluded that the long

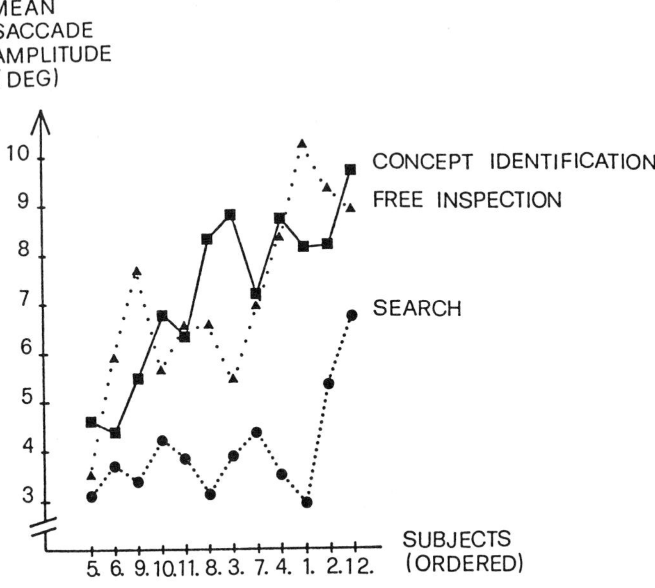

Figure 4 : The influence of tasks and subjects on mean saccadic amplitude

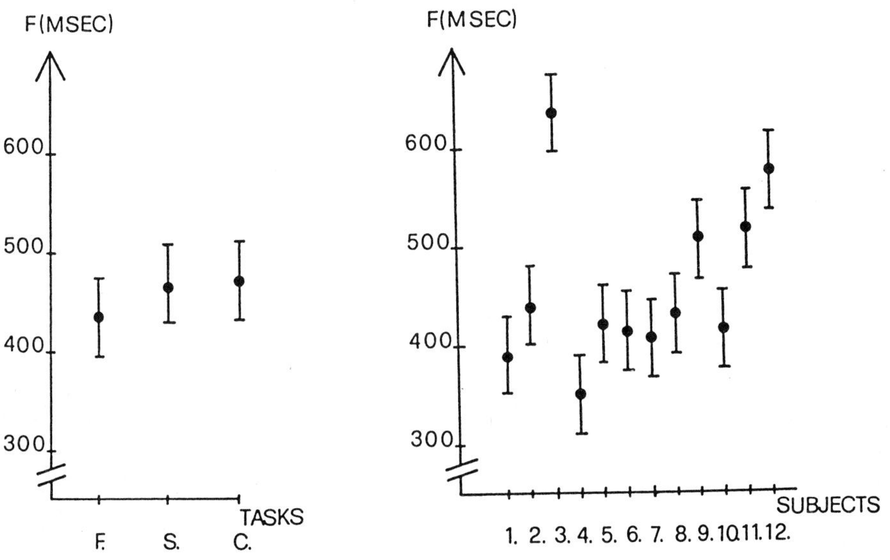

Figure 5 : Mean fixation duration ($\pm$ 1 SD) over tasks (left) and subjects (r.)

fixations indicate intensive cognitive processing, and the high variability within and between subjects reflects a wealth of different subprocesses involved.

For the analysis of local scanpaths, as a first step sequences of dwells in different subsquares were identified and divided into overlapping subsequences of three dwells called 'triplets' (e.g. the sequence 3-5-4-5-6... gives the triplets 3-5-4, 5-4-5, 4-5-6, ...). Their frequency was counted, and out of all observed triplets, the 15 with the highest frequencies were selected for further analysis. Next, a four-dimensional contingency table was constructed of the triplet x stimulus x subject x task combinations and analyzed by the loglinear model of the BMDP software package (Dixon et al., 1981). The results of testing the partial association between the four experimental factors are summarized in Table 1.

Table 1: Analysis of local scanpaths, tests of partial association. Only significant results are reported (*** $p < .001$; ** $p < .01$; * $p < .05$)

Source	Chi-square	df	Significance Level
Triplets	86.14	14	***
Subjects	36.87	11	***
Tasks	78.50	2	***
Triplets x Subjects	216.32	154	***
Triplets x Tasks	51.34	28	**
Subjects x Tasks	45.62	22	**

This is again a quite complex result. The main effect for the triplets could be expected, since although the 15 most frequent triplets had been selected for analysis, there is a frequency ratio of almost 3:1 (precisely 145 : 54) between the two extremes. The two other main effects are rather trivial, indicating that different subjects have also different total numbers of triplets due to unequal lengths of fixation paths; and that tasks also differ with respect to their number of triplets. Of greater interest is the result that different subjects maintain their specific local scanpaths (interaction triplets x subjects) and that different tasks evoke their characteristic local scanpaths (interaction triplets x tasks). The remaining result (subjects x tasks) reflects the fact that different subjects have unequal total frequencies of triplets with different tasks.

The scanpath hypothesis as proposed by Noton & Stark (1971) would predict that the same subject would generate identical scanpaths only with the same stimulus and task, which should result in a significant four-way interaction triplet x subject x stimulus x task. At least under the present conditions the results with local scanpaths can be accounted by a simpler model which states that subjects exhibit their characteristic scanpaths (independent of the other conditions, at least in the range of variation as introduced in this experiment) and that different tasks produce characteristic scanpaths (independent of subjects and stimuli).

In contrast to local scanpaths which indicate the immediate succession of consecutive fixations, global scanpaths reflect the distribution of fixations on a larger time scale. The temporal resolution is in principle arbitrary and in pilot studies different temporal grids should be tried. In the present study a partition into three intervals of equal length (start, middle, end) seemed useful, the same as had been used in our earlier study with faces (Groner, Walder & Groner, 1984). Figure 6 gives an example of such a partition in global scanpaths.

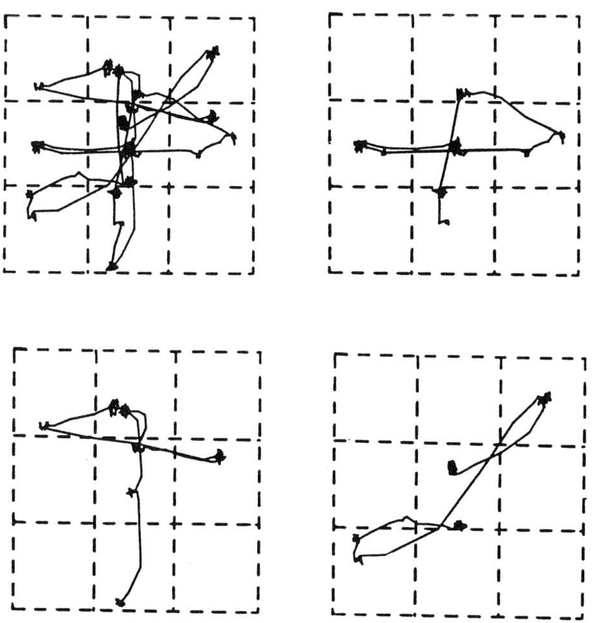

Figure 6 : A total scanpath (upper left) is divided into three equal intervals: start (upper right), middle (lower left), and end lower right (lower right), and the frequency distributions of fixations are counted in each time interval. The contingency table of fixation numbers and time interval represents the global scanpath.

This procedure resulted in a 5-dimensional contingency table of all combinations of subject x task x stimulus x gaze area x time . It again was analyzed by means of the loglinear model. Table 2 gives the results. We restrict the interpretation to those results connected with global scanpaths, i.e. the interactions of gaze x time x ... First of all, the two-way interaction gaze x time indicates that over all subjects and tasks, there exists a general tendency towards global scanpaths; however, it is quite weak compared with the size of the other effects. The task seems to exert a specific influence on global scanpaths (three-way interaction gaze x task x

Table 2 : Analysis of global scanpaths, tests of partial association. Only significant results are given (*** $p < .001$; ** $p < .01$; * $p < .05$)

Source	Chi-square	df	Significance
Gaze	1409.53	8	***
Subjects	216.27	11	***
Tasks	407.80	2	***
Gaze x Time	70.15	16	***
Gaze x Stimulus	63.35	8	***
Gaze x Subjects	394.65	88	***
Gaze x Tasks	162.38	16	***
Subjects x Tasks	170.50	22	***
Gaze x Time x Tasks	51.32	32	*
Gaze x Subjects x Stimulus	178.57	88	***
Gaze x Task x Stimulus	35.06	16	**
Gaze x Subjects x Tasks	437.54	176	***

stimulus). This effect is in accordance with our earlier hypothesis that global scanpaths are monitored by a top-down mode of information processing (= task driven).

In order to locate the incidences of either type of scanpaths over the 12 different subjects, the following strategy was applied with respect to the loglinear model : In a first step a reduced model was estimated which included all parameters for the main effects and interactions of all factors except for the factor of subjects. Then the chi-squared difference between observed and expected frequency was computed according to the reduced model, and the significant deviations ($p < .001$) were identified and counted over each subject. Although such a method has the faults of a post-hoc procedure, the conservative significance criterion reduces the number of spurious results. Table 3 presents the results of this test, and Figure 7 gives a graphic illustration of the findings. As might be noticed, the occurrence of either type of scanpaths is more or less independent of each other and all kinds of combinations could be observed : there are four subjects who clearly displayed both kinds of scanpaths, two who could be assigned only to either local or global scanpaths but not both, one subject with neither tendency, with the remainder falling in between these classes.
This result is in agreement with the earlier findings in Groner, Walder and Groner (1984), where in addition some interesting relations to performance measures in recognition memory were found.

Table 3 : Number of significant incidences ($p < .001$) of local and global scanpaths in the subjects.

Subject Number	1	2	3	4	5	6	7	8	9	10	11	12
Frequency of												
Local Scanpaths	2	0	1	3	7	8	3	4	7	8	0	0
Global Scanpaths	1	9	0	3	2	3	2	5	0	5	0	2

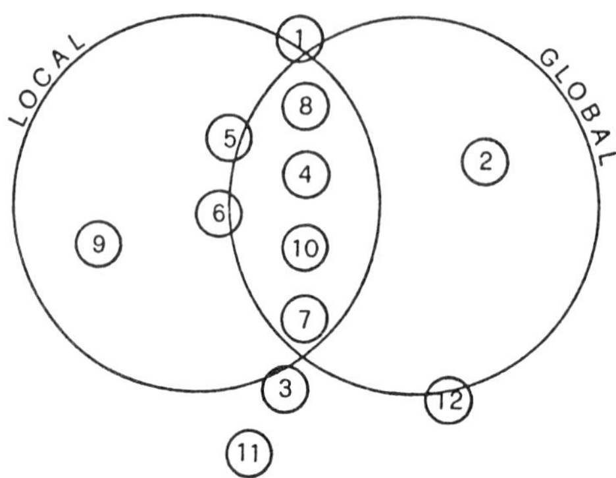

Figure 7 : Venn diagram of the contingencies between local and global scanpaths. Large circles represent the region of occurence, small circles subjects.

DISCUSSION

The complete factorial design used in this experiment made it possible to detect quite complex relationships between the three independent variables, however, in a first step on a purely descriptive level. First, there was the startling result with fixation durations, that except of the main effect of individual differences, there was no significant result due to the large variances. This variability reflects changes of fixation durations over short periods of time, and might be either due to purely random fluctuations or to systematic influences. In the second case there are again two possibilities: (1.) different samples of the visual input require different amount of subsequent cognitive precessing (=bottom-up hypothesis) or (2.) the search plan and information processing strategy while fixating involves various operations of different durations (= top-down hypothesis). It is also possible (and even quite plausible) that a mixed strategy is actually used where information is collected according to some search plan or hypothesis, but modified when some critical information is encountered (= interactive hypothesis). Although it is impossible to discriminate decisively between these alternatives on the basis of our experiment, it might be argued in favour of one or the other hypothesis.

With respect to local scanpaths one could expect that effects of the stimulus variable would indicate bottom-up processing, a prediction which could not be verified by our data. Possibly the present kind of stimulus material introduced too little variation to be effective as peripheral search guidance. However, it still should be noted that in the global scanpath analysis, significant effects of the stimulus variable could be shown, although here the interpretation of stimulus driven bottom-up processing does not make sense since these fixations are not connected with each other. It could rather be argued that for the visual scanning process as a whole, the stimulus characteristics had specific influence for different tasks and individuals. It is clear that there is no easy and straightforward way to interpret these interactions, but in future experiments one should be careful with averaging over different subjects and tasks or with overgeneralizing the finding from single instances.

The complexity of the results in this study and the difficulty to fit them into a simple model suggest that one should rather use another methological framework which has been successful in other domains (e.g. Groner, 1978; Groner & Groner, 1982, 1983): starting from models which are sufficient to generate performance by a sequence of information processing operations, comparing their predictions with behavioral data. If such a hypothetico-deductive approach is successful, the independent variables can be set in relation to each other in a more satisfactory way. Our present results would provide a framework for such an enterprise.

REFERENCES

Barlow, H.B. The efficiency of detecting changes of density in random dot patterns. Vision Research, 1978, 18, 637-650.

Berlyne, D.E. The influence of complexity and novelty in visual figures on orienting responses. Journal of Experimental Psychology, 1958, 55, 289 - 296.

Buswell, G.T. How People Look at Pictures. Chicago: University of Chicago Press, 1935.

Dixon, W.J. et al. (eds.) BMDP statistical software 1981. Berkeley: University of California Press, 1981.

French, R.S. Pattern recognition in the presence of noise. Journal of Experimental Psychology, 1954, 47, 27-31.

Goodman, L.A. Analyzing qualitative categorical data. Cambridge, Mass.: Abt Associates, 1981.

Groner, R. Hypothesen im Denkprozess. Bern, Stuttgart & Wien : Huber, 1978.

Groner, R., & Groner, M. Towards a hypothetico-deductive model of cognitive activity. In R. Groner & P. Fraisse (Eds.) Cognition and eye movements. Amsterdam: North Holland, 1982.

Groner, R., & Groner, M. A stochastic hypothesis testing model for multi-term series problems based on eye fixations. In R. Groner, C. Menz, D.F. Fisher & R.A. Monty (Eds.) Eye movements and psychological functions: international views. Hillsdale N.J.: Lawrence Erlbaum, 1983.

Groner, R., Walder, F., & Groner, M. Looking at faces: local and global aspects of scanpaths. In A.G. Gale & F. Johnson (Eds.) Theoretical and applied aspects of scanpaths. Amsterdam : Elsevier (North Holland), 1984.

Julesz, B. Binocular depth perception without familiarity cues. Science, 1964, 145, 356-362.

Locher, P.J., & Nodine, C.F. The role of scanpaths in the recognition of random shapes. Perception and Psychophysics, 1974, 15, 308-314.

Mackworth, N.H., & Morandi, A. The gaze selects informative details within pictures. Perception and Psychophysics, 1967, 2, 547-552.

Menz, Ch., & Groner, R. "Zweitlesenlernen" - die experimentelle Analyse der okulomotorischen und artikulatorischen Koordination bei einer komplexen Dekodierleistung. In K. Foppa & R. Groner (Eds.) Kognitive Strukturen und ihre Entwicklung. Bern, Stuttgart & Wien: Huber, 1981.

Menz, Ch., & Groner, R. The analysis of some componential skills of reading acquisition. In R. Groner & P. Fraisse (Eds.) Cognition and eye movements. Amsterdam: North Holland, 1982.

Noton, D., & Stark, L. Scanpaths in saccadic eye movements while viewing and recognizing patterns. Vision Research, 1971, 11, 929 - 942.

Reusser, M., & Groner, R. Informationssuchprozesse bei Globalisationsaufgaben. K. Foppa & R. Groner (Eds.) Kognitive Strukturen und ihre Entwicklung. Bern, Stuttgart & Wien: Huber, 1981.

Snow, R.E. Eye fixation and strategy analyses of individual differences in cognitive aptitudes. In A.M. Lesgold, J.W. Pellegrino, S.D. Fokkema, & R. Glaser (Eds.) Cognitive Psychology and Instruction. New York: Plenum, 1978.

Stark, L., & Ellis, S.R. Scanpaths revisited: cognitive models direct active looking. In D.F. Fisher, R.A. Monty & J.W. Senders (Eds.) Eye movements: cognition and visual perception. Hillsdale N.J.: Lawrence Erlbaum, 1981.

Wagner, I. & Cimiotti, E. Impulsive und reflexive Kinder prüfen Hypothesen. Zeitschrift für Entwicklungs- und Pädagogische Psychologie, 1957, 7, 1-15.

Witruk, E. Eye movements as a process indicator of interindividual differences in cognitive information processing. In R. Groner & P. Fraisse (Eds.) Cognition and eye movements. Amsterdam: North Holland, 1982.

Yarbus, A. L. Eye movements and vision. New York: Plenum Press, 1967.

ACKNOWLEDGEMENT

This work was supported by the Swiss National Science Foundation (1.374-.81) We would like to thank our subjects for their (unpaid) participation, and Daniela Krneta and Mario Truffer for drawing some figures; Marina Groner, Walter F. Bischof, Daniel Hofer and Kazuo Koga for interesting discussions.

Eye Movements and Human Information Processing
R. Groner, G.W. McConkie and C. Menz (eds.)

ON THE INTERPRETATION OF EYE FIXATIONS

Esther G. Gonzalez and Paul A. Kolers
Department of Psychology
University of Toronto
Toronto, Ontario

Eye movements are often taken as indicators of cognitive activity, the assumption being that what the eye is looking at testifies to what the mind is making of what the eye is looking at. To put it in other terms, the implication is that the location of a fixation testifies to the semantic aspects of the processing of the material fixated. An alternative view proposes that the location of fixations merely identifies the regions of the scene from which stimulation is derived, whereas the semantic or interpretative components are carried out subsequently on those inputs; acquisitive and interpretative processes are distinguished. Empirical tests provide some support for the second model.

Pictures and texts are subjected to considerable amounts of visual inspection, and most research on eye movements has been undertaken with such stimuli. Data obtained from the investigations are not always consistent; the lack of consistency creates a fundamental problem for theory. In reading texts people tend, largely, to move their eyes along a line of print and down the successive lines of the page, with occasional regressions and a few anticipatory progressive movements (Buswell, 1937). Thus, we may speak of the syntactic structure of texts as affecting the movements of the eyes made in reading. In examining pictures, the eyes move somewhat freely about the surface, and are less predictable, picture to picture, than they are page to page for text. Examination of pictures seems to be constrained more by semantic aspects of task and picture; people look at the regions of pictures where they can find the information that is focal to identity or that is focal to answering some question they have in mind regarding the picture (Kolers, 1972). This is not to say that the semantic aspects of text are unimportant to reading, but only that texts are possessed of a syntactic structure that plays a large role in predicting the form that sentences will take and thus the way that eyes will move to examine them, and pictures usually lack this structure.

This difference in the structure of the medium and the correlated difference in the procedures that the eyes use to examine the media raise a question about modelling: does the nervous system contain two distinct procedures for controlling the eyes' movements, one for text and the other for pictures or natural objects; or, rather, are the eyes' movements controlled by what is fundamentally one system with different characteristics adapted to the different tasks? Let us consider some evidence.

The strongest claims have been made for the control of fixations during reading. Perhaps the principal claim is that comprehension of text is accomplished "on line" in something approximating a word-by-word analysis. In this claim it is assumed that the eyes' fixation on a word represent perfectly, or index, the time spent comprehending or interpreting a word; hence the eye does not leave a word until it is intellectually satisfied with the analysis accomplished. Duration of fixation therefore tends to be associated with familiarity, frequency, length and related features of the word. (See Rayner, 1983, for discussion of aspects of the issue.)

Models of this form do seem to suppose an exquisitely precise control of fixations--for the eye is assumed to go to exact locations and to stay fixated just for that length of time that the mind is acquiring the information to be had at the position fixated. Exquisite control is not out of the question to achieve; the eye can be made to move precisely to locations or to find locations once fixated, with rather good accuracy (Carpenter, 1977). We do not doubt the possibility of such control; but let us consider one of its implications.

The implication of chief interest is this: suppose the same information is required from a location but is to be obtained in three different tasks involving judgment. We should then find a substantial positive correlation between the characteristics of the eyes' fixations on a region of a picture, and judgments of importance or salience of the information derived from that region. The experiment that we report on failed to confirm that correlation. We conclude from that that the location and duration of fixations are not necessarily an index of the interpretative or related cognitive activities that the viewer engages in.

The experiment required people to make judgments of similarity or of difference of pairs of animal-like shapes; meanwhile, we monitored their eyes' movements. Subsequently we required the people to scale the relative importance to their judgment of regions of the pictures, that is, body parts of the figures. The rationale behind these tasks was that if eye movements were indices of cognitive processing--that is, judgment, evaluation, interpretation--they should be sensitive to the same control as that governing the judgments, and therefore we should find a very high positive correlation between the extent of fixation on a region of a picture and the scaled weight assigned to that region. Pursuing the matter, we should find the same high correlation between fixations and regions of the picture that were diagnostic of similarity or dissimilarity between the pairs.

Figure 1 illustrates the eight creatures on which judgments were made. The creatures are modified from the set of "caminalcules" used in studies of numerical taxonomy (Sokal, 1966). The set we used was composed of seven binary features: head shape, pectoral marking, type of body, etc. Each of the eight creatures was paired with every other one and itself once, making (((64-8)/2)+8)=36 pairs--that is, the lower triangle plus the diagonal of the matrix of possible comparisons. Five subjects rated similarity of each pair on a scale from 1 to 5, and another five rated difference. During the inspection prior to judgment, eye movements were monitored.

After completing the set of 36 judgments, the subjects rated the importance to their judgment of each of the 7 features for each pair. Eye movements were measured in terms of number of fixations and total fixation time per feature; and these quantities were correlated with the ratings of importance assigned to features as well as the weights

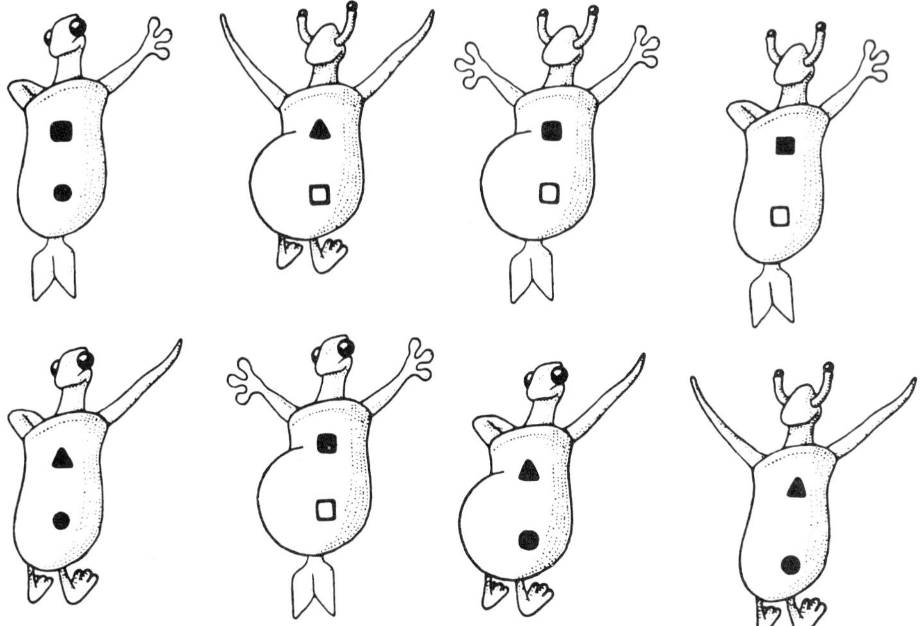

Figure 1. The eight creatures whose similarity was judged

inferred from the scale values.

The two groups of subjects did not differ in the correlation of number of fixations and their assignments of importance, r=.78 and r=.76 for the two groups respectively. The average correlation of r=.77, based on 250 df per subject, is reliably different from zero, $p<.01$. The correlation of total fixation duration and verbal weights was approximately the same. These high reliable positive correlations between region fixated and characteristics of fixation support the view that the eye looks at what the mind is thinking about.

The view is contradicted by more detailed analysis. Recall that the two groups of subjects were engaged in complementary tasks, one group judging similarity of a pair of creatures and the other group judging dissimilarity. Thus the number of features in common (or different) must be important to the judgments. Because different subjects made different numbers of fixations, the data were expressed as proportions. In Figure 2 the fixations made to common features is shown as a proportion of the number made to common plus differents, for the two

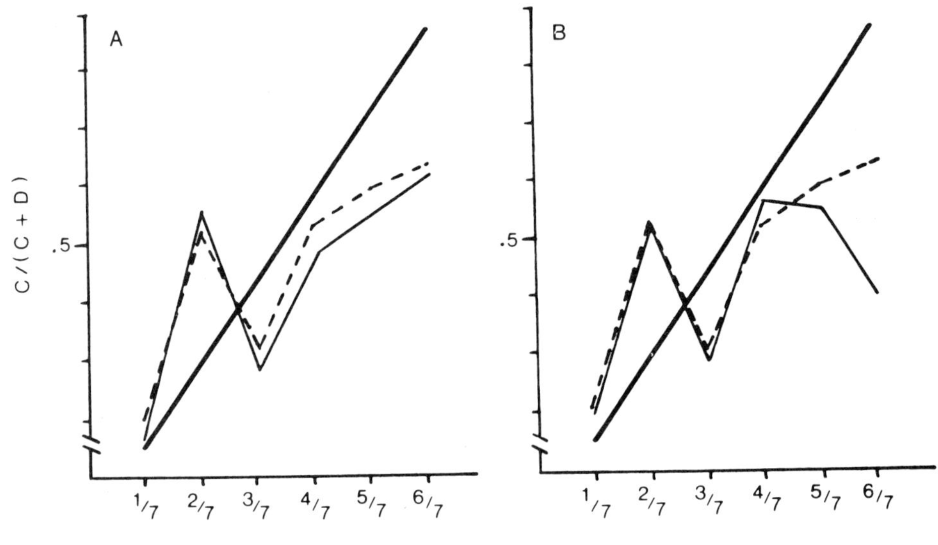

Figure 2. Ratios of fixations on common to common plus distinguishing features--C/(C+D)--for the Similarity (A) and Difference (B) groups (solid lines). The bold lines show the ratio in the slides and the broken lines the fixation data as predicted by the proportion of fixations per feature regardless of its being common or distinguishing.

groups of subjects separately. The base of the graphs is the proportion of features in common. The heavy solid line shows the proportion to be obtained if fixations were perfectly correlated with similarity. The light continuous line is the obtained proportion of responses. Statistically, the two lines are very different from each other, showing thereby that the fixations are not related to the formal similarity of the pairs of creatures.

Another way to assess expectation is to tally the fixations made to features across the whole set of creatures, regardless of whether they are shared or different in any pair. Thus we may tally the number of fixations made to heads, the number made to arms, to feet, and so on. Then, for any pair, if a feature is shared by the two creatures, the number of fixations that feature elicited would appear in both numerator and denominator of the ratio; whereas if that feature was different in the two creatures, its fixations appeared only in the denominator of the ratio. The broken line of Figure 2 shows the expected values of the proportion of fixations, calculated on this basis of individual features rather than on the basis of the commonness in the pairs. The fit between expected value and obtained value seems rather good to us.

Figure 3 shows the data for the verbal judgments of the importance of the features made by the two groups of subjects. The people distributed 100 points across 7 features in each pair of comparisons. The lefthand graph shows that the subjects judging similarity assigned about 10 points to each of the 7 features when they were shared (solid rectangles) but assigned between 8 and 25 points to each feature when they were not shared,

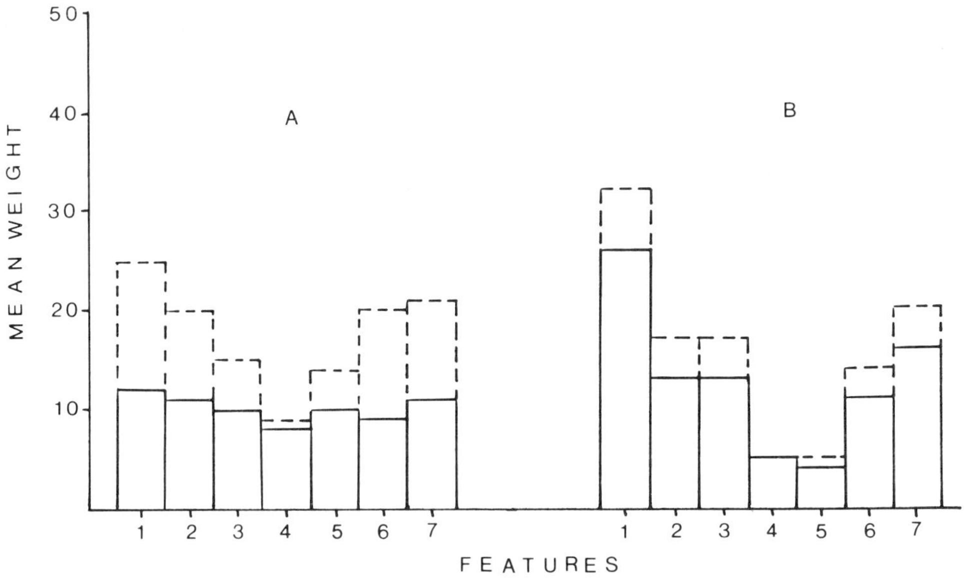

Figure 3. Mean verbal weights for shared (solid lines) and distinguishing (broken lines) stimulus features for the Similarity (A) and Difference (B) groups. Features are: head (1), left arm (2), right arm (3), pectoral mark (4), abdominal mark (5), feet or tail (6), and type of body (7).

that is, were distinguishing features (broken rectangles). The groups judging dissimilarity differentiated among their judgments both for common and distinguishing features. Both groups of subjects, notably, assigned greater weight to distinguishing features than to common features. We can conclude from this figure that the subjects discriminated among common and distinguishing features and assigned different weights to them for their judgments.

There are at least two structurally different models available to account for the data: People assume similarity and take distinguishing features into account, or people assume dissimilarity and take common features into account. Our data agree with neither of these models. Figure 4 shows that the rated similarity increased in perfect correspondence with an increase in the number of common features, that is, the subjects judged the pairs of creatures in perfect correspondence with their formal similarity; but their eye fixations did not correspond with those processes of judgment or with the judgments themselves (Figure 2). Thus the eye fixations were associated with the features individually judged to be important, but the fixations were not associated with judgments made about those features. We may distinguish therefore two different aspects of cognitive processing: salience or importance of a region as a source of information, and judgment or interpretations made about the information obtained from the region. We find eye fixations to be correlated with regions that are rich sources of information, but they are not associated with interpretations or judgments based on the information obtained from those regions. In this way we distinguish between acquisitive and interpretative aspects of information processing, and show that eye fixations identify the former but not necessarily the latter.

In our view, the eye performs largely logistical functions in pointing to places that are important sources of information, and acquiring information from those places. Mind can do much more with the information obtained than is done while the eye is fixated on those regions, however: it can reflect upon, reconsider, relate, extrapolate, compare, and perform many other functions also on the data that the eye has acquired. It would be remarkably cumbersome and inefficient if mind could do those thing only while the eye was looking at the regions that the mind was thinking about, comparing, relating, considering, and the like.

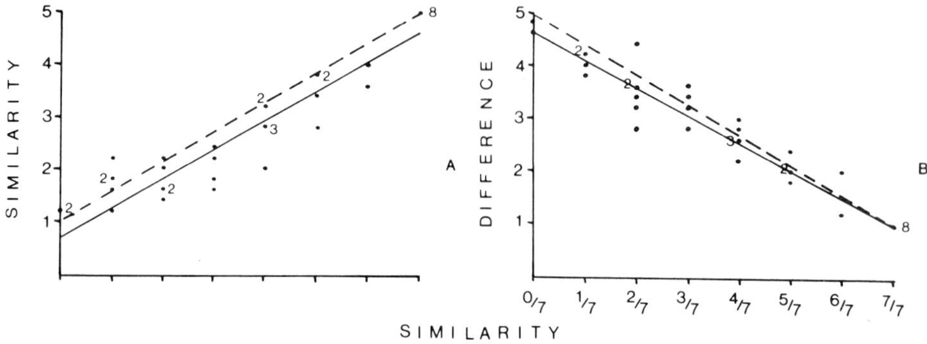

Figure 4. Similarity (A) and Difference (B) judgments as a function of a priori (experimenter computed) similarity values. Solid lines are lines of best fit, broken lines show optimal scaling.

The claim that the eye fixation is a perfect index of the mind's comprehension seems to us both unwarranted and implausible.

Actually, localization of information and operations upon the information are distinguished at many levels of function. Many students of animal behavior have developed econometric models, called Optimal Foraging models, to describe their ideas (for example, Krebs, Stephens, & Sutherland, 1983). Consider the behavior of a bee or of a bird seeking nectar or pollen. The animal forages in the field seeking sources of energy, samples from a target when it finds one, and spends time at the target proportional to the riches found there, then goes off to another target. The analogy we wish to bring out is to the difference between the acquisition of sources of energy and the metabolism of their product by the foraging animal. We have stressed the difference between acquisition of information by the eyes' fixations and the interpretation or subsequent processing the person engages in. Of course one does not want to press the analogy to optimal foraging too far; the theory is based on straightforward assumptions of energy processing, whereas people read and look at pictures or other objects for many reasons. The analogy will have served its purpose for us, however, if it succeeds in emphasizing the difference between localization of a source and other processes directed at its contents.

ACKNOWLEDGMENT

This work was supported by Grant A7655 from Natural Sciences and Engineering Research Council Canada to the second author.

REFERENCES

Buswell, G.T. (1937). How adults read. Supplementary Educational Monograph, No. 45, Chicago, Ill.: University of Chicago Press.

Carpenter, R.H.S. (1977). Movements of the eyes. London: Pion Limited.

Kolers, P.A. (1972). Reading pictures: Some cognitive aspects of visual perception. In T. Huang and O. Tretiak (Eds.), Picture bandwidth compression. New York: Gordon and Breach.

Krebs, J.R., Stephens, D.W., & Sutherland, W.J. (1983). Perspectives in optimal foraging. In G.A. Clark & A.H. Bush (Eds.) Perspectives in ornithology. Cambridge: Cambridge University Press.

Rayner, K. (Ed.). (1983) Eye movements in reading. New York: Academic Press, Inc.

Sokal, R.R. (1966). Numerical taxonomy. Scientific American, 215, 106-116.

Eye Movements and Human Information Processing
R. Groner, G.W. McConkie and C. Menz (eds.)

EYE MOVEMENTS AND FEATURE IMPORTANCE IN TAXONOMIC JUDGEMENTS: THE EFFICIENCY OF CLASSIFICATION HYPOTHESIS

Roger Hansell,[1] Paul Kolers[2] and Polly Sousan[1]
Departments of Zoology[1] and Psychology,[2] University of Toronto,
Toronto, Ontario, Canada, M5S 1A1

ABSTRACT

We test the hypothesis of efficient classification by examining the total number of eye fixations made in relation to the measured difficulty of the taxonomic decision. Subjects were asked to decide whether illustrations of animalcule 'A' or 'B' were more similar to animalcule 'X'. Eye movements were recorded by Dual Purkine Eye Tracker and the subjects were subsequently asked to identify features of the animalcules, numerically evaluate their similarity to 'X', and finally to evaluate the importance of these features. Weighting schemes were identified by measuring the degree of support of the numerical value of each feature for each taxonomic decision. Our results demonstrate that the number of fixations taken decreases with the disparity in similarity of the two animalcules being compared to 'X'. That is, the number of fixations decreases with the 'ease of classification'. We conclude that cognitive character weighting leads to fewer required fixations in perception during the process of classification.

INTRODUCTION

Algorithms for computer classification (Sokal and Sneath, 1963; Sneath and Sokal, 1973) utilize many taxonomic characters (object features) and give each equal weight in forming the classification hierarchy. This process is expensive in both human effort and computer time. Comparisons of subjective classification with machine classifications produced by the same subjects reveal interesting contrasts. Moss (1971) demonstrated that classificatory decisions based on subjective evaluation of similarity between organisms showed similar organisms more similar and distant organisms more distant than in the equivalent machine classifications. Moss and Hansell (1980) demonstrated that the differences in similarities between objects obtained by subjective and numerical methods could be explained by unequal weighting of object features by the subjects. The effect can be modelled by a local scaling of the subjective taxonomic space, and may be thought of as the placing of emphasis on a subset of the available features in forming the subjective taxonomies.

Hansell and Ewing (1974), Hansell and Chant (1974) developed methods for evaluating the degree to which measured or coded features support classificatory decisions of the type: object A is more similar to object X than B is to X. Traditional biological classifications were shown to be based on a few heavily emphasized features.

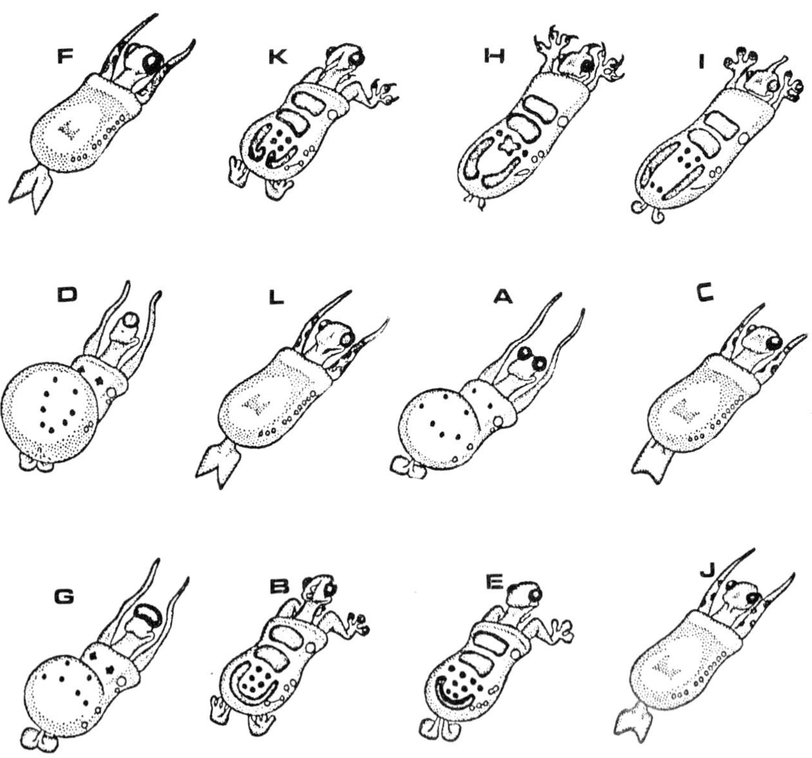

FIGURE 1. CAMINALCULES USED IN INDSCAL ORDINATION EXPERIMENTS.

In this study we test the hypothesis of Moss and Hansell (1980) that cognitive weighting of features improves the efficiency of the process of classification by emphasizing the discreteness of clusters of similar objects. This hypothesis implies that in general fewer features need be scanned in the data gathering process of perception, and has as a necessary condition that as the differential similarity of A and B to X increases, fewer eye fixations need be made before the classificatory decision is made.

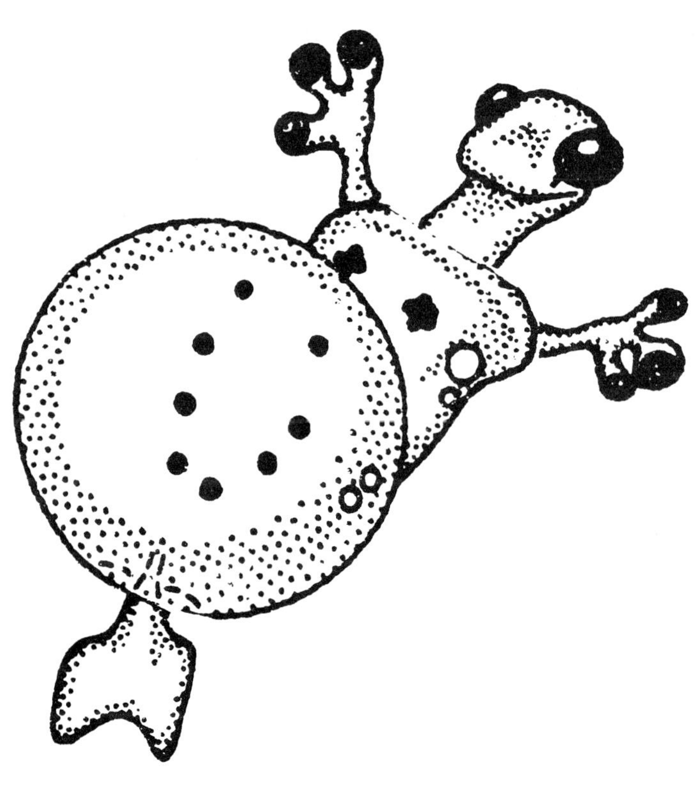

FIGURE 2. MODIFIED CAMINALCULE "X" USED IN PERCEPTION EXPERIMENT.

METHODS

The objects used in these experiments are modified 'Caminalcules' (Figure 1), originally created by the late Dr. Joseph Camin of the University of Kansas (Camin and Sokal, 1965). In the initial experiments we test the first result of Moss and Hansell (1980) that sets of similarities between objects based on subjective evaluation show unequal weighting of features compared to the equivalent machine based similarities. Subjects were asked to fill out a lower triangular matrix of similarities between caminalcules. Then they were asked to choose features and numerically evaluate the objects for these features. This data was then converted into taxonomic similarity using the simple matching coefficient of Sokal and Michener (Sneath and Sokal, 1973). The resulting 28 12 by 12 similarity matrices were analyzed using the INDSCAL program of Carrol and Chang (1970). We take the INDSCAL ordination of these objects to be a model for the subjects' cognitive maps. We subsequently designed a new 'Caminalcule' which incorporated features of all other clusters of the objects. This test object (Figure 2) was made to be intermediate in similarity among the scaled objects. We expected that taxonomic decisions about the resemblance of this object to others would involve cognitive decisions about the importance of features of the object involved, that is, about the weights constraining the cognitive map. Perception experiments to determine the position of eye fixation while carrying out taxonomic tasks were performed using the Stanford Research Institute Dual Purkine Image Eye Tracker. Accuracy of localization was about 10 minutes of visual angle during these experiments.

The subjects were seated 85 cm from the images, with their heads immobilized by biting on a fixed dental bar and with their foreheads resting on a plate. The DPI eyetracker, on line to a P.D.P. 11/45 computer at the University of Toronto Computer Research Facility, was utilized to collect data on the location and duration of eye positions.

The following series of tests was carried out: 1 - Calibration chart; 2 to 11 - Comparisons of pairs of objects against the third test object which was held constant throughout ten tests; 12 - A repeat of the calibration chart.

In Tests 2 to 11 the subject was asked to decide which of two illustrations of the objects was most similar to the third. The subject signified his decision by raising one or two fingers, and his decision was recorded by the experimenter. The end of test signal recognized by the computer was the act of closing the eyes.

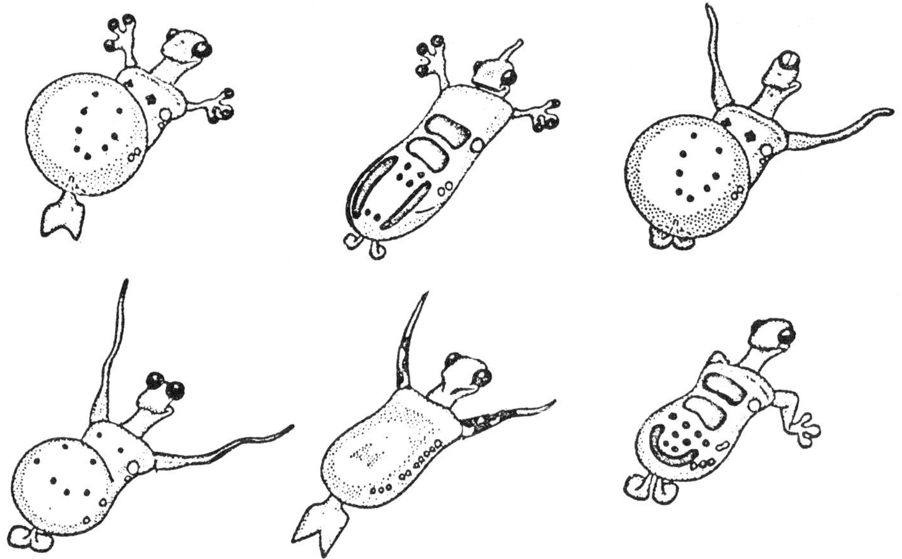

FIGURE 3. CAMINALCULES USED IN PERCEPTION EXPERIMENTS.

Following the perception experiment, the subjects answered a series of taxonomic questions about the same set of objects used in the perception experiment (Figure 3). First they were asked to list features describing the objects, and to form the character into coded states. They were then asked to describe how similar each object was to the referent X object. This was repeated using each character described by the subject. Finally the subjects were asked to cluster the objects into groups.

The information on similarity of each object to X on each character was used to determine the estimated relative weight attached to each feature in the decisions made in the perception experiment. The method (Hansell and Ewing, 1974) consists in using the degree to which a taxonomic character (feature) supports a taxonomic decision. If a subject decides that A is more similar to X than B is similar to X, then clearly characters to which he has given strong emphasis in making his decision will also show A more similar to X than B is similar to X.

Support $S = \left|V_X - V_B\right| - \left|X_X - V_A\right|$

Where V_X is the value of the character for object X.

In our experiments, five objects were compared in pairs to X. By summing the support S over all 10 such comparisons, we obtain an estimate of the degree to which the subject relied upon this feature. The significance of Σ S was tested by obtaining the particular probability distribution of this event for the character values coded by the subject for that character. These monte-carlo distributions were run on the IBM P.C. and were based on repetitions of random assignment of A or B more similar to X for the 10 object comparisons. This was repeated to test individually all characters for all subjects.

To validate the experimental procedure we then tested whether feature weightings from taxonomic decisions made in the eye tracking experiments were positively associated with feature weightings implicit in their subsequent assignment of taxa to groups.

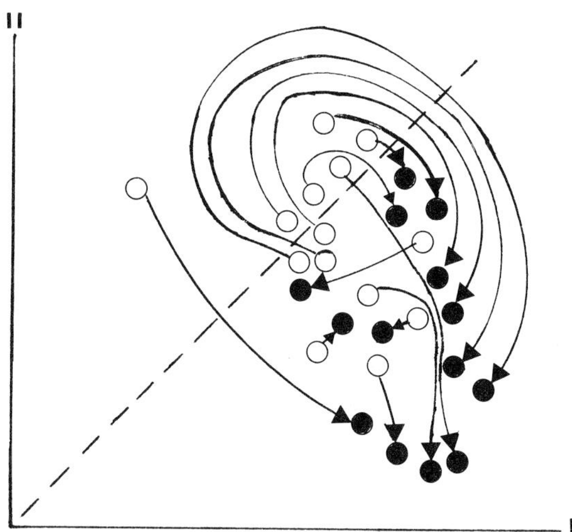

FIGURE 4. INDSCAL ANALYSIS OF SUBJECTIVE WEIGHTS OF NUMERICAL AND SUBJECTIVE TAXONOMIES (SEE TEXT).

RESULTS AND DISCUSSION

The INDSCAL analysis of similarity matrices (Figure 4) shows numerical evaluations (○ dots) with the equivalent subjective matrices (● dots) connected by arrows. In most of the 14 paired cases, the numerical solutions fall closer to the 45° diagonal, indicating that the axes tend to be given equal weight. These axes can be interpreted from Figure (5) which shows the objects ordinated on the same axes. Body shape is a major determinant of the first axis while structure of arms and legs influence the second. These results confirm the finding of Moss and Hansell (1980) that relative scaling of axes or character weighting can explain the difference between numerical and subjective measure of similarity. Gonzalez and Kolers (this volume) have demonstrated that similarity and distance measures by subjects involve differential weighting of those characters which better differentiate between pairs of objects being compared.

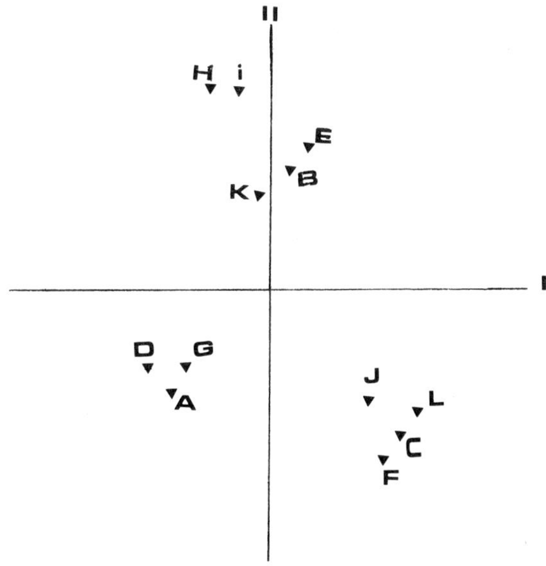

FIGURE 5. INDSCAL ORDINATION OF OBJECTS FROM FIGURE 1.

Turning now to the experiments which test the more direct classificatory problem of deciding whether object A or B is more similar to our 'intermediate' test object X, we have analyzed in detail the results of five subjects. The number of significantly weighted characters is given in Table 1. Clearly, from the features which the subjects have chosen, there are a number which each has significantly discounted in his decision. Also there is a subset of characters which have been given significant positive weight in the process. The number of significantly weighted characters is greater than would be expected by chance.

TABLE 1. SIGNIFICANCE OF CHARACTER WEIGHTINGS

Subject	Significant +ve	Significant -ve	Not Significant	Total
1	6	3	6	15
2	2	3	2	7
3	2	0	9	11
4	7	6	10	23
5	3	3	11	17
Totals	20	15	38	73

e.g. Character 1. Body Shape

	Object X	1	2	3	4	5
Codes	10	2	10	8	3	3

Decision 1, Object "2" more similar to "X" than "1" is to "X".
Character support $S_1 = |10 - 2| - |10 - 10| = + 8$
Sum of character support over all comparisons $\Sigma S = + 36$
Tested for significance $p = .008$

The features weighted in the eye movement experiments are highly associated with the features weighted when the subjects were asked to cluster the objects into groups.

TABLE 2. SCALED SIMILARITIES TO 'X'

Subject	Before Weighting						After Weighting					
	Object						Object					
	1	2	3	4	5	<.1*	1	2	3	4	5	<.1*
1	.90	.67	.66	.57	.83	4	.85	.00	.01	.65	.81	2
2	.84	.79	.81	.76	1.0	6	1.0	.00	.15	.75	1.0	1
3	.98	.48	.35	.83	.80	1	.50	.05	.10	.60	1.0	2
4	.67	.81	.73	.71	.69	9	.90	.00	.44	.70	.55	0
5	.80	.50	.54	.83	.80	4	.33	.16	.16	.00	1.0	1
6	.84	.78	.65	.65	.73	3	.00	1.0	.77	.46	.18	0
7	.67	.58	.58	.70	.60	10	1.0	.67	.47	.13	1.0	1
8	.67	.47	.47	.53	.53	6	.56	.69	.41	.00	.28	0
9	.55	.75	.40	.46	.38	5	1.0	.21	.16	.51	.48	2
Totals						48						9

*Comparisons.

We have established that characters are actively discounted or emphasized in the process of making taxonomic decisions. Is it also the case that this weighting reduces the number of difficult decisions to be made?

Table 2 shows the effect of character weighting on the average similarities of each object to the referent 'X'. Column 1 shows the measure taken over all characters chosen by each subject. Column 2 shows the measure taken over the positively weighted characters. In the former case, the similarity values fall closer together than in the second case. We may think of a decision based, say for subject 1, on all characters showing resemblance of object 1 to X at a value of .84 and 2 to X at a value of .79 to be a more difficult decision than one based on weighted features showing 1 to X at a value of 1.0 and 2 to X at a value of 0.0. We have tabulated the number of decisions based on the scaled values differing by .1 or less for each case. Over the 9 subjects evaluated, there were 48 such 'difficult' decisions based on all features, but only 9 such difficult decisions based on weighted features.

A process such as weighting features tends to make classificatory decisions easier. The existence of the analogue of such a process in humans suggests that some evolutionary advantage or efficiency should be involved. It may well be that the time taken to make a classificatory decision is under such evolutionary constraint: the ability to make rapid yet successful decisions on the relatedness of objects being a component of the evolutionary fitness of the subjects.

In Figure (6) we show the relationship between number of fixations taken and the average degree of character support for that decision for each subject over all decisions. When character support is high the decision is easily made, while when average character support is low, then the decision is in some sense difficult, either object might be considered more similar to X.

The negative relationship between support and fixations in all five subjects for which we have this data (probability $<.05$) indicates that the more difficult the decisions the more fixations are made, and the greater the time taken. Considering now the problem of efficiently classifying a number of objects, we note that a procedure of giving importance to a few features which emphasize the perceived cluster structure of the data reduces the number of difficult decisions faced by the classifier.

In the three object case, this reduces to a procedure of giving importance to features which resolve the problem of A or B more similar to X, thus reducing the number of fixations needed for the decision. In the two object case, features which differentiate between the objects are emphasized (Gonzalez and Kolers, this volume).

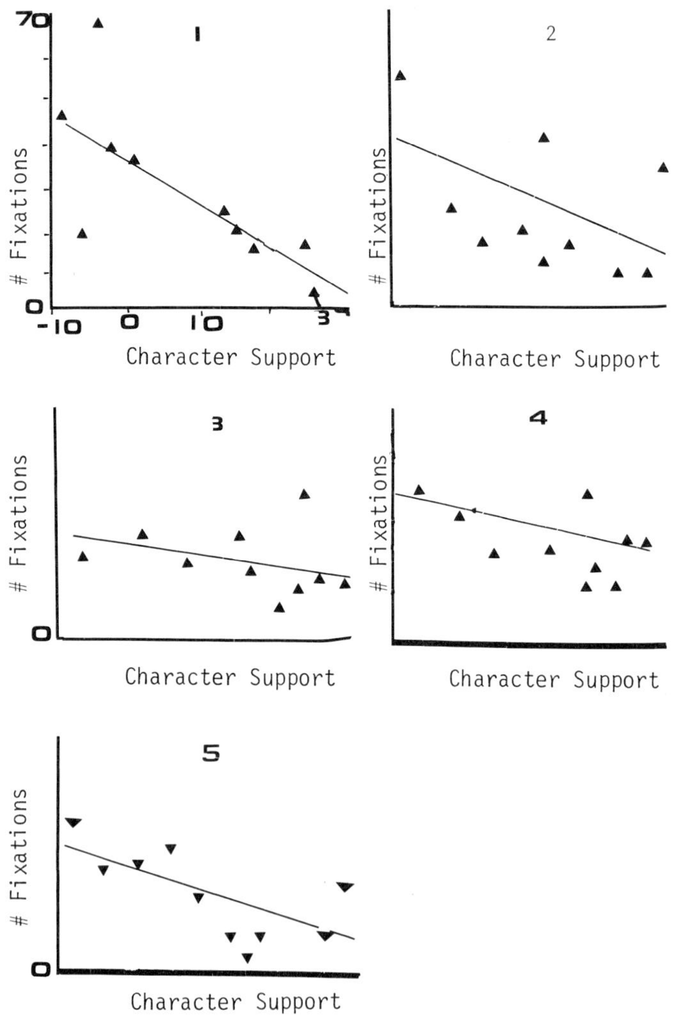

FIGURE 6. RELATION OF # OF FIXATIONS TO EASE OF CLASSIFICATION IN 5 SUBJECTS FOR 10 DECISIONS EACH.

An interesting problem underlies this 'efficiency of classification' phenomenon: the scaling of the cognitive map appears to occur with a short response time and is followed by eye fixations dealing with regional problems. Is there an initial time independent process of pattern recognition which is the basis for a cognitive directing of eye fixation location? In cases where object A is very dissimilar from B and X, A often receives no fixations until late in the decision process--almost as if the subjects follow the dictum: don't waste time on the obvious. We may postulate a primary gestalt process which may be in part a peripheral vision phenomenon followed by a secondary central vision information gathering process under cognitive control.

ACKNOWLEDGEMENTS

We thank our subjects, both professional taxonomists and students. Wayne Moss, Dennis Carmody and Esther Gonzalez contributed helpful discussions of these ideas. We thank Patricia Bennett for typing the manuscript.

REFERENCES

Camin, J., & Sokal, R. R. A method for deducing branching sequences in phylogeny, Evolution, 1965, 19, 311-326.

Carrol, J. D., & Chang, J. J. Analysis of individual differences in multidimensional scaling. Psychometrika, 1970, 35, 283-319.

Gonzalez, E., & Kolers, P. A. On the interpretation of eye movements. (This volume), 1984.

Hansell, R. I. C., & Chant, D. A. Taxonomic methods: Relative weights applied to characters by classical taxonomists in the Genus Iphiseius Berlese (Acarina: Phytoseiidae). Can. Ent., 1973, 105, 775-785.

Hansell, R. I. C., & Ewing, B. The detection and estimation of character weighting in classifications. J. Theor. Biol., 1973, 39, 297-314.

Moss, W. W. Taxonomic repeatability. Syst. Zool., 1971, 20, 309-330.

Moss, W. W., & Hansell, R. I. C. Subjective classification: The effects of character weighting on decision space. Class. Soc. Bull., 1980, 4,(4), 2-6.

Sneath, P. H. A., & Sokal, R. R. Numerical Taxonomy. San Francisco: W. H. Freeman, 1973.

Sokal, R. R., & Sneath, P. H. A. Numerical Taxonomy, San Francisco: W. H. Freeman, 1963.

Eye Movements and Human Information Processing
R. Groner, G.W. McConkie and C. Menz (eds.)

SEARCHING HIGH AND LOW: THE DEVELOPMENT OF EFFICIENT VISUAL SEARCH IN HEARING, DEAF AND LEARNING DISABLED CHILDREN

Lesley C. Hall

Division of Cognitive Science and Psychology
Deakin University
Australia.

The development of the directive role of language on visual search was studied by comparing the performance of various groups of hearing, deaf and learning disabled children on a pictorial visual search task which varied in terms of (1) the presence or absence of linguistic information about target location, (2) the positive/negative form of that information and (3) the spatial location of the target picture. The results indicated that linguistic control over visual search takes many years to perfect, even for hearing children, with other groups of children showing developmental delay. However for all children language served some directive function which, with age, acquired a greater capacity to organize visual input.

INTRODUCTION

This research addresses the questions raised by Bruner (1968) when he asked: "through what means does the child gain control of his own visual attention? How does the child learn to visually orient and search in a way that reflects the needs of problem solving rather than the mere tracking of sensory change?" For the sighted child, nearly all learning situations require that the child use her or his visual attention to seek out and maintain attention on those parts of the visual world that are relevant for the task at hand. Crucial also, for many learning situations is the ability to integrate information provided verbally with that which is available visually. Such integration underlies situations as basic as that which occurs when a teacher talks about a visual array, be it a picture or text in a book or on the blackboard or T.V. It seems reasonable to suggest that with age, language and its cognitive/semantic underpinnings will begin, however inadequately to serve this function. This is not to suggest that language necessarily determines the perceptual experience but rather to propose that it may, depending on the situation, influence the order and nature of the visual information which is acquired as sensory input for the perceptual systems.

Luria (1959), along with other Russian researchers, emphasized the importance of language for the development of voluntary behaviour. He has described the development of this function from the early stages in infancy, where language can serve to produce an orienting response, through to the 5½ to 6 year old child who is able to inhibit certain behaviours while executing others - without the need for external speech of his own or from someone else. However Luria's studies on the effect of language on voluntary behaviour only examined the control of manual behaviour such as pressing or not pressing a hand-held bulb. The effect of language on visual search, which provides the child with so much more precise and yet comprehensive information about the world, has not yet been studied extensively nor systematically.

The development of visual search strategies in normal children, viewed within the larger context of the development of mechanisms of selective attention, has been the subject of an increasing amount of research in recent years. However, as indicated by Day's (1975) review, there have been very few studies which have looked at the regulative role of language and cognitive development by controlling specific linguistic variables and using precise eye movement measures.

Some studies like that of Mackworth and Bruner (1972) have been concerned with search patterns in a fairly unconstrained task, such as identifying objects on a blurred slide. Others have been more concerned to use eye movements and fixations as a measure of the child's comprehension of particular concepts: e.g. O'Bryan and Boersma's (1971) study of the eye movements of conserving and non-conserving children and Vurpillot's (1968) use of visual search as a measure of children's comprehension of the terms 'some' and 'different'.

But there are few studies which look at the ability of children to use linguistic information about known objects and concepts to organize subsequent visual search. There is evidence from Cooper (1974) that adults will spontaneously and rapidly direct their fixations to those pictures in a visual display which are most closely related to the meaning of the concurrent spoken input. But what of the development of this ability? The ability to use spoken, manual and written language systems to direct efficient searches for visual information is obviously an important one. Learning problems may arise from making the false assumption that all children can quickly direct their attention to something being talked about and can efficiently extract the information relevant for a given task.

Some clues, albeit with respect to a manual/visual search task comes from a study by Sophian and Wellman (1980), who reported that children as young as three were able to integrate two sources of information about an object's location when both were relevant and that they were able to ignore irrelevant knowledge about an object's normal location when verbal information was logically superordinate. The task used in this study required the children to locate small toys that were placed at normal and unusual room locations in a doll's house. On different trials children were provided with either no information, partial information ('upstairs'/ 'downstairs') or full information ('it's in the downstairs bedroom') about the location of the toy. The three year olds were able to improve their performance from 37% to 63% successful searches when partial information was provided while the four year olds improved from 35% to 69% and the seven year olds from 41% to 85%. This study provides a useful background against which to consider the development search processes operating solely at the visual level.

It is often suggested that problems in attentive behaviour characterize children who are labelled as learning disabled (Doyle, Anderson & Halcomb 1976; Tarver & Hallahan 1974). However Koppel (1979) argues that more research is needed in order to differentiate between various kinds of explanations which might explain the performance deficits found in learning disabled children. For instance to what extent do deficits arise with respect to the initial location of task-relevant information, to the maintenance of attention on task-relevant information, to the ability to successfully process both relevant and irrelevant task information and to the ability to terminate processing by selecting the appropriate response when sufficient information is available to complete the task?

There is additional question of whether learning disabled children are characterized by a developmental lag in selective attention rather than a more permanent defect in learning. Tarver, Hallahan, Cohen and Kauffman (1977) addressed this question in a study which contrasted the central versus incidental recall of pictures of learning disabled boys varying in age from 8, 10, 13 to 15 years. Their findings, as did the one by Bauer (1977), supported the idea of a developmental delay in the use of verbal rehearsal strategies in learning disabled children.

A more direct measure of these hypotheses is possible by using visual search measures to examine the nature of attentional processes throughout a task which requires selective attention and allows children to use verbal rehearsal on some occasions but not on others.

With respect to deaf children, almost no direct information is available concerning linguistic control of visual search, although some studies have examined the relationship between verbal language and impulse control (Binder, 1970; Harris, 1978). Yet the reliance of deaf children on the co-ordination of various sources of visual information to supplement or replace auditory information makes this an important area. For such children the acquisition and development of spoken/written language is often delayed (Brooks, 1978). Does such a delay mean that the integration of the language system with the perceptual and motor systems is also delayed, so that language fails to serve the kind of regulative role seen developing in hearing children? Alternatively it may be that deaf children develop compensatory mechanisms which enhance the efficiency of their visual search by using whatever linguistic information is available to them. Most studies of language abilities in deaf children (Blanton 1968; Lieben 1978) focus on weaknesses to be found in their syntax, morphology and vocabulary in spoken and written language. Research questions have not been asked with respect to how the deaf child puts to good functional use those aspects of language over which they have achieved some command.

By systematically varying the kind of linguistic and perceptual input provided to the viewer, this study sought to examine the ability of children to use linguistic information about familiar objects and concepts (top/bottom) to organize a visual search. Thus, what was of interest was the ability of children to use known concepts, rather than the comprehension of the concepts themselves. The extent to which children can use language to rapidly locate and process visual information may depend upon the form of the linguistic information and the specific spatial configuration of the visual arrays. The position of the target was varied between the top and bottom since other studies (Levy-Schoen and Pouthas, 1971) have found that from an early age, search is normally directed first to the top of a display in unstructured "exploratory" search. The effect of this perceptual bias on the performance of the task was examined in order to assess if and how the perceptual and cognitive/linguistic aspects of a search task interact at different points during the developmental process. Luria's (1959) work suggests that the younger the child the less able they will be to use negative information to inhibit search of the named location and to direct search to other relevant picture locations. It was predicted that with age, children would become more efficient in using language to direct and constrain search but that deaf children and learning disabled children would be delayed relative to hearing children.

METHOD

Subjects

The research to be discussed is based on a comparison of five groups of hearing, non-learning disabled children, two groups of learning disabled children and two groups of deaf children. Each of the groups consisted of twelve children. Table 1 provides information about the groups in terms of age, sex of children and the availability of WISC-R IQ scores. References to the groups throughout the paper will be in terms of the abbreviations listed in Table 1.

TABLE 1

Characteristics of Subject Groups

Group Reference	Group Type	Ages (Years; Months) Mean(SD)	Number Males/ Females	WISC-R PIQ Full Mean(SD)	WISC-R PIQ Partial Mean(SD)	WISC-R VIQ Mean(SD)
H1	Hearing	4;5(0;6)	6/6	-	-	-
H2	Hearing	7;9(1;5)	6/6	-	-	-
H3	Hearing	9;7(0;13)	6/6	100(10)	97(14)	100(10)
H4	Hearing	13;3(0;14)	6/6	102(13)	105(18)	101(9)
H5	Hearing	24;0(4;0)	6/6	-	-	-
LD1	Learning Disabled	7;5(0;8)	10/2	90(12)	-	97(12)
LD2	Learning Disabled	10;9(6;7)	10/2	109(10)	-	102(6)
D1	Deaf	9;8(1;3)	2/10	90(11)	94(14)	46(5)
D2	Deaf	13;2(1;3)	6/6	96(13)	97(15)	54(7)

Hearing groups H1, H2 and H5 had no known sensory, perceptual or learning disability. No IQ data was available for these subjects. An additional forty hearing children were tested on the WISC-R in order to select Hearing groups H3 and H4 to provide a match for the two deaf groups in terms of age and range of WISC-R performance scores.

Two groups of pre-lingually deaf children were selected from a school for the deaf which had adopted the total communication approach. The school used English signing, finger spelling, written and spoken English and a version of the Australian Sign Language AUSLAN. The children were placed at the school at age 6 to 7 years if they were judged as unable to benefit from a completely oral education. This judgement was based on the child's performance in a strictly oral pre-school program. The children selected ranged from severely to profoundly deaf. The mean hearing loss in the better ear exceeded 85db (SD 13) at frequencies of 250,500,1000,2,000 HZ, and the loss in the other ear exceeding 110db (SD 18) over the same frequency ranges. Information was available for 21 children on the WISC-R performance scale and 19 children of the verbal scale. These test scores had been collected over two years prior to the visual search data. However, an up to date partial performance score was available for all the children based on the coding and block design sub-tests of the WISC-R.

The children in the two learning disabled groups were identified by the educational services as being within the normal IQ range but as not performing at that level due to specific learning difficulties which were not related to sensory or emotional problems. In particular, the children experienced difficulties with reading, spelling and writing. Groups LD1 and LD2 showed an average delay of 10 and 28 months respectively on the Schonell Word Reading Test and an average delay of 16 and 36 months on Schonell Word Spelling Test. The children attended regular classes except for some special remediation lessons.

Experimental Task

On each of six practice trials and eighteen test trials a subject was asked to search an array consisting of six different pictures in order to find and signal when they could see a pre-designated target picture. See Figure 1 for an example of one visual array. The picture location numbers that are provided on this example array were not present on the arrays seen by the subjects. Prior to the presentation of each array, the particular target was named: "Find the picture of the (e.g. kangaroo) as quickly as you can. Press the button when you can see the kangaroo". The pictures in each array consisted of easily recognizable black line drawings of different objects arranged so that three were equally spaced (12^0 visual angle apart) along the top of the display and three similarly spaced along the bottom. The initial fixation point from which the subject began the search was placed in the centre of the display. The subject fixated this point on the screen until the slide appeared. The subject signalled the detection of the target by pressing a button held in the preferred hand. The button press resulted in a bell-like noise. For the deaf children the bell mechanism was placed in their laps so that vibration might provide tactile feedback of their response.

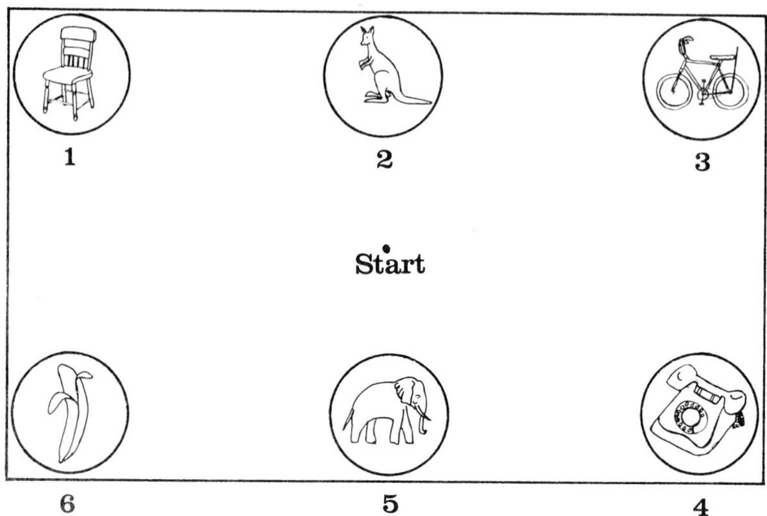

FIGURE 1
Example of Pictorial Array
(Picture location numbers were not present on arrays viewed by subjects)

In order to assess the ability of subjects to use language to direct their search, on six trials the subject was provided with no information concerning the location of the target, on six trials information was given in a positive form (e.g. "The chair is at the top/bottom"), and on six trials it was given in a negative form (e.g. "The cow is not at the top/bottom"). This information was always true of the array. It was provided in spoken form for hearing children and in written and signed English form for deaf children. The visual array appeared within two seconds of the delivery of the instructions.

For the deaf groups the general nature of the task was explained by the class teacher using speech, sign and finger spelling. In the test situation the instruction to look at the central fixation point until the visual array appeared was replaced with a small light flashing on and off to attract attention. The light was used in an attempt to attract and maintain the deaf children's attention on the initial fixation point since pilot work with the deaf children has revealed that the instructions "to look at the spot until the pictures come on" were not understood by the deaf children. Even when the light was used the deaf children made many anticipatory first eye movements so they they were fixating a picture instead of the spot when the visual array appeared. This meant that perceptual information from the top and bottom was not equally available at the start of the visual search. The consequences of this will be discussed later.

Experimental Design

On each trial the subject had to search for a different target (bed, spade, elephant, clock, table, banana, mouse, butterfly, teapot, rabbit, telephone, chair, fish, car, horse, gun). Each visual array had a different set of non-targets and within each array the non-targets were different. The eighteen arrays were designed so that each of the six locations contained a target on three occasions. For any one target location a positive instruction was given on one trial, a negative instruction on one trial and on another trial, no instruction. Thus there were six positive, six negative and six no instruction trials, with each set of six made up of one trial for each picture position at the top (1,2,3) and one at the bottom (4,5,6). Each subject searched for the same twelve targets and accompanying non-targets, but over all subjects within a group, a particular target picture was located an equal number of times at each position for each instruction type. Three different random orders of presentation were used with the constraint that no more than two trials from any one instruction condition could be given together. In each group of subjects, two subjects received each of these orders and two received the same orders with the first and second halves reversed.

The ability of subjects to recognize the target items was determined prior to the experimental session as well as establishing that all children were able to identify the "top/top row" and "bottom/bottom row" without any difficulty.

Procedures and Equipment

The same task, materials and basic procedures were used for each group of subjects. However the method of recording the child's visual search varied inasmuch as Groups H3 and H4 were tested using a Gulf and Western computer-based 1998 Eye View System. This system provided a video record of the subject's eye movements and fixations superimposed on top of the array being viewed. All of the other groups viewed the arrays by looking through a slot to a screen at the back of a viewing box. A video record of the subject's eyes was made by means of an overhead camera and a half-silvered mirror arrangement inside the box. Corneal reflections of marker lights were used to determine which pictures had been searched and in which orders. The experimenter presented the slide which triggered a reaction timer and also turned on a light so as to provide a video record of the slide onset. The pressing of the button by the subject to signal target location stopped the timer and also flashed a light inside the box. The visual display was not removed for some seconds to allow the subject the possibility of further inspection. The arrays subtended the same degree of visual field for both recording methods, the only difference being the absence of the viewing box for Groups H3 and H4.

With both methods it was possible to monitor the search during each trial and to detect (1) trials on which initial fixation was not maintained, (2) trials on which the button was pressed to signal target detection prior to the inspection of the appropriate picture location and (3) trials on which subjects did not locate the target or forgot to signal the target location.

Additional trials were run to replace all three types of trials for all hearing and learning disabled groups, since they occured reasonably infrequently. Only the latter two types of trials were replaced for the deaf subjects. For deaf subjects, trials where subjects anticipated the first eye movement were not replaced as these constituted 29% of trials of Group D1 (84% of these in the appropriate direction) and 56% trials for Group D2 (91% of these in the appropriate direction). Reliability checks for each group of subjects showed that both methods of recording the visual search patterns provided data which could be coded with almost complete reliability (98-100%).

Coding of Visual Search Measures

The video and computer records were scored from the onset of each slide to the point at which the subject signalled their detection of the target picture, in order to obtain the following measures of visual search. These different aspects of search are illustrated in Figure 2.

Appropriate First Eye Movement (AFEM) refers to the direction (anticipated or not) of the first eye movement from the initial fixation point. If this FEM was to the row containing the target, it was judged to be appropriate. It was hypothesized that this would be the aspect of search over which children would first gain control. It was also hypothesized that with increasing age, instructions (especially positive ones) and top target positions, the number of AFEMS would be greater.

Efficient (E) Search Patterns refer to all trials where the AFEM search was sustained in the appropriate direction and search did not proceed past the target picture until its location had been signalled. It was expected that more efficient searches would be made the older the subject, with positive instructions and with top target positions.

Efficient Target (E(T)) Search Patterns refer to a subset of efficient search trials where the target picture was the first one located and no other pictures were inspected before signalling target detection. This search pattern was scored in order to check that peripheral vision was not sufficient to guide search to guide search to the target, independently of the instructions.

Appropriate/Inappropriate (A/I) Search Patterns refer to trials where, despite an AFEM, one or more inappropriate picture locations were inspected before the target was located.

Redundant (R) Search Patterns refer to trials where additional pictures were inspected after the target had been inspected, but before signalling its detection.

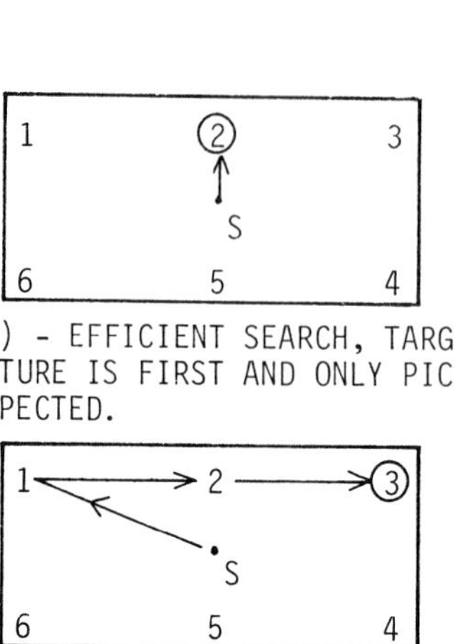

E(T) - EFFICIENT SEARCH, TARGET PICTURE IS FIRST AND ONLY PICTURE INSPECTED.

E - EFFICIENT SEARCH WHERE ONLY APPROPRIATE PICTURES ARE INSPECTED

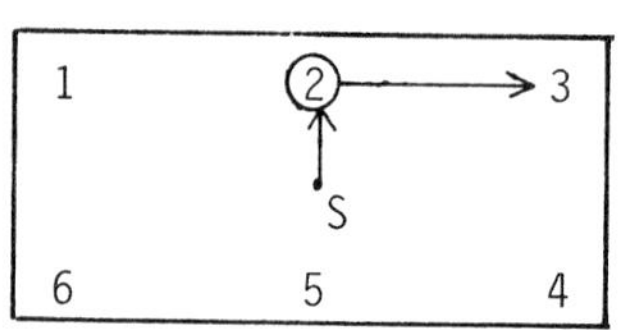

E(T)+1R (ONE REDUNDANT SEARCH)

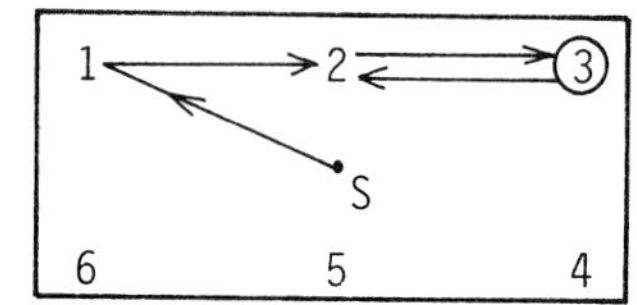

E +1R (ONE REDUNDANT SEARCH)

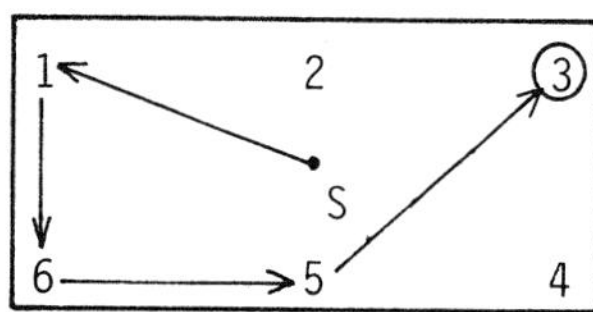

A/I - APPROPRIATE FIRST EYE MOVEMENT BUT INAPPROPRIATE PICTURES SEARCHED BEFORE TARGET

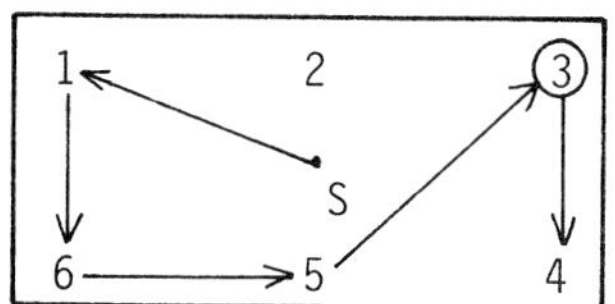

A/I+1R (ONE REDUNDANT SEARCH)

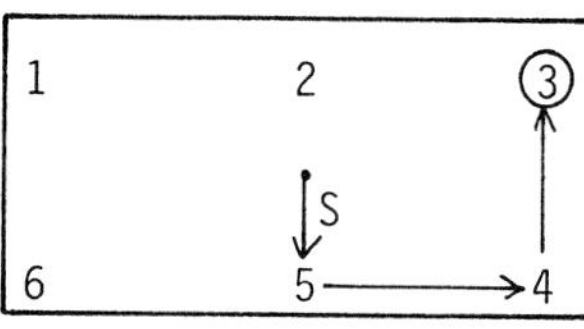

I/A - INAPPROPRIATE PICTURES ARE SEARCHED BEFORE APPROPRIATE ONES

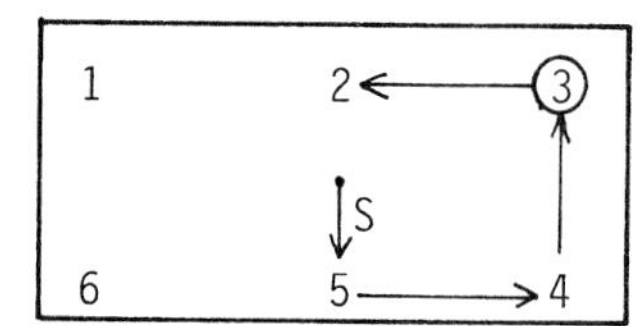

I/A+1R (ONE REDUNDANT SEARCH)

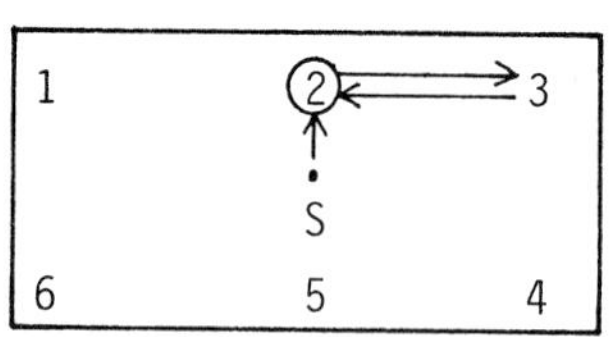

E(T)+2R(1T) - EXAMPLE OF REDUNDANT SEARCHES WITH RETURN TO TARGET PICTURE

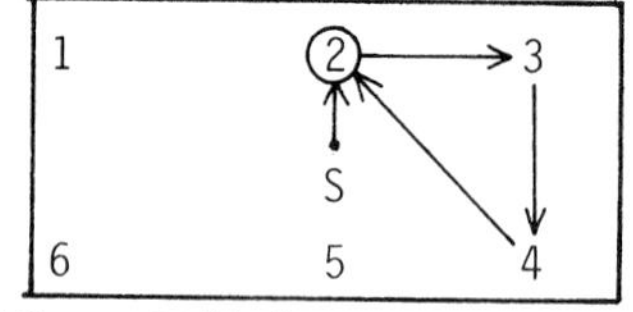

E(T)+ > 2R(1T) - EXAMPLE OF MORE THAN TWO REDUNDANT SEARCHES

FIGURE 2

Categories of Search Patterns

(Target picture location is circled)

Number of Pictures Inspected (No. Pic.) refers to all pictures inspected from the onset on the slide to the subject's pressing the button. Each return to a picture counted as a separate inspection: It was not possible to score fixations occurring within each picture inspection.

Search Reaction Times (RT) refer to the time by the subject from the onset of the slide to pressing the button to signal target detection.

RESULTS AND DISCUSSION

Task Validity

The first point to establish is that the task actually required a visual search in order to locate the target picture and that peripheral vision was not sufficient to allow the viewer to locate the target from the initial central fixation spot. Table 2 provides a comparison of the mean percentage of trials on which subjects in each group made either E(T) or E(T)+R searches with Instruction and Noinstruction trials considered separately.

TABLE 2

Mean Percentage of E(T) and E(T)+R Trials for Each Subject Group

Groups	H1	H2	H3	H4	H5	D1	D2	LD1	LD2
Instruction Trials	26	31	31	36	35	27	29	25	36
No Instruction	18	18	19	20	22	19	18	26	23

It can be seen that for most trials peripheral vision did not enable subjects to locate the target without a visual search. As expected, subjects were more likely to immediately locate the target on Instruction trials but they have not done so at a level higher than that to be expected by chance (33%, provided that the instructions constrained the initial search direction.) The overall percentages of E(T) trials occurring under No Instruction trials are somewhat misleading in that most of these trials occurred when the target was at picture location 2 (centre top) and to a much lesser extent at picture location 5 (centre bottom). E(T) trials almost never occurred for the other target locations. This bias reflects the fact that for No Instruction trials, 56% of first eye movements were directed to picture location 2 and 27% were directed to picture location 5. Thus, targets at these locations were more likely to be immediately located than targets at other locations, but peripheral vision does not seem to be implicated since these locations were also likely to be searched first when no target was present.

The second point to establish is whether the task succeeded in eliciting from the subjects, searches that were related to the target. In other words, did the subjects respond to the instructions to signal their detection of the target as quickly as they could or did they tend to search all picture locations, or alternatively, did they signal their response prior to location of the target? Table 3 provides a break-down for each subject group of the number of trials which were replaced because the subject failed to make a decision or else signalled the detection of the target prior to an inspection of the appropriate picture location. With respect to the latter type of response it is interesting to note that for H3, H4, LD2 and D2 groups these anticipatory response trials included some where the subject gave evidence of some sort of rapid deductive reasoning. For instance on a trial where target location was specified as the top row, a subject would inspect locations 2 and 1, and then signal target detection before making an eye movement to inspect the target at location 3.

TABLE 3
Number of Replacement Trials for Each Subject Group
(out of 144 trials)

	H1	H2	H3	H4	H5	D1	D2	LD1	LD2
Total Trials Replaced	6	6	7	8	2	11	16	12	7
Deductive Anticipations	0	0	2	3	0	0	9	0	2
Number of Subjects	5	4	4	4	2	3	7	5	3

Allowing for the deductive anticipation trials, the number of trials where children respond inappropriately is relatively small and indicates comprehension of the requirements of the task. It is the younger of the learning disabled and deaf groups which make most inappropriate responses.

The extent to which location of the target led to prompt response execution was examined by comparing the percentages of trials on which each group signalled the target location (1) while inspecting the target location for the first time (2) while inspecting the target location on a repeated occasion (3) having inspected one or two pictures subsequent to target location but without returning to the target location. As Table 4 shows only group H1 showed a tendency to signal target location while inspecting a non-target location.

TABLE 4

Percentages of Trials Showing Different Response Patterns With Respect to Target Location

Groups	H1	H2	H3	H4	H5	D1	D2	LD1	LD2
Response Made at 1st Target Inspection	50	73	81	77	81	64	69	60	74
Response Made at Repeat Target Inspection	31	23	16	14	13	30	17	30	23
Response Made Without Return to Target	19	4	3	7	6	6	14	10	3

Search Patterns

Table 5 provides a general overview of the kinds of search patterns which occurred most frequently for the nine subject groups. Over all groups, an average of only 54.1% of trials were totally efficient in their execution (E and E(T) patterns). Where then did subjects experience difficulty? Failure to initiate search in the appropriate direction (I/A and I/A+R patterns) accounted for 17.3% of the inefficient search patterns although some of these searches were inefficient for other reasons as well. Failure to sustain search in the appropriate direction, once initiated (A/I and A/I+R patterns) was not a major contributor to inefficient search (6.2%) and will not be discussed in the following analyses. However it is interesting to note that for the hearing children this kind of search pattern had actually disappeared by age 9;7 years, whereas 12% of the searches by deaf children of 9;8 years were of this sort, as were 6% of the searches by the LD1 group (10;7 years).

TABLE 5

Percentages of Search Pattern Types for Each Subject Group

Subject Groups	E	E+R	E(T)	E(T)+R	A/I	A/I+R	I/A	I/A+R
H1	15	13	8	17	9	4	18	16
H2	31	12	21	10	8	1	13	5
H3	49	8	25	11	1	0	6	0
H4	52	7	18	13	0	0	7	3
H5	56	8	24	11	1	0	0	0
LD1	24	8	8	15	6	4	22	13
LD2	40	6	22	14	5	1	7	5
D1	22	7	17	10	8	4	17	15
D2	43	8	17	12	3	1	6	10
Means	36.5	8.4	17.6	13.4	4.5	1.7	10.6	7.3

Comparison of Subject Groups

Planned contrast ANOVAs were carried out on various combinations of subject groups in order to examine subject group differences and task factor differences (Target Position, Positive/Negative form of instructions) for each visual search measure. For the AFEM and Number of Pictures Inspected measures an additional comparison was made between the No Instruction and Instruction trials. The influence of task factors on visual search will be considered in a separate section.

Subject group differences for each of the visual search measures of AFEM, E searches, R searches, Number of Pictures and RTs can be seen in Figures 3, 4, 5, 6 and 7. The same basic pattern emerges with respect to each measure,with age differences within each type of subject group reflecting increased efficiency in search, but with the younger learning disabled and deaf groups performing less efficiently than the younger hearing groups. This can be seen most clearly by looking at the mean ranking of the subject groups on all search measures, as shown in Table 6.

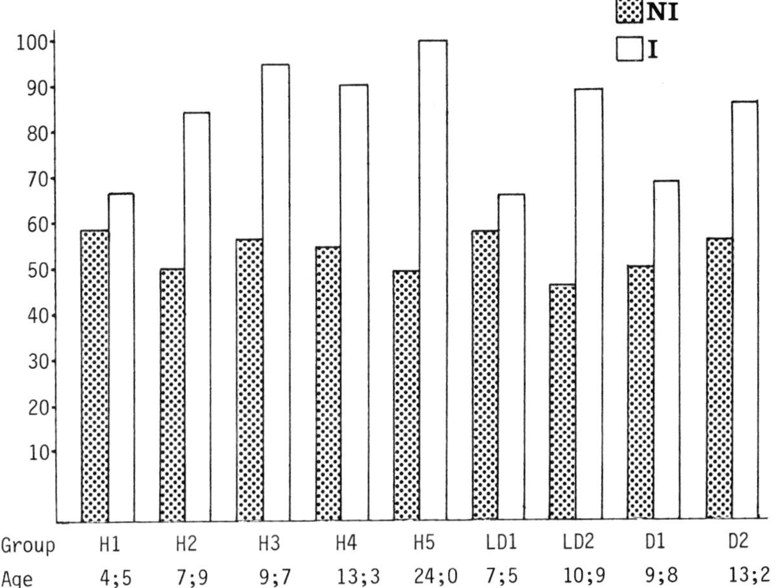

FIGURE 3
Mean Percentage of Trials on Which AFEMs Occurred for Each Subject Group

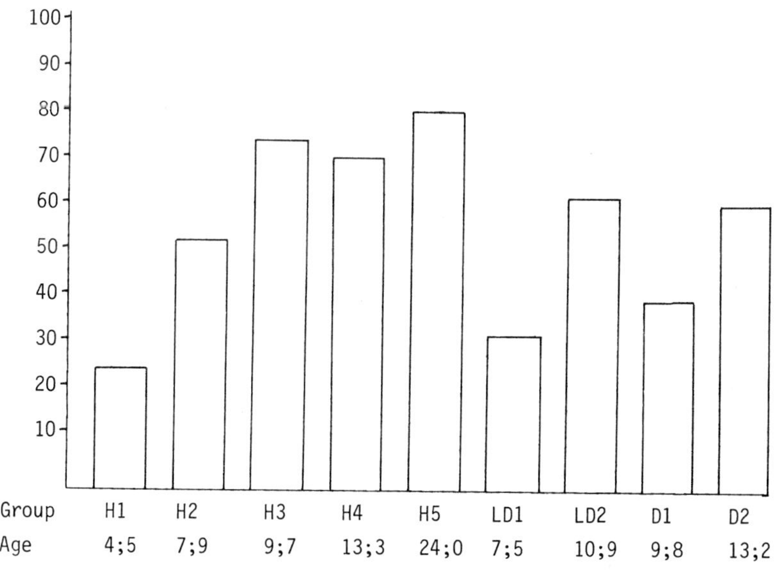

FIGURE 4
Mean Percentage of Trials on Which Efficient Search Patterns Occurred for Each Subject Group

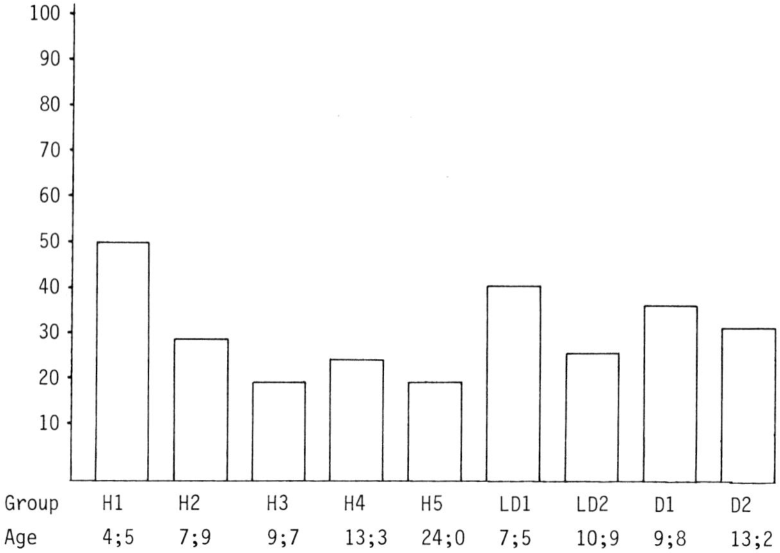

FIGURE 5
Mean Percentage of Trials on Which Redundant Searches Occurred for Each Subject Group

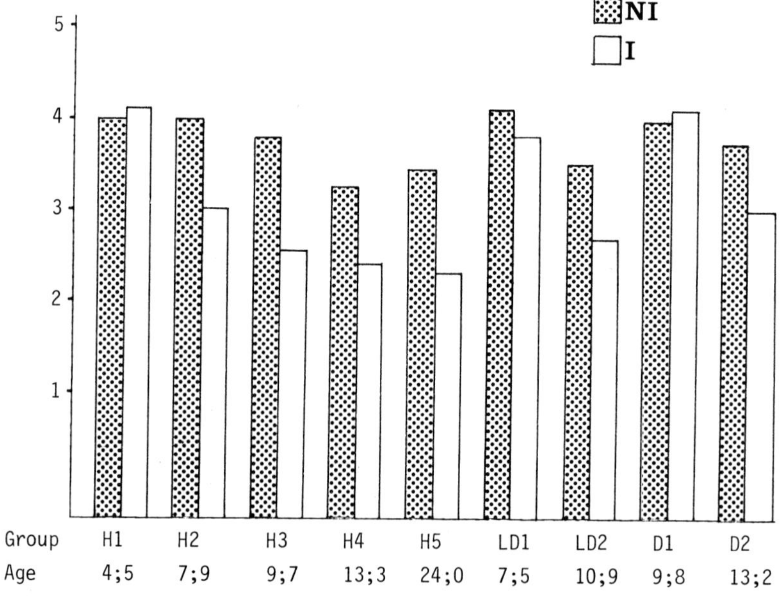

FIGURE 6
Mean Number of Pictures Inspected Per Trial for Each Subject Group

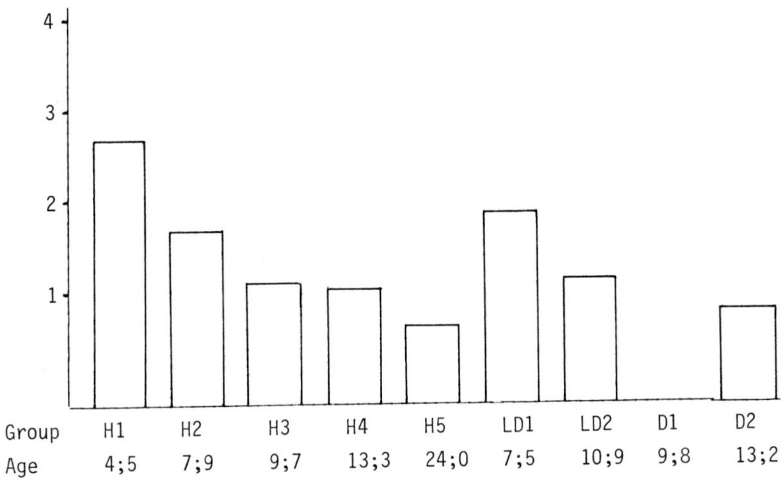

FIGURE 7

Mean Reaction Times (Seconds)

TABLE 6

Average Ranking of Subject Groups Across all Search Measures

Groups	H5	H4	H3	LD2	D2	H2	H1	D1	LD1
Age	24;0	13;3	9;7	10;9	13;2	7;9	4;5	9;8	7;5
Rank	1.1	2.4	3.7	4.1	4.9	6.1	7	7.4	7.8

(1 = most efficient
7 = least efficient)

A Kendall Tau Correlation Matrix showed the rankings on each measure to be significantly correlated to the rankings obtained on each of the other measures.

Hearing Groups (H1, H2, H5)

With respect to hearing groups H1, H2 and H5, for whom no IQ data was available, Group H2 searched more efficiently than Group H1 with respect to AFEM ($F(1,33)$, = 4.648, $p<.05$), E searches ($F(1,33)$, = 12.638, $p<.01$), R searches ($F(1,33)$, = 8834, $p<.01$), Number Pictures ($F(1,33)$, = 9.248, $p<.01$) and RTs ($F(1,33)$, = 9.242, $p<.01$).

Although the seven year olds had improved their efficiency compared to the four year olds, there was still room for further improvement as indicated by the following significant differences found between the H2 and H5 groups: AFEM ($F(1,33)$, = 10.051, $p<.01$), E searches ($F(1,33)$, = 13.933, $p<.01$), Number Pictures ($F(1,33)$, = 9.970, $p<.01$) and RTs ($F(1,33)$, = 19.790, $p<.01$).

Comparison of Deaf and Hearing Groups (H3, H4, D1, D2)

Because the age matched hearing and deaf groups differed in their full performance IQ scores, the effect of performance IQ was partialled out by means of a hierarchical multiple regression carried out for each dependent variable of AFEM, E and R searches and for Mean Number of Pictures Inspected per trial. Significant differences were found between the matched hearing and deaf groups in terms of AFEM ($F(1,46)$, = 4.57, $p<.05$), E searches ($F(1,46)$, = 3.51, $p<.05$), Number of Pictures ($F(1,46)$, = 6.4, $p<.05$) and R searches ($t(46)$, = 2.47, $p<.05$). Similar significant differences were found when partial PIQ was partialled out. No RT measure analysis was carried out as a result of missing data for Group D1 due to equipment failure. Moreover the reaction times available for the D2 group were underestimates of total search times because of the 56% of trials on which subjects made anticipatory FEMs. For the purposes of a general comparison, the mean RT of the D2 group was calculated and found to be slightly less than that of its matched hearing group (1.05). The RTs of the two groups appear equivalent if an allowance of 200-250 milliseconds is made for the anticipatory FEMs of the D2 group.

Differences between the deaf and hearing groups were most striking for the youngest deaf group (9;8 years) whose performance was significantly less efficient than a hearing group of the same age with respect to AFEM ($F(1,44)$, = 7.668, $p<.01$), E searches ($F(1,44)$, = 11.456, $p<.01$), R searches ($F(1,44)$, = 6.237, $p<.01$), and Number of Pictures ($F(1,44)$, = 14.167, $p<.01$).

The older deaf group did not differ significantly from its age equivalent hearing group. However the D2 group did differ from the hearing adults in search efficiency, whereas Hearing groups H3 and H4 did not. This suggests that the 13 year old deaf group still has some little way to go before reaching the search efficiency shown by hearing adults.

Various planned contrast ANOVAs were carried out to examine the effect of task factors (target position and positive/negative instructions) and age differences on the performance of the hearing and two deaf groups for each visual search measure. For the AFEM and Number of Pictures measures an additional comparison was made between the No Instruction and Instruction trials.

Comparison of Learning Disabled Hearing Groups (LD1, LD2, H3, H4)

In order to place the performance of the learning disabled groups with respect to the hearing groups, while taking into account the effect of any differences in IQ between the groups, groups LD1 and LD2 were compared to groups H3 and H4 for each visual search measure. When the effects of age and IQ differences between the groups were partialled out, the hearing and learning disabled groups differed significantly in terms of AFEMs ($t(46) = 2.1$, $p<.05$) and E searches ($F(1,46) = 2,39$, $p<.05$). These differences are mainly due to the poor search performance of the younger LD group. A comparison of the two LD groups, carried out as part of a larger analysis of serveral additional LD groups, revealed that there were significant differences between the two groups in terms of AFEM ($F(1,41), = 5.901$, $p<.05$), E searches ($F(1,41), = 11.150$, $p<.01$), Number of Pictures Inspected ($F(1,41), = 8.878$, $p<.01$) and RTs ($F(1,41), = 16.970$, $p<.01$), and also the ability of the older group to benefit more from instructions than the younger LD group ($F(1,41), = 20.20$, $p<.01$).

Any developmental lag shown by the younger LD children seems to have been overcome by the age of eleven years since the older LD group is performing almost at the same level as the H3 (9;8 years) group with respect to AFEMs, Number Pictures, RT and Redundant searches.

Comparison of Deaf and Learning Disabled Groups (LD1, LD2, D1, D2)

The average search efficiency ranking provided in Table 6 showed that groups LD1 and D1 ranked lower than even the H1 group. A comparison of LD1 and LD2 with D1 and D2 with the effects of performance IQ removed, revealed no significant differences between these two kinds of groups. Since the LD groups were younger than the D groups, this suggests that the developmental lag of the LD groups is overcome sooner than is that of the D groups.

The Effects Task Factors on Visual Search

Instructions

As can be seen from Figure 3 there were no significant differences between the groups on terms of AFEMs on No Instruction trials. However all groups showed significant increases in AFEMs on Instruction trials. For the comparison of the H1, H2 and H5 groups the effect of Instruction was significant ($F(1,33)$, = 80.15, $p<.001$) with Group H2 benefitting more from Instructions than Group H1 ($F(1,33)$, = 8.58, $p<.01$). The deaf/hearing matched group comparison similarly showed an overall effect of Instruction ($F(1,44)$, = 76.43, $p<.001$), with instructions resulting in a greater increase in AFEMs for Bottom Target Position trials than the Top Position trials ($F(1,44)$, = 18.43, $p<.001$) this being more true for Group H3 than for Group D1 ($F(1,44)$, = 5.005, $p<.05$). The effect of Instruction was significant for both LD groups ($F(1,44)$, = 17.54, $p<.01$) with Group LD2 showing more improvement on Instruction trials than Group LD1 ($F(1,44)$, = 28.3, $p<.001$).

The effect of Instructions on the Number of Pictures Inspected measure was a similarly striking one. However the only Group by Instruction/No Instruction interaction effect to be significant was one comparing Group H3 and D1 where Instructions were more useful in constraining search for hearing than deaf subjects.

Having demonstrated that instructions do allow all children to improve their visual search performance, the effect of the form of the instructions will now be considered.

Positive/Negative Target Location Information

For groups H1 and H2 the form of the instruction had a significant effect on AFEMs (F(1,33), = 6.203, p<.01) and on E searches (F(1,33), = 7.122, p<.01) with positive instructions resulting in more AFEMs and E searches. For the older hearing groups, both forms of instructions were effective in directing efficient search. Groups LD1 and LD2 also showed an overall effect of Positive/Negative instructions on AFEMs (F(1,40), = 4.86, p<.05) and RTs (F(1,40), = 5.15; p<.05), with positive instructions leading to faster searches, but the deaf groups did not appear to be sensitive to the form of the instruction on any measures. In this they ressembled the older hearing groups, but the older hearing groups were efficient for both kinds of instruction whereas the deaf groups were relatively inefficient for both kinds of instructions.

Top/Bottom Target Position

Figure 8 shows the bias for all groups to search the top first when no target position information is provided. That this bias is not fully overcome by instructions until age eight or nine is indicated by the fact that a significant Target Position effect was found on the AFEM measure for each of the following comparisons: H1, H2 and H3 (F(1,33), = 29.11, p<.01); H1, H2, D1, D2 (F(1,44), = 10.684), with Top Target Position trials receiving more AFEMs than Bottom Target Position trials. Groups H3, H4 and H5 showed no effect of Target Position.

The effect of Target Position on other search measures was not as consistent across subject groups, but they all indicated the difficulty of making efficient searches to Bottom Target Positions, particularly for groups D1 and LD1. For example Group D1 only made efficient searches on 28% of Bottom Target Position trials as compared to 50% of Top Target Position Trials.

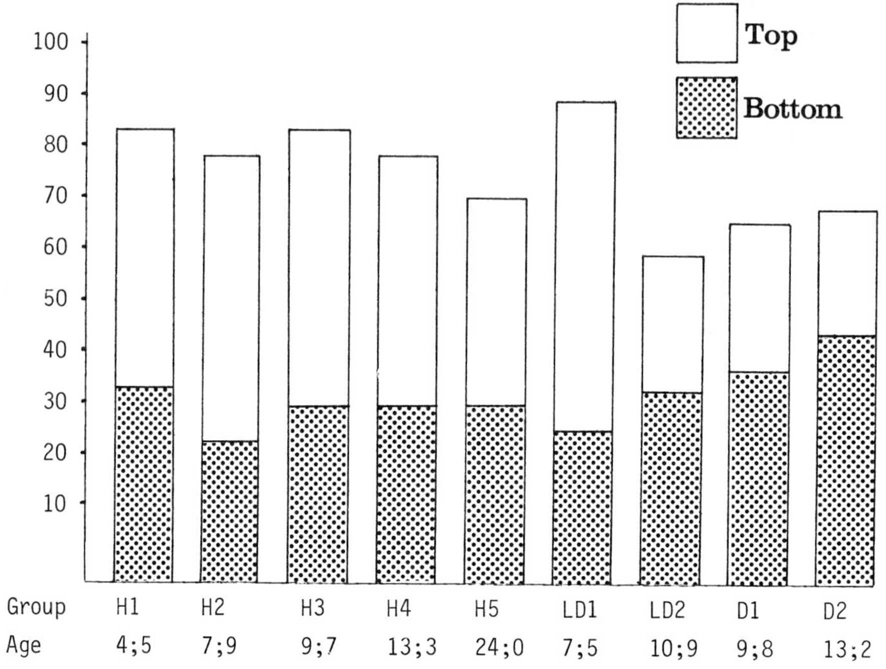

FIGURE 8
The Effect of Target Location on Mean Percentages of AFEMs For No Instruction Trials

SUMMARY

The results indicate that linguistically mediated cognitive control of visual search takes many years to perfect. In the absence of instructions, the search patterns of the subject groups were similar, but when information was provided, the older children and adults were able to search more efficiently. The pre-school and younger deaf and learning disabled children were least able to use instructions to plan and execute a search without being distracted by irrelevant and redundant stimuli. They were also least able to use negative information and least able to overcome a perceptual bias to search the top row first, regardless of instructions. However, instructions couched in positive terms did enable even the youngest children to begin to search in appropriate direction. The ability to signal the recognition of a target before continuing an onward search was still being perfected even by adults.

In summary, the findings suggest that even for the youngest subjects, the deaf and the learning disabled, language has begun, however imperfectly, to serve a directive function, and with age it acquires a greater capacity to organize visual input as well as to report upon it. In the case of the young profoundly deaf children it must be remembered that their relatively poor ability use written and signed English instructions to organize visual search does not preclude the possibility that an early acquired signed language would take on the regulative function of spoken language for hearing children. Questions about the role of second language systems in the regulation of visual search remain to be explored. This research indicates the potential of eye movement measures in discovering the kind of processing changes that occur with the perceptual, cognitive and linguistic growth of the child. However, much more remains to be done using eye fixation times as well as locations to reveal how the visual system acquires functional flexibility as well as efficiency.

ACKNOWLEDGEMENTS

This research was carried out with the assistance of a grant from the Australian Research Grants Commission. The cooperation of the Victorian and Western Australian Education Departments is also gratefully acknowledged.

REFERENCES

Bauer, R.H., Short-term memory in learning disabled and nondisabled children. Journal of the Psychonomic Society, 1977, Vol. 10, 2, 128-130.

Bruner, J.S., Processes in cognitive growth: Infancy in The Heinz Werner Lecture Series, 1968, Clark University Press.

Cooper, R.M., The control of eye fixation by the meaning of spoken language. Journal of Cognitive Psychology, 1974, 6, 84-107.

Day, M.C., Developmental trends in visual scanning. Advances in Child Development and Behaviour, Vol. 10, 1975, Academic Press.

Doyle, R.B., Anderson, R.P., Halcomb, C.G. Attention deficits and the effects of visual distraction. Journal of Learning Disabilities, 1976, 9, 48-54.

Koppell, S., Testing Attentional Deficits. Journal of Learning Disabilities, Vol. 12, 1, January 1979.

Levy-Schoen, A., and Pouthas, V., Une etude experimentale du champ d'activite oculaire de l'enfant d'age pre-scolaire. Bulletin de Psychologie, 1971-72, 301, XXV, 14-17.

Luria, A.R., The role of speech in the regulation of normal and abnormal behavior. 1961, Pergamon Press Ltd.

Luria, A.R., The directive function of speech in development and dissolution, Part 1, Word, 1959, 15, 341-352.

Mackworth, N.H., and Bruner, J.S., How adults and children search and recognize pictures. Human Development, 1970, 13, 149-177.

O'Bryan, K.G., and Boersma, F., Eye movements, perceptual activity and cognitive development. Journal of Experimental Child Psychology, 1971, 12, 157-169.

Sophian, C. and Wellman, H.M., Selective information use in the development of search behavior. Journal of Developmental Psychology, 1980, 4, 323-331.

Tarver, S.G., Hallahan, D.P., Cohen, S.B., Kauffman, J.M., The development of visual selective attention andverbal rehearsal in learning disabled boys. Journal of Learning Disabilities, 1977, Vol. 10, 8, October 1977.

Vurpillot, E., The development of scanning startegies and their relation to visual differentiation. Journal of Experimental Child Psychology, 1968, 6, 632-650.

Eye Movements and Human Information Processing
R. Groner, G.W. McConkie and C. Menz (eds.)

Sequences of Eye-Movements in a Problem Solving Situation[1]

Gerd Lüer, Ronald Hübner, Uta Lass
University of Göttingen
West Germany

This study describes some aspects of subjects' behavior in a complex problem solving situation. Ss were asked to play the role of a manager who had to direct a shirt producing factory. The information about conditions in the factory for each of 15 subsequent trials was presented in a 5 by 5 matrix format on a screen in front of the S. Eye-movements were measured during the first 5 trials while the S was deciding on economic measures to be taken. Then, using spectral analytical methods, we analyzed differences between successful and unsuccessful problem solvers (N = 10) in the way they scanned the information matrix. The results indicate that successful subjects use a more harmonious information gathering strategy while unsuccessful subjects do not primarily rely on systematic information gathering strategies.

INTRODUCTION

In psychology problem solving is usually described as goal-directed behavior. In typical experimental situations problem solvers are confronted with tasks in which they have to reach a goal as a solution to an unsolved problem. In most of the studies published to date these goals were clearly described and defined for the problem solver (e.g. Newell and Simon 1972). The subject was expected to construct relationships among the conditions of the problem solving situation (problem environment), his own knowledge and his possibilities to perform. An internal representation of the problem environment had to take place in the mind of the problem solver in a so-called problem space.

In Germany during the last few years problem solving especially has been studied in complex and uncertain situations. In a typical study Ss are given computer-simulated systems as problem situations (e.g. Dörner et al. 1983, Putz-Osterloh 1983). They are asked to control the dynamically developing system and to avoid catastrophes and negative developments. Goals are not precisely specified, instead only very general characteristics of a possible solution are offered.

The Ss' first step in such a situation is to find out and formulate goals which they want to reach. This can only be done in interaction with their own knowledge and the requirements of the problem solving situation with which they are confronted. The process of gathering information about the problem environment seems to us to be of central importance. We therefore decided to study this process by the registration of eye-movements.

METHOD

In the present experiment Ss were asked to play the role of the manager of a shirt producing factory. The factory was simulated by a computer program consisting of 24 variables[2]. 11 of them could be influenced directly by the Ss. Some of the variables followed a dynamic development, changing their values without Ss' interventions. Others fluctuated stochastically.

At the start of the experiment the subject was given some initial knowledge about the situation in the simulated factory, and was then asked to improve conditions there by deciding on economic measures to increase the factory's profits. The Ss gave their decisions orally to the experimenter who fed the data into the computer. The computer then delivered the new simulated results to the subject who was again asked to decide on new interventions. In all, 15 trials were performed for each S in our study.

The information about the state of the factory in each of the 15 trials was presented in a 5 x 5 matrix format on a screen in front of the S. In this matrix we tried to avoid all combinations of variables between neighbouring cells which could be used to deduce meaningful dependent relationships.

Eye-movements were measured only during the first five trials. The x- and y-coordinates were calculated every 40 milliseconds and recorded and monitored by computer (system DEBIC 80). The eye-movements were measured by tracking the corneal reflection center with respect to the pupil center via a video camera (cf. Young and Sheena 1975).

Viewed from the S's position the midpoint of each cell of the information matrix was separated by a visual angle of 5°. Thus during fixation of one cell, adjacent cells were out of focus. A gaze was defined as an uninterrupted sequence of fixations on the same cell, defined as a circle around the midpoint of the cell.

SUBJECTS

Out of sample of 30, the data from 10 were chosen for analysis: the five classified as very successful in running the factory and the five classified as least successful.

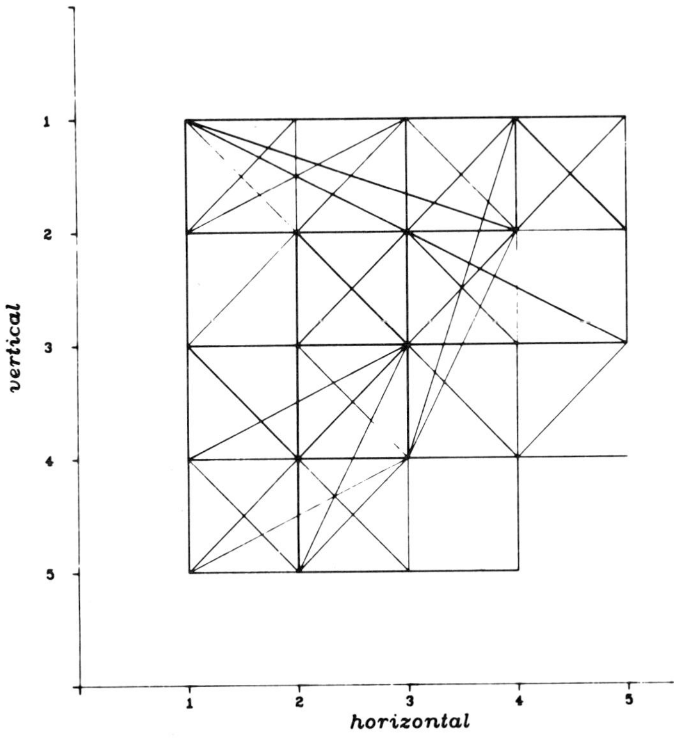

Figure 1
Eye-movements taken from a successful problem solver (+)

DATA ANALYSIS AND RESULTS

The results now presented are at the descriptive level. In a first inspection of the data we examined drawings of sequences of eye-movements. Successful Ss showed quite balanced distributions over nearly all fields of the information matrix. Unsuccessful Ss established focal points, to which they returned quite often during their visual exploration. Examples of this fact are seen in Figure 1 und 2.

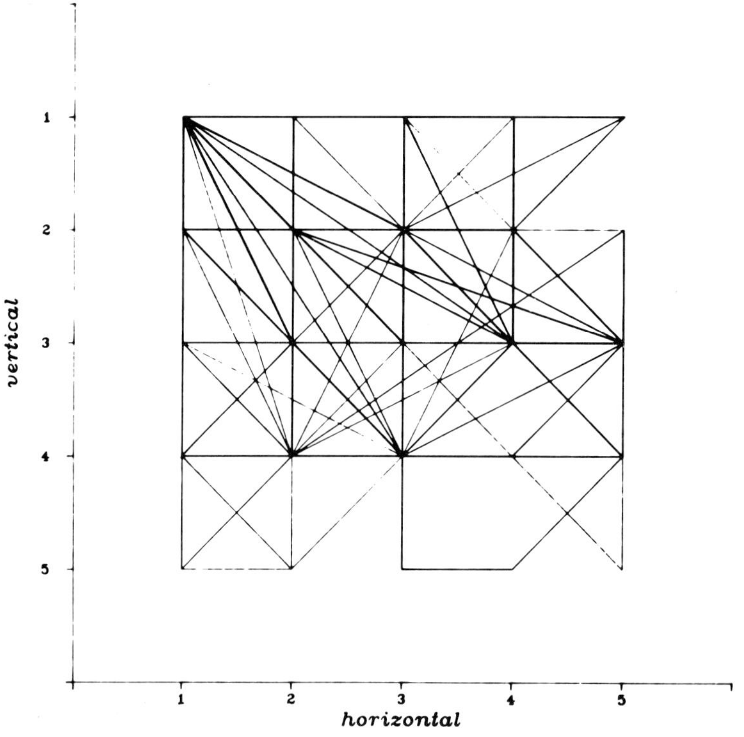

Figure 2
Eye-movements taken from an unsuccessful problem solver (-)

In a next step we looked for a method which would uncover systematic patterns in the sequences of gazes and which would take into account the whole process of the visual inspection of the information matrix. We decided to apply spectral analytical methods (Gottman 1981), and, in order to do this, we separated horizontal from vertical eye-movements, as seen in Figure 3.

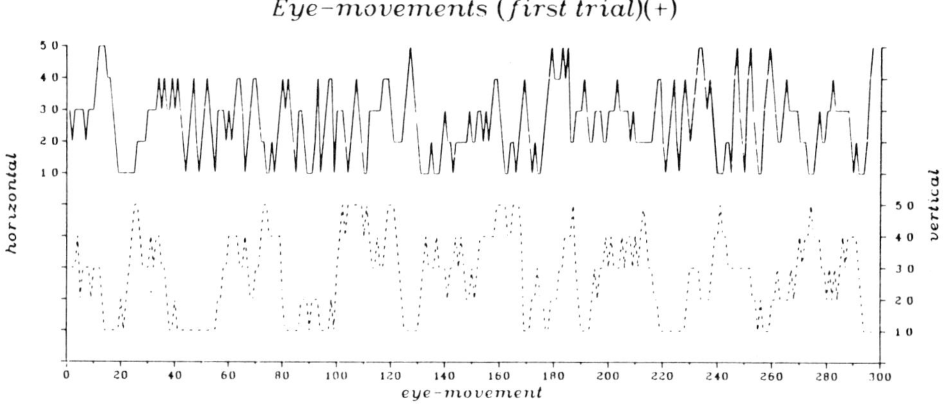

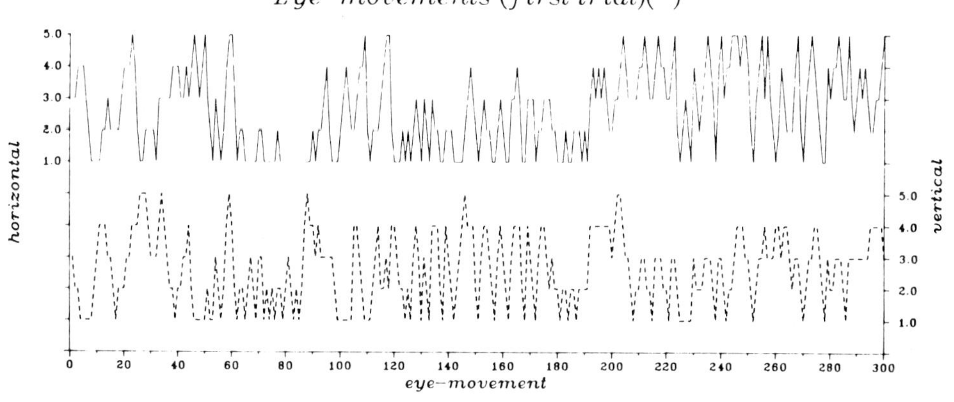

Figure 3

Horizontal and vertical eye-movements taken from a successful problem solver (+) and an unsuccessful problem solver (-)

To estimate the spectral density functions, each of the series was decomposed into orthogonal frequency components by means of a Fourier transform of the autocorrelation functions up to 50 lags. The Parzen window was chosen to smooth out the resulting power spectra. The power spectra were averaged for each group and for each of the 5 trials.

The most important results are listed below:

(1) Generally most of the variance of the series can be accounted for by waves of slow frequency. Hence, if patterns exist, they should have relatively long periodicies. This could, however, also, in part, be an effect of the separation of horizontal and vertical eye-movements.

(2) In respect to successful problem solvers:
The peaks of the power spectra do not differ remarkably in their magnitude over the first five trials. Therefore, a characterization of the successful problem solver could be as follows: The beginning of the process of problem solving is characterized by a balanced eye-movement behavior in order to scan and to select visually presented information.

In respect to unsuccessful problem solvers:
The peaks of the power spectra of this group show great differences in their magnitude. We interpret these very noticeable changes as insecurity in using large amounts of information.
A second and more interesting result is the difference in the location of the peaks. Over the first two trials the spectra of unsuccessful problem solvers peak at frequency 0. This fact indicates a linear trend in the data.
On the other hand, if we inspect the spectra of the successful problem solvers we notice a peak frequency of about 0.02 on the first trials. This means that a reoccuring pattern, which repeats itself about every 50 eye-movements, contributes the greatest portion of variance.
These results indicate a lack of pattern in the eye-movements of the unsuccessful problem solvers in contrast to the successful problem solvers who showed a greater amount of short waves in the beginning.

(3) The spectra of horizontal and vertical eye-movements have been averaged in the next figures (Figure 4 and Figure 5). Both differences already mentioned appear again in these representations, namely: (1) No remarkable differences appear in the magnitude of the peaks over the 5 trials with successful problem solvers, while distinctive differences

are noticeable in the group of unsuccessful subjects. (2) In most of the trials the spectra of the unsuccessful problem solvers indicate remarkable linear trends while the spectra of successful subjects show a greater contribution of waves with lower frequencies.

Power of eye-movements (+)

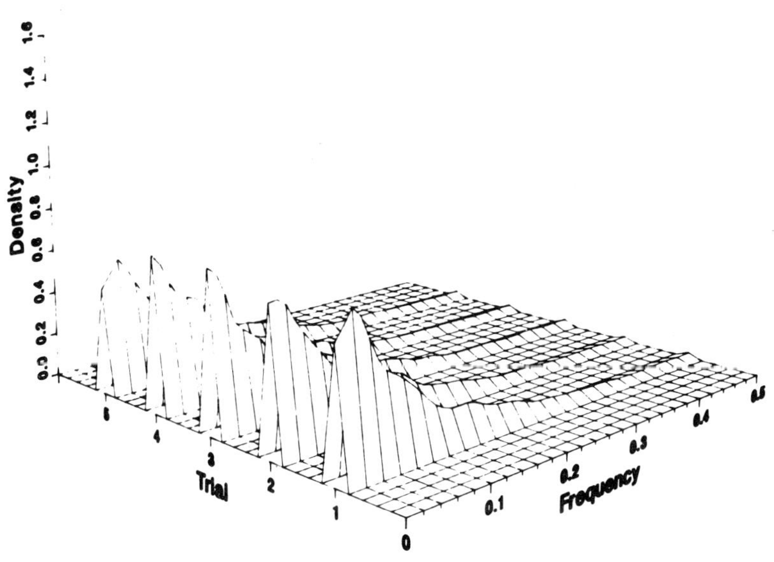

Figure 4
Power spectra of horizontal and vertical eye-movements (averaged) from 5 successful problem solvers (+)

Power of eye-movements (-)

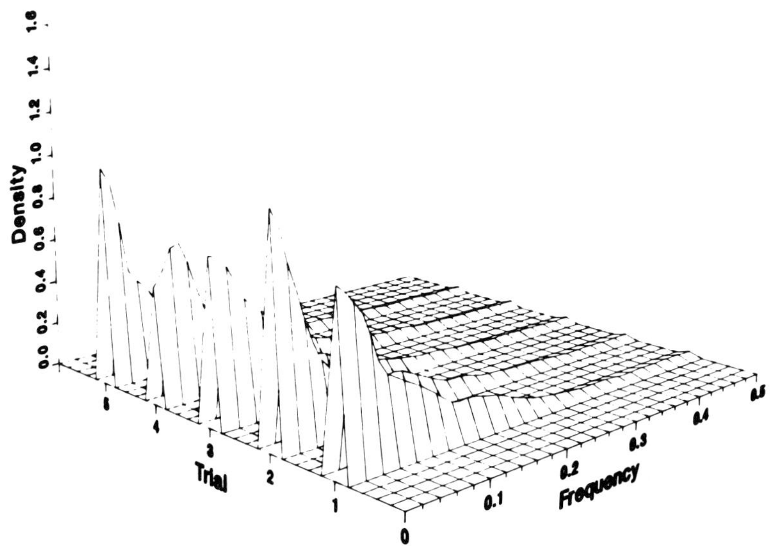

Figure 5
Power spectra of horizontal and vertical eye-movements (averaged) from 5 unsuccessful problem solvers (-)

Taken together these results could be interpreted as an indication that successful subjects use a more harmonious information gathering strategy while unsuccessful subjects do not primarily rely on systematic information gathering strategies.

CONCLUDING REMARKS

If problem solving depends on the subject's capacity to build up an internal representation of the problem environment, eye-movement research can help to understand the development of this process, as we have tried to demonstrate here. Our experiment seems to indicate that systematic and balanced explorative visual behavior is a more successful strategy for acquiring large amounts of information, useful in problem solving, than less systematic strategies.

---

[1] The study was supported by the Deutsche Forschungsgemeinschaft, Bonn-Bad Godesberg, West Germany. We would like to thank H.W.Schroiff and D.Sommer for their help in running the experiment.

[2] This program was developed by D.Dörner, University of Bamberg, West Germany.

REFERENCES

(1) Dörner, D., Kreuzig, H.W., Reither, F. and Stäudel, T. (eds.), Lohhausen. Vom Umgang mit Unbestimmtheit und Komplexität (Huber, Bern - Stuttgart - Wien, 1983).

(2) Gottmann, J.M., Time-series analysis (Cambridge University Press, Cambridge, 1981).

(3) Newell, A. and Simon, H.A., Human Problem Solving (Prentice-Hall, Englewood Cliffs N.J., 1972).

(4) Putz-Osterloh, W., Über Determinanten komplexer Problemlöseleistungen und Möglichkeiten zu ihrer Erfassung, Sprache & Kognition 2 (1983), 100 - 116.

(5) Young, L.R. and Sheena, D., Survey of eye movement recording methods, Behavior Research Methods and Instrumentation 7 (1975), 397 - 429.

Eye Movements and Human Information Processing
R. Groner, G.W. McConkie and C. Menz (eds.)

DATA ON SOLUTION STRATEGIES FROM EYE-MOVEMENT RECORDINGS

Gerhard Deffner
Department of Psychology
University of Hamburg
Federal Republic of Germany

Theoretical task analyses are presented which show that items from a test of spatial ability can be solved by the use of several strategies that require such ability to different degrees. In order to explore the use of these strategies during the performance of tasks, eye-movement data were collected from 48 subjects. Working on the assumption that there is a close link between gaze direction and attention, a computer program was developed which performs analyses of the recorded sequences of gazes in accordance with principles derived from the task analysis. In this paper, a description of these principles is given and the performance and possibilities of this approach are discussed.

INTRODUCTION

The basic idea behind intelligence tests which consist of a battery of subtests to assess different aspects of intelligence (e.g. abstract reasoning, memory, spatial reasoning, etc.) is the concept that all people working on the particular subtask will do so by using the same kinds of cognitive operations in about the same general approach to the task. That is, all subjects are assumed to be using one and the same strategy in solving the task, so that one particular set of cognitive operations needs to be performed in very much the same sequence by each and every subject. In the development of intelligence tests working with such a subtask-structure, this assumption has always been acknowledged to be crucial. The traditional approach towards evaluating this assumption has been through correlational and factor-analytic studies. Consequently, the requirement for a good subtask was that the items of any particular scale should have high loadings on one and the same factor. But this approach has one basic flaw: in computing correlations among items of a subtask and items or scales which have previously been established to measure a certain intellectual skill or ability, one does not gain additional information on the strategies used. If these previously established items or scales do not fulfill the requirement that only one strategy be possible then there is no way of telling whether the new items fulfill the same requirement. In order to avoid this circularity it is necessary to get more information about the strategies which are employed towards the solution of a given task, and it is also necessary to obtain data on the actual use of these strategies when the task is performed. This paper is meant to provide an example of such an approach using eye-movement recordings.

METHOD

Materials. The task which was used in the present study was taken from a German intelligence test (IST, Amthauer, 1953) and consists of items from the spatial subtask 'Figurenauswahl'. For the purposes of running eye-movement experiments, the layout of these tasks was changed slightly so as to present alternative solutions and a single item in one display (see Figure 1). The task of the subject is to imagine putting together the

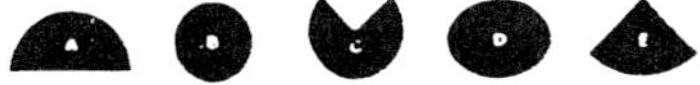

Figure 1
Experimental task

scattered geometrical shapes given as items and then judge which of the five possible solutions presented in the top row is the result of performing that assembly. Three such tasks of different degrees of difficulty (easy, intermediate, and hard) were used in the experiment, in which the task of intermediate difficulty was used for explanation and training.

Task analysis. Following Newell's (1973) injunction to "know the method the subject is using" (p. 294), preliminary trials were conducted in which subjects (psychology undergraduates from the University of Hamburg) solved these tasks as paper-and-pencil tests. After that, these subjects were asked to describe retrospectively their solution attempts. These descriptions served as a basis for the following summary of three different strategies of performing the task.

1. 'Assembly and Selection' (A+S). In this strategy, the task is performed by first concentrating all attention on the small pieces at the bottom. These pieces are assembled (by imagery) with the aim of arriving at a well-formed closed shape. Only when this has been achieved will the shapes in the row of possible solutions be examined for a match with the new shape which has been formed by imagery. This match will be selected as the solution.

2. 'Directed Assembly' (DA). There are two variations of this strategy, which share the basic feature of using shapes from the row of possible solutions to guide the assembly of pieces. In the first version of this strategy, a shape from the top row is used to 'put pieces into'. The other version of the strategy employs the same basic operation of directed assembly , but this time the pieces at the bottom are put together 'in place', that is, they are rearranged at the bottom to make a new shape on the basis of one of the shapes in the row of possible solutions.

3. 'Analytical Strategy' (AN). In this approach, the five shapes in the row of possible solutions are searched for special features that differ in frequency of occurence (i.e. the number of right angles, number or length of curved lines, etc.). By checking for the presence of these features in the small pieces at the bottom, the solution is found by eliminating those shapes in the top row which do not match the features at the bottom.

When these three strategies are compared, it is important to note that they rely on imagery to different degrees. Subjects who use strategy A+S (Assembly and Selection) claim to have a vivid picture in their mind which enables them to perform the task without any additional guidance from the possible solutions. Subjects who use strategy DA (Directed Assembly) do use information from the row of possible solutions but they claim to image the assembly of small pieces into one of the shapes. Those subjects who use strategy AN (Analytical Strategy), on the other hand, often admit that they cannot image putting these pieces together at all, and that they solve the task on the basis of comparisons of only parts of the shapes without ever forming an image of a completed figure made up from small pieces.

These large differences make it extremely important to know which strategies are used by subjects performing such a task, if tasks of this kind are to be used in the assessment of spatial ability. The reason for this is that any score based on the number of correct solutions in a given period of time could conceivably be an indication of such distinct dimensions as spatial/imagery ability <u>or</u> analytical ability. It will be shown how the above task analysis can be used for the identification of strategies.

<u>Experiment</u>. Eye-movement recordings of subjects solving the experimental tasks were obtained in the context of a larger experiment in which three other types of tasks were used as well (Deffner, 1984a). In that experiment, subjects (N = 48) were randomly assigned to one of two conditions: they either performed the tasks with concurrent thinking aloud or performed them silently. The subjects were psychology undergraduates from the University of Hamburg. There were no time constraints, subjects were simply instructed to "take as much time as is necessary for performing well". Thinking aloud subjects received additional non-directive verbalization instructions prior to each task. A task of intermediate difficulty was presented first, and questions were answered. After this, the easy and the difficult task were presented in that order. There was no interference from the experimenter during task performance. Eye-movements were monitored with a NAC IV Eye Marker and recorded on video tape. Also, a counter of video-frames (units of 1/25 second) was recorded simultaneously.

<u>Description of data</u>. The video tapes were analyzed by scoring successive video frames. Due to the low accuracy of the NAC IV Eye Marker, this was done according to a rough grid that corresponded to the areas of the different geometrical shapes in the display. This grid was drawn on transparent plastic and was obtained for each individual subject on the basis of a recorded scanning of the display (for details see Deffner, 1983). Since this mode of evaluating video-taped eye-movement recordings results in a loss of information about small saccades, the final outcome must be

understood as a sequence of 'gazes' (cf. Carpenter & Just, 1976), the duration of which could be determined from the counter in the video recording. An extremely short example of such a sequence is given in the upper part of Figure 2, where each gaze is a pair consisting of gaze direction and video frame at the beginning of that gaze. Gaze direction is expressed in terms of letter names for the five shapes in the row of possible solutions (A to E) and the letter 'F' is used to denote gazes on that part of the display where the small pieces are shown. The lower part of Figure 2 shows the same sequence after computation of gaze duration:

B24 F28 C38 D44 E48 B56 F68 B72 F76 C84 F89 C105 F117 C186 D197
B204 C212 F216 C223 D229 E234 D244 C251 B255 A261 F273 C316 B327
E331 A336 E339 END344

(B 4)(F 10)(C 6)(D 4)(E 8)(B 12)(F 4)(B 4)(F 8)(C 5)(F 16)(C 12)
(F 69)(C 11)(D 7)(B 8)(C 4)(F 7)(C 6)(D 5)(E 10)(D 7)(C 4)(B 6)
(A 12)(F 43)(C 11)(B 4)(E 5)(A 4)(E 5)

Figure 2

Example of data before and after computation of gaze durations

IDENTIFICATION OF STRATEGIES

Relating sequences to mental operations and to strategies. An important assumption must be stated upon which all of the following is based: That any sequence of gazes is closely related to concurrent central cognitive activity, so that gaze direction can be understood as an indication of what is at the focus of attention at each particular instance. That is, gaze direction is not merely taken to be a peripheral phenomenon which is part of the perceptual process. This is, of course, an assumption which is controversial, but a discussion of the issue of 'control of eye-movements' is beyond the scope of this paper.

The first step towards the development of computer programs to yield information about solution strategies was to take a closer look at the kind of eye-movements that had occurred during the solution of the experimental tasks. Generally speaking, three types could be observed: 1) Sequences of several shorter gazes in the row of possible solutions, 2) Sequences of fixations on the small parts at the bottom of the display - on the level of accuracy achieved by the NAC IV Eye Marker, these appear as one long gaze in our data; and 3) Sequences of alternating gazes between the top row and the parts at the bottom of the display. Upon closer analysis, the latter sequences could further be subdivided into three kinds: 3a) Alternations with longer gazes on the elements in the top row, 3b) Alternations with longer gazes at the small parts at the bottom, and 3c) Alternations in which gazes at the top row as well as the parts at the bottom were short. On the basis of several intensive post-experimental interviews, these five types of sequences were then related to particular mental operations during the performance of the task. Table 1 gives an overview of these operations and the symbols introduced to denote the particular eye-movement sequence.

1) Search of alternatives	=	S
2) Assembly	=	ASS
3) Alternation:		
a) assembly into top row	=	ALT/top
b) assembly at the bottom	=	ALT/bottom
c) for comparison	=	ALT

Table 1
Types of operations as related to gaze sequences

On the basis of this classification, sequences can be related to the three strategies which were described earlier in the paper; Table 2 presents that correspondence:

A+S	-	'ASS'-, and short 'S'-sequences
DA	-	'ALT/top'-, 'ALT/bottom'-, and short 'S'-sequences
AN	-	'ALT'-, and long 'S'-sequences; short 'S'-sequences if succeeded by 'ALT'-sequences; 'ASS'-sequences if succeeded by long 'S'-sequences

Table 2
Strategies as related to gaze sequences

One additional rule was added during the development of the program: if the overall sequence of gazes should begin with a sequence of type 'S', then that sequence would be labelled 'FS' on the grounds that it constitutes a first scan of the task.

Computer implementation. The program performs three steps: 1) It reduces the original sequence of gazes to sequence of gaze-sequences ('S', 'ASS', 'ALT/top', 'ALT/bottom' or 'ALT'), 2) It reduces such sequences to sequences of strategies ('A+S', 'DA', or 'AN'), and 3) It computes statistics that describe each subject's use of strategies. These three steps are described next.

Step 1: Reduction to sequences of gaze-sequences.
In this first step, the program scans the original sequence of gazes and segments this sequence in accordance with a set of rules that specify the distinctions between the five types of sequences described earlier ('S', 'ASS', 'ALT/top', 'ALT/bottom', and 'ALT'). This is performed by looking at each individual gaze and making a decision as to what sequence it could belong to. In order to make that decision it is necessary for the program to keep track of whatever sequence is currently being found, and also it is necessary to look ahead in the sequence of eye-movements. Table 3 gives a comprehensive listing of the definitions and rules that underlie these decisions. One term used in the table needs to be explained: Sequences of gazes are defined as 'alternations' if at least three gazes in an immediate sequence conform to a pattern of top/bottom/top or bottom/top/bottom (the understanding being that the 'top' element remains the same).

'S': Sequences of gazes at any element in the row of possible solutions and short gazes at the parts at the bottom. Any duration of a gaze at the lower parts of the display qualifies as 'short' if it is no more than 20 units (20 frames = .8 seconds) longer than the mean duration of gazes in type 'S'-sequences which have already been

Table 3
Definitions of gaze-sequences

identified in the overall sequence. If there are no sequences of that type as yet, then an initial mean value of 10 units is used until a true mean duration can be computed. This mean gaze duration in typs 'S' sequences is updated whenever a new sequence of that type has been identified.

'ASS': Gazes at the to-be-assembled parts at the bottom of the display that have a duration of more than 20 units above the mean duration of gazes in type 'S' sequences.

'ALT/top': Alternations of gazes in which the mean duration of gazes at the element in the top row is longer than the duration of gazes at the bottom elements (within that alternation) and also longer than the mean duration in type 'S' sequences.

'ALT/bottom' Alternations of gazes in which the mean duration of gazes at the elements at the bottom of the display is longer than the duration of gazes at the elements in the top row (within that alteration) and also longer than the mean gaze duration in type 'S' sequences.

'ALT': Alternations of gazes in which the conditions for 'ALT/top' or 'ALT/bottom' are not fulfilled, that is, in which all gazes are short.

Table 3
Definitions of gaze-sequences (continued)

At the beginning of the search through each sequence, there is a good chance that no mean duration of gazes in type 'S' sequences has been computed, because there may not have been such a sequence up to that point in the sequence of gazes. In such cases, alternations are labelled as either 'ALT/top' or 'ALT/bottom' depending on whether gaze durations within that sequence are longer for the top elements or for the bottom ones.

One problem of this approach is that some of the criteria for classification overlap (e.g. type 'ALT/bottom' sequences contain type 'ASS' gazes). For this reason, a fixed priority ordering was incorporated into the program: it tries to find alternations before classifying any sequence or gazes as either 'S' or 'ASS'. Figure 3 gives an example of a sequence of gazes and the result of reducing that sequence on the basis of the above definitions in Table 3.

Input to Step 1:
(B 4)(F 10)(C 6)(D 4)(E 8)(B 12)(F 4)(B 4)(F 8)(C 5)(F 16)(C 12)
(F 69)(C 11)(D 7)(B 8)(C 4)(F 7)(C 6)(D 5)(E 10)(D 7)(C 4)(B 6)
(A 12)(F 43)(C 11)(B 4)(E 5)(A 4)(E 5)

Output of Step 1:
(S 32 5)(ALT-TOP 28 4)(ALT-BOTTOM 113 5)(S 15 2)(ALT 17 3)
(S 44 6)(ASS 43 1)(S 29 5)

Figure 3
Example of Step 1

The sequence in the bottom part of Figure 3 consists of parentheses that contain the label for that particular type of sequence, the duration of that sequence (in units of 1/25 of a second) and the number of gazes in that sequence.

Step 2: Relating sequence types to strategies.
As was outlined in Table 2, the different sequences can be related to the different solution strategies. The rationale for this is that only certain sequences of gazes are compatible with each particular strategy. Expressing Table 2 as rules that can be used by the program in order to relate sequences to strategies is quite straightforward: It only requires definite criteria for decisions on whether type 'S' sequences are 'short' or 'long'. The criterion used in the program is: sequences containing up to three gazes are called 'short' and sequences containing more than three gazes are 'long'.

In performing this second step, the program takes as input the sequence of gaze-sequences produced in Step 1 and then successively groups all those sequences which conform to one and the same strategy. Also, one change is made at this stage: if there should be a first sequence of type 'S' (search) then that sequence is dropped from further analysis on the grounds that it is not really part of any strategy, but rather a first scan of the display to understand the task. For this reason, the type 'S' sequence at the beginning of the sequence output from Step 1 is dropped prior to further identification of strategies. A continuation of the example is presented in Figure 4, which shows the input and output of Step 2.

```
Input to Step 2:
(ALT-TOP 28 4)(ALT-BOTTOM 113 5)(S 15 2)(ALT 17 3)(S 44 6)
(ASS 43 1)(S 29 5)

Output of Step 2:
(DA  (ALT-TOP 28 4)(ALT-BOTTOM 113 5))
(AN  (S 15 2)(ALT 17 3)(S 44 6)(ASS 43 1)(S 29 5))
```

Figure 4
Example of Step 2

As can be seen from Figure 4, all that happens during Step 2 is that sequences which belong to the same strategy are combined into a list with the name of the strategy at the beginning of that list. Thus, the output of the example can be interpreted such that the task was first approached according to the 'Directed Assembly' strategy, and after that, the 'Analytical Strategy' was employed.

Step 3: Statistics to describe strategy use.
For the purposes of traditional statistical data analysis, the program outputs numerical values that describe the use of strategies. These values give information about how much of the total solution time was spent using each of the three strategies. Also, the number of strategy shifts is recorded. In order to provide information which can be used in between subject comparisons, relative measures are used. That is, the proportion of total solution time is computed for each strategy and the number of strategy shifts is given as strategy shifts per fixed amount of time. But apart from using these numerical descriptions, it is also possible to obtain the output of Step 2 if information about the sequence

of strategies is of interest.

Validity of strategy identification. The crucial question is, of course, how much importance can be attached to the analysis described in this paper. This question is a tricky one, because it requires something to compare the output of the program to. Unfortunately, there are very few options, which can be grouped under the two headings of: 1) circumstantial evidence, and 2) verbal reports. An earlier attempt at using circumstantial evidence was reported in Deffner (1984a). There, solution time was correlated with the output of the program for the 24 subjects of the silent group. The underlying idea was that strategies differ with respect to the time required for their execution and thus there should be correlations between solution times and the use of fast or slow strategies. The flaw in this reasoning was uncovered in a more recent, as yet unpublished study (Deffner, 1984b), in which subjects were trained in the use of one of the strategies described above. The results indicate an interaction of ability with selection of strategy. This finding can be interpreted such that subjects who can perform these tasks quickly will be those who can, for each experimental task, select that strategy which is best suited to their individual ability, i.e. choose an analytical strategy if they have higher analytical than spatial ability and vice versa. Correlating proportions of strategy use with solution times therefore confounds the time requirements of the various strategies with individual ability. For this reason, the following, more sophisticated argument is suggested:

Solution times can be examined under conditions where the use of strategies was induced by experimental variation that affected all subjects. In such a case, different levels of ability or different skills in the selection of strategies would contribute random error. This idea can be pursued on the basis of data from the thinking-aloud vs. thinking-in-silence variations: There was a tendency for the thinking-aloud group to spend a higher proportion of their solution time using the 'Directed Assembly' strategy. This finding was interpreted to be an indication that think-aloud subjects tend to be more thorough (Deffner, 1984a), although because of the very high variances, this difference is a weak one. Also, solution time was longer in the think-aloud group. If these findings are taken together, it can be argued that task performance with an experimentally induced higher proportion of the 'Directed Assembly' strategy is slower. This fits in well with introspective reports from subjects and own experience with these tasks. But it is necessary to make some qualifications of this: the longer solution times of the thinking-aloud group may not have been related to the use of a more time-consuming strategy but to some other effects brought about by thinking-aloud - the argument therefore admittedly is somewhat circular.

In the other approach, verbal reports were compared to the program output. This presents problems too, for the validity of verbal reports has been questioned (cf. Nisbett and Wilson, 1977). A discussion of this is beyond the scope of this paper, and it must be sufficient to say that 'verbal reports' in this context do <u>not</u> mean subjects' reports about their use of strategies but protocols of concurrent thinking-aloud of a kind which is discussed by Ericsson and Simon (1984). The comparison was performed for protocols from the performance of the difficult task, because only these were sufficiently long. For purposes of comparison, two extreme sets were selected: six protocols from task performances for which the proportion of use of the 'DA' strategy was in the upper quartile of the respective numerical program output and six protocols for which the proportion of use of the 'AN' strategy was in the upper quartile. Only these two strategies were considered, because the use of the third strategy (A+S) was not very frequent. These protocols were then evaluated as to which of the strategies was the dominant one. Table 4 shows the results:

	dominant strategy in protocol			
	A+S	DA	AN	unclear
six cases of high % DA	0	4	1	1
six cases of high % AN	1	0	5	0

Table 4

Program output vs. strategies in protocols

As can be seen, there is considerable overlap between the evaluation of protocols and the output of the program.

DISCUSSION

The procedure outlined in this paper is not understood to be a general, well proven technique which can readily be used. Rather, it is at an experimental stage, and therefore should be seen as an example of what may prove to be a fruitful type of analysis. Like many other techniques which are used to uncover the psychological relevance behind empirical data, it requires two main ingredients, one theoretical and one technical: 1) the basic assumption about the relation of gaze direction to attention, and 2) the computer implementation of principles derived from task analyses. Both issues should be scrutinized thoroughly, because the use of the technique entails the acceptance of the decisions made on these issues. What is important about the method in its present form is that it explores at least one possible route towards the in-depth study of what subjects do when they perform tasks of this kind, which are typically found in routine psychological assessment. Seen in this light, the main purpose of this study is to demonstrate the feasibility of research on solution strategies.

REFERENCES

Amthauer, R. (1953). Intelligenz-Struktur-Test. Göttingen: Hogrefe.

Carpenter, P.A. & Just, M.A. (1976). Eye fixations and cognitive processes. Cognitive Psychology, 8, 441-480.

Deffner, G. (1983). Verbesserung der Messgenauigkeit der NAC IV [Improving the accuracy of the NAC IV eye-movement recorder]. (Arbeiten aus dem Fachbreich Psychologie der Universität Hamburg, No 55) Hamburg: Department of Psychology.

Deffner, G. (1984a). Lautes Denken - Untersuchung zur Qualität eines Datenerhebungsverfahrens [Thinking-aloud - a study of the quality of a research instrument]. Frankfurt: Lang.

Deffner, G. (1984b). Spatial tasks: Strategy and ability. (Manuscript in preparation).

Ericsson, K.A. & Simon, H.A. (1984). Protocol analysis. Cambridge: MIT Press.

Newell, A. (1973). You can't play 20 questions with nature and win. In W.G. Chase (ed.), Visual information processing. New York: Academic.

Nisbett, R.E. & Wilson, T.D. (1977). Telling more than we can know: Verbal reports on mental processes. Psychological Review, 84, 231-259.

III.

APPLIED AREAS

Eye Movements and Human Information Processing
R. Groner, G.W. McConkie and C. Menz (eds.)

APPLIED AREAS

Introduction

This final part of the book provides a selection of five contributions involving the eye movement methodology in various applied areas. Some contributions are promising examples that eye movement recording is a well applicable technique to investigate even highly complex processes in their constituent parts of information acquisition. By the same token research data from applied areas show clearly that many essential links between theory and results are still missing in foundamental research.

The first paper by S.I. Andersson attempts to separate two clinical groups, psychotic patients and alcohol abusers from each other and from normal controls according to their eye tracking behavior. The small number of individuals in each group and their comparatively large individual differences make it a priori clear that any results of such a study are to be considered preliminary and should be crossvalidated. This study provides a good example of the situation where there exists a large body of data of only a few subjects which must be compressed to statistics and processed by various methods of data analysis.

The following papers are concerned with the functioning of the saccadic system in some search and reading tasks. The inspection of radiographs with their comparatively high rate of misses is a challenging area for applied eye movement research. The goal is to provide explanations for suboptimal behavior as well as suggestions for improving search performance. In his paper, D.P. Carmody starts from a careful review of earlier studies using different techniques and then proceeds to related research with other tasks. The final model is consistent with Hochberg's ideas of two interacting systems, the cognitive search guidance, based on a schematic map of expected information, and the peripheral search guidance, based on additional information from peripheral vision.

A very interesting stimulus which combines pictorial, symbolic and verbal information is given by a geographic map. The processes involved in map reading are the object of a study by J.R. Antes, K.T. Chang, T. Lenzen and C. Mullis. In a first experiment, they compared the eye movements in well balanced and poorly balanced thematic maps. They found that areas in the poorly balanced maps received fewer fixations than the corresponding parts of the well balanced maps. This difference was only found during the first part of the global scanpath. In a second experiment experienced and inexperienced users of topographic maps were compared. The authors conclude that the selective aspect of visual attention is influenced primarily by the informativeness of a stimulus part, and the intensive aspect is influenced mainly by the complexity of that part. But neither informativeness nor complexity can be defined without taking into account the particular subject and given task. These conclusions agree with the results of the paper by Groner & Menz on scanning patterns (section II.B) where exactly this kind of interactions was found.

Movies with subtitles provide information for three input channels with the pictures, the sound and the subtitling. The main purpose of the paper by d'Ydewalle, Muylle and van Rensbergen is to examine the attention shift in situations with considerable information overlap. They varied presentation time and amount of text in subtitles. They found that the proportion of time spent in the subtitled area decreases with increasing presentation time. More time is spent on the two text lines compared to one line. The viewing times, on the other hand, were increasing with an increase in projection time of subtitles. An inspection of the eye movement patterns showed that reading is reduced to an encoding of single keywords. They concluded that the encoding of information resolves around an interactive perceptual cycle where peripheral vision is an important issue. Information from the story structure and from understanding parts of the audio channel guides the efficient processing of keywords in subtitles.

The paper by H.T. Zwahlen, A.L. Hartmann, S.L. Rangarajulu and L.M. Escontrela is concerned with ergonomics and video display terminals. Two exploratory experiments were conducted measuring the scanning behavior and performance of experienced typists. High visual activity was observed for tasks characterized by much information acquisition and processing demands. Long dwell times were required for the document representing the data entry and for the screen where errors had to be detected and corrected. Short dwell times were spent on the keyboard. A variety of visual strategies were applied. But a relation between the manifold visual strategies and specific task requirements could not be found.

Are there results in this book that are consistent enough to be considered as the basic elements of a more general model of visual information selection? Are there results that allow predictions for new application areas? Reviewing the chapters in this book with these questions in mind one sees that finding a synopsis for all these data is preserved to the reader and to future research.

Eye Movements and Human Information Processing
R. Groner, G.W. McConkie and C. Menz (eds.)

EYE TRACKING PERFORMANCE AND ATTENTION IN ALCOHOL ABUSERS, PSYCHOTIC PATIENTS AND NORMALS - TOWARDS A MULTIDIMENSIONAL MODEL

SVEN INGMAR ANDERSSON
Department of Psychology, Lund University
S-223 50 Lund
and
Health Sciences Centre, Lund University
S-240 10 Dalby
SWEDEN

Pendular eye tracking performance of alcohol abusers (n=3), psychotics (n=4) and normals (n=7) was studied, using electrooculography, the alcohol abusers being tested 3, 9 and 10 times, respectively, over an extended period. An electronic pendulum involving a "moving" light of constant speed was employed, there being two tasks, one less and the other more attention-demanding (red light only vs. having to press a button each time the light changed to green). Noise/signal ratio, deviation area and microtremor rate were calculated. Results indicate psychotic patients to be high on both noise/signal ratio and deviation area compared with normals. Alcohol abusers appeared to be low in microtremor rate when in a sober condition but to show a marked increase in microtremor rate to a level well above that of normals and psychotics when under the influence of alcohol. In the alcohol abuser group, an increase in cognitive strain was found to produce an improvement in performance in terms of noise/signal ratio and a decrement in performance in terms of deviation area. This apparent discrepancy was interpreted as indicating cognitive strain to increase deviations from correct following at a level intermediate between the coarser deviations measured by noise/signal ratio and the finer ones measured by microtremor. Evidence from one of the normals tested when in a highly stressed state, who showed a drastic increase in microtremor rate over time, suggested effects of stress on microtremor. Analyzing separately the results of each subject's most recent testing, a special computer program developed so as to more systematically study the various types of deviation from smooth eye tracking was employed. From the eye position curve the program computed sliding means over 16- and 128-point intervals, respectively, so as to produce two smoothed curves interpreted as being fine and coarse representations of subjective stimulus. Registering deviations of the recordings upwards or downwards from these two curves allowed a detailed analysis of differences between the subject groups in their manner of following the stimulus position. Cluster analysis of the results succeeded quite well in distinguishing on the three-cluster level between three groups, representing the two alcohol abusers who were acutely intoxicated, the four psychotics, and the seven normals together with an alcohol abuser who had been sober for some time. At the five-cluster level the latter subject and one of the normals formed a cluster. Analysis of the results for the various measures, considered separately, also suggested marked differences in eye tracking between the subject groups.

Introduction

Several studies have shown eye tracking impairments to be more characteristic of schizophrenics than of other diagnostic groups (for a review see Lipton et al. 1983). However, impairments similar to those found in schizophrenia have been reported to occur in other diseases, as well as in certain drug-induced states (e.g., Corvera et al. 1973, Drischel 1968, Flom et al. 1976, Holzman et al. 1975, Levy et al. 1981). In eye tracking studies involving 19 psychotic patients (predominantly schizophrenics and cycloid psychotics, Andersson 1983b) and 20 alcohol abusers (Andersson 1984), the present author found none of the overall macro-level noise/signal ratio and deviation area measures employed to distinguish between the two groups. Both types of measures were responsive to situational changes, however, performance being found to be better under more than under less attention-demanding conditions, a result obtained for both groups in terms of noise/signal ratio, but for the alcohol abuser and not the psychotic patient group in terms of deviation area. Macro squarewave jerks were found to be more frequent in alcohol abusers than in psychiatric patients. Regarding microtremor level, Andersson 1983a found hebephrenics to have a significantly higher microtremor rate than non-hebephrenic schizophrenics and cycloid psychotics, a small reference group of normals (n=4) falling within the range of the latter two groups. In a more recent investigation, Andersson 1984 found microtremor rate to be categorically higher in psychotic patients generally than in alcohol abusers. The results just cited call for further study in order to clarify the apparent relationships involved and explore various questions they raise.

STUDY I

Test-retest data reported in Andersson (1983b and 1984) suggested certain eye tracking dysfunctions at the microlevel to be characteristic of psychotics generally. Nevertheless, the question of the stability over time of the microtremor rate results obtained, remains. To explore this question, particularly in the alcohol abuser group, two of the 20 alcohol abusers studied earlier and reported on in Andersson (1984) were followed for a period of approximately a month, one of the subjects being tested nine times and the other ten times during this period. In addition, about three months later these same two subjects were tested again together with a third person, who was also from the group of alcohol abusers tested originally. Results from these three subjects were compared with those of four psychotic outpatients (three of whom were diagnosed as schizophrenics) and of seven normal subjects. Microtremor rate was of primary interest, although measures of noise/signal ratio and deviation area were also obtained for each of the subjects.

Method

Recording Procedure Details of the testing procedures are given in Andersson (1983b). Eye movements were registered in the AC mode, using a mingograph. Silver-silver chloride electrodes were placed at the outer canthi for horizontal recording and above and below the right eye for recording blinks. A ground electrode was attached to the middle of the forehead. Placement of electrodes for horizontal recording aimed at controlling blinks in the recordings. Calibration was facilitated by having subjects shift their gaze several times between the two endpoints of the pendulum. The mingographic preamplifier drove a Tandberg FM tape recorder; it was RC-coupled to balance out DC voltage, with a high pass and low pass filter (cut-off frequencies 0.16 and 30 Hz, respectively) for noise reduction.

The electronic pendulum involved a "moving" light of constant speed, provided by special light diodes which lit up either red or green. The tracking task consisted of three parts. In the first part (60 sec) the target light was red. In the second part, involving 180 secs of tracking following a 60 sec pause, the light changed temporarily to green at short irregular intervals. Subjects were to press a button each time the light changed to green; a green segment, when occurring, comprised a one quarter "swing" of the pendulum in the one direction or the other. The third tracking part, 60 sec in length following a 30-sec pause, involved a red stimulus only.

Measures Obtained Data processing for any given subject followed Andersson (1983b, 1984) and was carried out for each of the four slightly over 30-sec segments of the total tracking task separately, such a segment comprising slightly more than 12 pendular cycles. Period 1 represented the initial segment of the first red-light only tasks, Period 2 the initial segment of the two red-and-green tasks, Period 3 a segment of the latter task commencing 90 seconds after the end of Period 2, and Period 4 the initial segment of the second red-light only tracking task. Tape-recorded signals were digitized at a rate of 8,192 sampling points for each segment. Data-processing involved computing eye position from electrical voltage at each of the sampling points; a correction was employed for drift, consisting of subtracting from the electrical voltage its mean value within each cycle. Each recording segment was shortened to exactly 12 cycles, a preliminary Fourier analysis being used in identifying cycles.

The following measures were obtained for each of the four periods: (1) Noise/signal ratio: the ratio between the sum of the squared amplitudes of the 2nd to 6th harmonics, and the squared amplitude of the major wave (1st harmonic). A low value, as regards this measure, indicates the subject to be following the pendulum closely. (2) Deviation area: the area between the two curves, describing the movements of the pendulum and of the subject's eyes, respectively. A low value here too indicates the subject to be following the pendulum closely. (3) Microtremor rate: (d(tot)-d(eff))/d(eff), where d(tot) represents the total distance and d(eff) the "effective" distance the eye covered, d(tot) and d(eff) representing the sum of all small eye movements as measured by recording eye position at 3.66 msec intervals, and at intervals nine times larger (33 msec), respectively.

For each measure above, a summary measure of subject's overall tracking performance (OTP) was calculated, as were two difference scores. Dif-1, which is the difference (1+4)-(2+3), where the numbers refer to the successive periods, indicates the effect of changing from the less attention-demanding conditions (red-light only) to the more demanding (changing light color). Dif-2, which is the difference (1+2)-(3+4), represents the effect of practice.

Subjects Of the alcohol abusers reported on in Andersson (1984), two subjects, designated (just as they were in Andersson 1984) as subjects 5 and 6 (aged 34 and 32 years, respectively), were selected randomly from the group of alcohol abusers available in the clinic at the time and were asked to appear in the clinic at least twice each week for continued testing. Prior to this arrangement, both subjects had been tested twice (Andersson, op. cit.), subject 5 being re-tested on the first and subject 6 on the second day after the initial testing; both subjects had imbibed heavily prior to the initial testing but had not consumed alcohol since then. The extended period of testing embraced one month for subject 5, and 16 days for subject 6, the former subject being tested seven times and the latter eight times during that period. For both subjects, the extended period of testing became terminated through their relapse into a new period of abuse. Subject 6 was tested once at the end of this period of heavy alcohol abuse, during which he reported having drunk at least 75 cl 40% ethanol daily. Subject 5, who had been administered a single dose of benzodiazepine derivates on the second testing occasion, received no medicine until four days prior to the ninth testing, when another dose of benzodiazepine derivates was administered. Subject 6 who had been without medicine during at least a week prior to the first testing, was administered klomeliazole and benzodiazepine derivates two days prior to the second testing and was still on benzodiazepine derivates when tested the third time; prior to the fourth testing, he had been without the drug for three days, no medication being given him then until just prior to the tenth testing, when he was put back on benzodiazepine derivates .

After an extended period without testing, some 3 months after testing had commenced, subjects 5 and 6 were tested once more. At this time, subject 6 declared he had drunk no alcohol for a week, whereas subject 5 reported having drunk at least 20 cl of 40% ethanol just a few hours before testing. The latter was accompanied by subject 3 (age 43 years), who had been tested twice before; though cooperative, this subject was even more acutely intoxicated by ethanol than subject 5, declaring he had drunk about 35 cl of 40% ethanol just one hour before. None of the three subjects were on additional drugs at this testing occasion.

Of the four psychiatric out-care patients (referred to here as subjects 21-24) subject 21 (male, age 32 years) was diagnosed as a schizophrenic of the simplex type, subject 22 (female, age 42.6 years) as a psychotic of the undifferentiated type, subject 23 (male, age 55.3 years) as a schizophrenic of the undifferentiated type, and subject 24 (female, age 28.8 years) as a schizophrenic of the hebephrenic type. Subjects 21, 23 and 24 were on phenothiazine-derivates, whereas subject 22 was on a tricyclic antidepressive. In addition, subject 21 was receiving an anticholinergic.

As to the seven normals (subjects 25-31, mean age = 37.6 years, s.d. = 6.9), all were recruited among the personnel of the health care center at which the investigation was carried out. Six of these subjects were male and one (subject 29) was female. None of them reported use of drugs at the time of testing. One of the normals, subject 31, appeared at the laboratory in a very stressed condition, due to having to get to another appointment afterwards. As time passed he appeared increasingly worried about being late, although the experiment was not interrupted.

Results

OTP-scores: Table 1 shows results for overall tracking performance on each testing occasion for the three alcohol abusers (subject 3, 5 and 6 tested three, nine and ten times, respectively), the four psychotic patients (tested once) and the seven normals (tested once).

Each of the psychotic patients and one of the alcohol abusers (subject 5) scored higher on noise/signal ratio than did any of the normals, the superiority of this latter subject compared to each of the normals being found on each of the ten testing occasions. The latter subject´s scores on this variable were at their lowest level when the subject was directly under the influence of ethanol (testing 5:10). A similar tendency was evident in subject 3, who only scored within the range of the normals when highly intoxicated (testing 3:3), scoring higher than all of the normals on the other two testings.

Deviation area was found to be higher in all four psychotic patients than in any of the seven normals, whereas in alcohol abusers that measure showed considerable fluctuations. Those two alcohol abusers who were tested repeatedly over an extended period of time and were partially on benzodiazepine medication (subjects 5 and 6) were found in intraindividual comparisons to show consistently lower

TABLE 1

OTP-scores, Dif-1- and Dif-2-values
of alcohol abusers, psychotic patients and normals

No. of subject and testing	Noise/signal ratio			Deviation area			Microtremor rate		
	OTP-score	Dif-1-score	Dif-2-score	OTP-score	Dif-1-score	Dif-2-score	OTP-score	Dif-1-score	Dif-2-score
ALCOHOL ABUSERS									
3:1	.523	+.243	-.117	1.379	+.213	-.317	5.030	-.182	+.152
:2	.448	+.112	-.026	1.684	+.392	+.164	3.837	-.183	+.085
:3	.363	-.047	-.039	2.600	-.344	+.062	9.806	-.554	+.772
5:1	.664	+.270	+.046	1.460	+.486	-.140	2.013	-.277	+.129
:2	1.057	-.091	-.185	1.354	-.272	-.078	2.855	+.043	-.053
:3	.730	+.218	-.174	1.971	+.253	-.525	2.258	-.272	+.176
:4	.604	+.224	-.062	2.169	-.019	-.257	7.753	-.737	-.681
:5	.804	-.064	+.110	1.874	-.178	+.146	1.742	+.020	-.004
:6	.652	+.170	-.026	1.874	-.054	-.360	5.063	+.059	-.020
:7	.674	+.050	-.042	1.749	-.273	-.295	3.858	+.024	+.024
:8	.531	+.095	-.011	1.642	-.262	-.044	2.632	-.134	-.036
:9	.547	+.071	+.125	1.405	-.021	+.052	2.994	-.118	-.118
:10	.522	+.072	-.050	1.699	-.027	-.079	10.637	-.259	-.197
6:1	.437	+.081	+.001	1.392	+.290	-.014	2.533	+.003	-.075
:2	.329	+.017	-.029	.910	-.058	+.196	2.974	-.068	+.094
:3	.328	+.094	-.038	.942	-.010	-.236	2.218	-.086	+.128
:4	.485	+.069	-.095	.935	-.049	-.099	2.122	-.014	+.204
:5	.366	-.008	-.008	.806	-.082	-.082	2.945	+.089	+.361
:6	.408	+.050	-.006	.954	-.090	-.068	2.984	-.003	-.122
:7	.580	+.002	+.052	1.210	-.062	-.078	3.046	+.094	+.244
:8	.385	+.017	+.003	.761	-.083	-.069	3.577	-.110	+.159
:9	.430	+.014	-.016	.897	-.089	+.079	4.937	+.109	+.317
:10	.408	-.008	-.012	1.052	+.028	-.032	2.936	-.100	-.214
:11	.388	+.024	-.022	1.460	+.104	+.196	4.884	+.022	+.302
PSYCHOTIC PATIENTS									
21:1	.485	+.177	-.061	1.661	+.631	-.419	8.483	-.465	+1.051
22:1	.457	-.021	-.061	1.840	-.504	-.142	7.765	-.877	-.149
23:1	.466	-.036	+.040	2.459	+.167	+.781	6.466	+.598	+.862
24:1	.418	+.066	+.026	1.854	+.391	-.013	5.812	-.010	-.012
NORMALS									
25:1	.330	+.032	±.000	1.169	+.055	-.205	7.865	+.039	+.109
26:1	.382	+.012	+.012	1.073	+.155	+.109	6.916	-.006	+.098
27:1	.319	+.029	+.007	1.277	-.017	+.081	6.521	+.013	+.303
28:1	.416	+.018	+.010	1.168	-.102	-.272	6.171	+.155	+.065
29:1	.294	+.022	-.008	1.461	-.305	-.063	7.363	-.087	+.257
30:1	.311	-.017	-.033	1.189	+.029	-.031	7.259	-.409	+.515
31:1	.274	+.037	+.015	1.266	+.036	-.184	8.416	-.176	-1.246

deviation area scores while on the medication.

No differences were found between psychotic patients and normals on OTP-measures of microtremor rate. Microtremor rate in alcohol abusers showed considerable fluctuations over testing occasions but was generally relatively low except under conditions of acute intoxication, also being low when the subjects were on benzodiazepine derivates (subjects 5 and 6 at testings 5:2, 5:9, 6:2 and 6:3). In alcohol abusers who were acutely intoxicated (subjects 3 and 10, testings 3:3 and 5:10, respectively), however, microtremor rate increased to levels well above those registered in psychotic patients and normals. When tested about a day after a drinking period had ended, subjects 5 and 6 alike scored comparatively low on this measure (testings 5:1, 6:1 and 6:10). A similarly low microtremor rate was also found in those alcohol abusers for whom there was no sign of their having consumed alcohol for several days or weeks.

Dif-1 and Dif-2 scores relating to noise/signal ratio. Noise/signal ratio performance of the alcohol abusers was better generally under the more than under the less attention-demanding conditions, as shown by the Dif-1 scores being predominantly positive. Similar results were also found for six of the seven normals, although their improvement under the more attention-demanding conditions was only slight. Of the four psychiatric patients, two showed marked improvement and two a slight decrease in performance under the more attention-demanding conditions. As to Dif-2, the three alcohol abusers showed performance impairment over time, 18 out of their 24 scores being negative, whereas for the normals and the psychotic patients no clear tendencies of this sort were found.

Dif-1 and Dif-2 scores relating to deviation area. No clear tendencies regarding Dif-1 scores were found for the normal and psychotic groups. In 17 of the 24 records of the alcohol abusers Dif-1 scores indicated performance in terms of deviation area to deteriorate under the more attention demanding condition. A tendency for performance to deteriorate over time (Dif-2 scores) was noted in the alcohol abusers, and such a tendency was also noted in 5 of the 7 normals and in 3 of the 4 psychotic patients.

Dif-2 scores relating to microtremor rate were found in the normal group to be predominantly positive (6+, 1-), indicating a decrease in microtremor rate over time. Subject 31, who appeared at the laboratory in a highly stressed state, was the only normal subject who increased his microtremor rate over time, his increase being quite drastic.

Discussion

Psychotic patients appear to be high on both noise/signal ratio and deviation area compared with normals, but do not differ from normals as regards microtremor rate. Alcohol abusers in turn appear to show low microtremor rate when in a sober condition but to show a marked increase in microtremor rate to approxiomately the level of normals and psychotics when under the influence of alcohol. Thus, different mechanisms appear to be involved in the eye-tracking deficiencies of psychotics and alcohol abusers. One can speculate that for alcohol abusers the rise in microtremor rate to about the level of normals, which the use of large quantities of alcohol has as an immediate effect, may serve some functional end. It would be of interest to know whether their low microtremor rate when not intoxicated is produced by their long-term alcohol abuse or is inherited.

All of the three types of measures just considered--noise/signal ratio, deviation area and microtremor rate--appear sensitive to the effects of an increase in cognitive strain and of fatigue, as shown by the respective Dif-1 and Dif-2 measures. In both the normal and alcohol abuser groups an increase in cognitive strain was found to yield an improvement in performance as far as the noise/signal ratio measure was concerned. In the case of deviation area measure the result for the alcohol abusers appeared to be just the opposite, performance showing a decrement under conditions of increased cognitive strain. The apparent discrepancy here can be interpreted as a difference in the type of performance decrements involved, where the decrements are of a more coarse nature in the case of noise/signal ratio, which takes account of the first six harmonics only, whereas deviation area can be said to include decrements of a greater number of types. In alcoholics, therefore, an increase in cognitive strain, although producing a decrease in coarser deviations from correct pursuit, appears to yield an increase in total deviations. The latter effect can be assumed to be based on an increase in deviations at an intermediate level between that of the first six harmonics and of microtremor.

The finding that for normals the improvement in performance shown on the noise/signal ratio measure under the more attention demanding conditions was only slight compared to that in the alcohol abusers, can be seen as based on the fact that for the normal subjects, who already tracked quite well under the less attention demanding conditions, there was less room for improvement. The result that the normal subject who was highly stressed showed the highest microtremor rate of any of the normals and that his microtremor rate increased dramatically over time, despite his noise/signal ratio scores indicating his tracking at the macrolevel to be the best among the normal subjects who were tested, suggested that stress tends to strongly affect specifically microtremor. The subject in question appeared to have achieved high performance at one level (macro-level) at the cost of increased activity at the microtremor level.

STUDY II

This study emanated from the need of a more extensive and multidimensional analysis of eye tracking records identifying the occurrence of various types of deviations.

Method

To this end, a program for a detailed analysis of various deviations from smooth eye tracking was developed, partly on the basis of a reanalysis of the records of four subjects reported on earlier (see Andersson 1983b, Figures 1-2; Andersson 1984, Figures 1-2), subjects considered illustative of eye tracking in psychotic patients and alcohol abusers, respectively. This program was then used to analyze again data from the most recent testing made of each of the 14 subjects reported on in Study I, the data for each subject being the same as that analyzed for the respective testing session in Study I and comprising, as there, four periods of about 30 sec each. The fact that the records of the analog signals had all been saved on a single tape and that the analog-to-digital conversion was performed on a single day can be seen as having tended to keep chance variations due to the equipment at a minimum. For each period of tracking analyzed, which comprised 12 waves each with an amplitude of approximately +/-21 degrees, smoothing was carried out with the aim of obtaining a representation of subjective stimulus position. An initial smoothing was accomplished by computing sliding means over 16-point intervals, one interval corresponding to 10 msec (16 intervals thus corresponding to 0.16 sec). The resulting curve will be referred to as the V4 curve; it closely resembles the eye position curve, but excludes certain apparently unconscious tremor, which will be referred to here as macrotremor to distinguish it from the microtremor described above.

A second smoothing involved quadratic interpolation over 128-point intervals, corresponding roughly to half a wave length, i.e. the distance from a wave crest to the following trough. This curve will be referred to as the V7 curve. Being close in form to the curve representing the movements of the target, this curve indicates readily the extent to which the gross following movements remained on target.

The two types of sliding curves, based respectively on 16-point and 128-point intervals, were seen as fine and coarse representations of the subjective stimulus position.

Macrotremor was computed by identifying and counting both the upwards and downwards deviations of the eye position curve from the V4 curve and then identifying bands of adjacent deviations. This analysis aimed at finding bands of deviations of roughly equal size; single large saccades were excluded automatically through a rule by which any deviation, the neighbors of which were less than half as large, being eliminated. For each tracking period the following computations were obtained: a) the number of macrotremor deviations, b) their mean size, c) their width, d) their speed and e) the percentage of the V4 curve involved.

The analysis of jerks took into account deviations of the V4 curve from the V7 curve. Deviations to either side which were sufficiently long and steep were classified as jerks. The criterion for steepness here was that the jerk be at least double the speed of the stimulus, the criterion for size being (somewhat arbitrarily) set to 3.15 degrees (corresponding to 0.15 of the maximal amplitude in Figure 1). Deviations larger than 2.1 degrees (corresponding to 0.1 unit in Figure 1) were analyzed in more detail. A deviation that began and ended with a jerk was classified as a macro squarewave if the line between the jerks was flat, horizontal, and of minimum temporal size. Flatness was defined as existing if the V4 curve deviated from the center point of a straight line between the jerks by less than 14% of the center point´s distance from the V7 curve. Horizontalness was defined as existing if the slope of the line was less than half the speed of the stimulus. Deviations bounded by two jerks but not fulfilling all the other criteria, as well as deviations bounded by a jerk on one side only but fulfilling the criteria above, were thus identified. In summary, the following computations of the V4 curve from the V7 curve were performed for each of the four periods of tracking: f) number of deviations of the V4 curve from the V7 curve, g) mean size of these deviations, h) number of deviations greater than 2.1 degrees as defined above, i) mean size of the greater deviations, j) number of jerks, k) mean size of jerks, l) mean slope of jerks, m) mean number of recoils, n) percentage of the V7 curve involved by recoils, o) number of plateaus and p) mean number of macro squarewaves.

OTP, Dif-1 and Dif-2 scores were obtained for each of the measures a) through p) above for any given subject, the rules followed being in accordance with those given in Study I. Separate cluster analyses employing Ward´s (1963) minimum variance method were performed for the OTP measures and for the combined OTP, Dif-1 and Dif-2 measures, not only regarding deviations of the eye position curve from the V4 curve, (i.e., regarding macrotremor) and of the V4 curve from

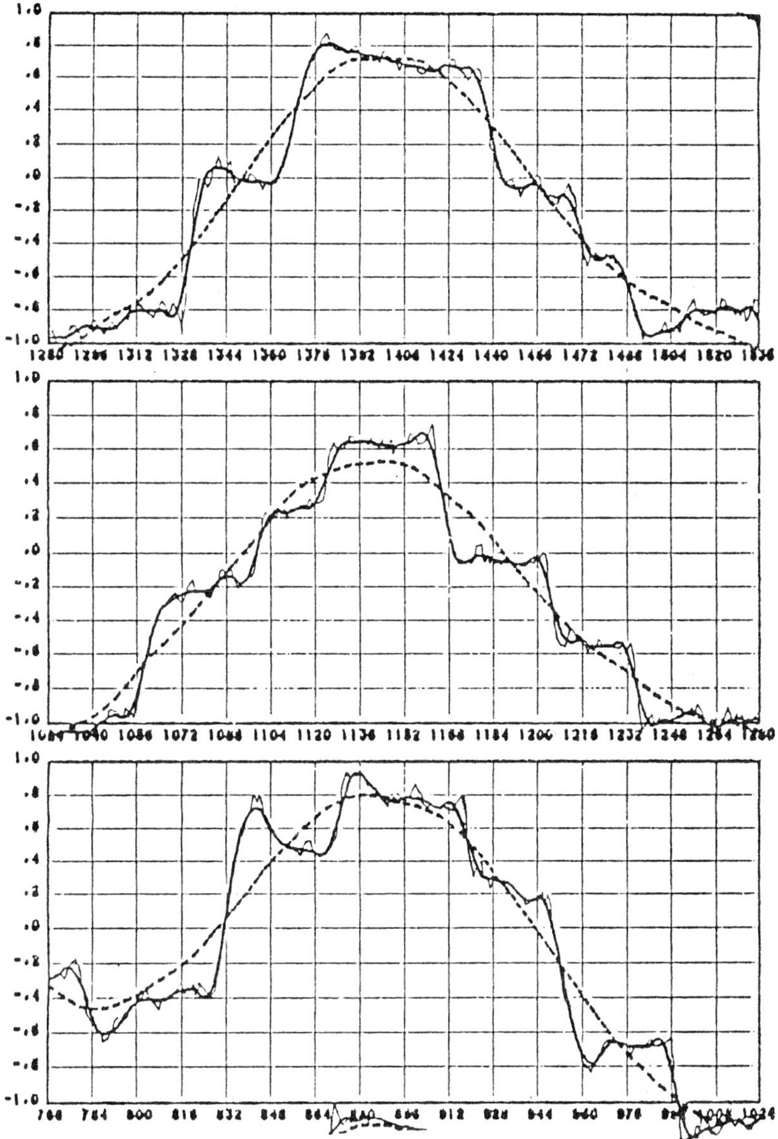

Figure 1. Eye-tracking segments (2.5 sec each) from the record of an acute alcohol abuser (no.03). The lighter line represents eye position, the darker line the V4-curve, and the dotted line the V7-curve.

the V7 curve (i.e. regarding V7-deviations), but also regarding OTP-measures for macrotremor and V7-deviations combined, and regarding the combined OTP, Dif-1 and Dif-2 measures for macrotremor and V7-deviations combined--resulting in six cluster analyses.

Results and Interpretation

Figure 1 presents eye-position, V4- and V7-curves obtained for three pendular cycles from the recording of one of the acutely intoxicated subjects (no. 3:3). Tracking here shows a typical step-wise pattern, although this does not prevent the V7 curve from appearing to follow the rhytmic oscillations of the target fairly closely.

Results of the cluster analyses are presented in Figure 2. Cluster analysis (6), which is based on all OTP, Dif-1 and Dif-2 scores obtained from computations (a) through (o) and thus involves all macrotremor and V7-deviation measures combined, succeeds quite well in distinguishing on the three-cluster level between the two acute alcohol abusers, the four psychotics and the seven normals, the sober alcohol abuser being found in the same cluster as the normals. Cluster analyses (1) and (2), based on macrotremor OTP-scores, processed separately and in conjunction with macrotremor Dif-1 and Dif-2 scores, respectively, differentiate on the two branch level between the acute alcohol abusers and the remaining subjects, though no very clear cleavage between subgroups is evident among the remaining subjects.

Cluster analysis (3), based on the V7-deviation OTP scores, shows a clear cleavage at the first branching, between the four psychotics and the two acute alcohol abusers, on the one hand, and the remaining group consisting of all the normals and the sober alcohol abuser on the other. On the five-cluster level here, one of the acute alcohol abusers, subject 05, is joined by subject 23 from the psychotic group, while subject 03, the other acute alcohol abuser, forms a cluster of his own. In cluster analysis (4), which involves, in addition to the V7-deviation OTP-scores, the V7-deviation Dif-1 and Dif-2 measures, separation of the psychotics from the acute alcohol abusers is more obvious. On the four cluster level here, one cluster is occupied by the psychotic subject 23 and a second by the remaining three psychotics, with the two alcohol abusers forming a cluster of their own, and all the normals and the sober alcohol abuser being included in the remaining cluster.

Cluster analysis (5), based on all the OTP-macrotremor and V7-deviation measures, results, at the three cluster level, in a clear separation between the chronic alcohol abusers, the four psychotics and the remaining subjects, the latter cluster embracing all the seven normals and the sober alcohol abuser. In cluster analysis (6), where Dif-1 and Dif-2 scores have been added to the variables just mentioned so that all measures of macrotremor and V7-deviation area are included, a similar cleavage is found, and in addition, at the five-cluster level, the sober alcohol abuser appears in a separate cluster together only one of the normals (subject 27).

On the OTP-scores for macrotremor. the number of deviations (measure (a)) was categorically lower in the two acute alcohol abusers than in any of the other subjects, the mean of the number of deviations per period being 346 and 459 respectively for the acute alcohol abusers 3 and 5, in contrast the mean number of deviations per period for the remaining subjects as a group being 621 (s.d.=37.3). Also, the two acute alcohol abusers were shown to be the lowest of all the subjects on mean size (b), mean velocity (d) and percentage of the V4 curve involved (e). In addition, mean width of deviation (c) was rather low in the acute alcohol abusers as compared with the other subjects. No categorical differences

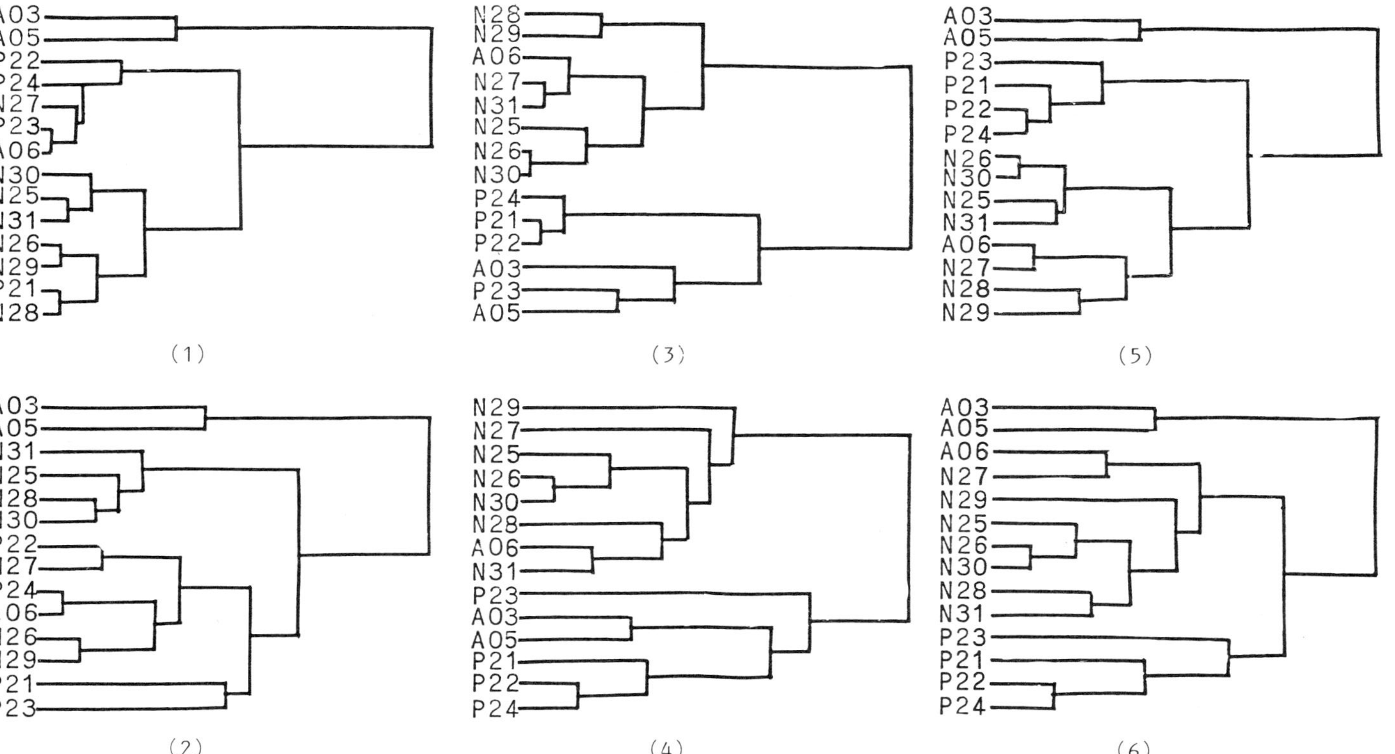

Figure 2. Cluster analyses (dendrograms) of the 14-subject group with inclusion of (1) macrotremor OTP scores, (2) macrotremor OTP, Dif-1 and Dif-2 scores, (3) V7-deviation OTP-scores, (4) V7-deviation OTP, Dif-1 and Dif-2 scores, (5) macrotremor and V7-deviation OTP scores, (6) macrotremor and V7-deviation OTP, Dif-1 and Dif-2 scores. The horizontal axis in each dendrogram represents prediction ratio (0 to 1, left to right).

such as those just mentioned were found between the normals and the psychotic patients, although three of the psychotics (subjects 22-24) scored higher than any of the normals on mean number of macrotremor deviations per period (a), the fourth psychotic (subject 21) being at about the level of the normals. Interestingly enough, that subject reported earlier periodic alcohol abuse. As regards the frequency of occurrence of macro squarewaves a visual analysis of the mingographic recordings suggested only comparatively few to be present, viz about 2-3 per person for the four periods considered.

No clear differences between the subject groups were found on macrotremor Dif-1 scores. Macrotremor Dif-2 scores for each of the measures included indicated the values for the two acute alcohol abusers to decrease over time. The same tended to be true of the normals, but their decreases were less marked. Results for the psychotics were the opposite, all macrotremor measures for this group showing an increase over time. Macrotremor Dif-1 and Dif-2 results for the sober alcohol abuser were similar to those of the normals.

OTP-scores for the V7 measure of total number of deviations (f) were lowest for the two alcohol abusers (the mean number per period being 239 and 207 for subjects 3 and 5, respectively) and for the psychotic patients (the mean number per period for these subjects, 21 and 22, being 165 and 164, respectively). In contrast, the sober alcohol abuser scored highest of all the subjects here (300). Mean size of all deviations (g) in the two acute alcohol abusers and in each of the psychotics was higher than in any of the other subjects. This was reflected in the fact that the number and size of deviations larger than 2.1 degrees was likewise categorically greater for the acute alcohol abusers than in the remaining subjects. Although the number of jerks (j) which occurred was about the same in all groups, the psychotics and the two acute alcohol abusers scored higher than normals on height of the jerks (k), the sober alcohol abuser scoring lowest of all the subjects. On mean slope of the jerks (l), however, a categorical difference was found between all the alcohol abusers and psychotics on the one hand and all normals on the other, the slope being steeper in the former group. The number of recoils (m) did not seem to differ between the groups. The two acute alcohol abusers and subject 23, a psychotic, were highest of all the subjects on percentage of the V7 curve involved in recoils (n) and on number of plateaus (o).

In terms of V7 Dif-1 scores, the number of deviations (f) on V7 was found to increase in the subjects generally under the more attention-demanding conditions. In terms of V7 Dif-2 scores, the same (f) measure was found to decrease generally over time in the alcohol abusers and the normals, and to increase over time in the psychotics.

V7 Dif-1 scores also indicated the number of deviations greater than 2.1 degrees (h) to increase in all three alcohol abusers and to decrease in all three schizophrenic psychotics (21, 23, 24) under the more attention demanding conditions, whereas the normals as a group showed no clear tendency in either direction. In the alcohol abusers V7 Dif-1 scores for number of jerks (j), recoils (m) and plateaus (o) all increased during the more attention demanding conditions. No consistent tendency of this sort was found for the other two groups as regards (j), whereas the normals showed a similar picture and the psychotics an opposite one as regards (m) and (o).

Discussion

Results indicate numerous possibilities for using eye tracking parameters to map out response profiles for the categories of subjects studied here. Although the groups were small, global measures such as noise/signal ratio, deviation area and microtremor rate appear to at least partly succeed in differentiating the eye tracking performance of normals, alcohol abusers and psychotics. Continued study calls for the on-line analysis of stimulus position, eye position and the subjective representation of the stimulus.

Lipton et al. (1983) have recommended using global measures of smooth pursuit (measures on a level with those of noise/signal ratio and deviation area employed in the present investigation) for studies attempting to characterize patient groups, and using specific parameters such as number of saccades to identify and specify the nature of smooth pursuit dysfunction. One might argue, on the other hand, that for matters much in need of basic research a multidimensional approach which does not exclude the parallel use of both global and more specific measures is best.

Levy et al. (1983) argue that a single finding such as that of abnormal smooth pursuit occurs in many CNS disorders and is thus not specific in itself. They recommend considering quite different measures such as those of oculomotor and vestibular reactivity and the like in conjunction with such a finding. Although by no means arguing against such an approach, one may note that abnormal smooth pursuit need by no means represent a single finding, and that a multidimensional analysis of eye tracking performance, even with a very limited number of recordings, can offer considerable potential for assessing somatic and attentional correlates of pathology of various kinds.

REFERENCES

Andersson, S.I., Smooth pursuit eye movements and attention in schizophrenia and cycloid psychoses. In Groner, R., Menz, C., Fisher, D.F. and Monty, R.A. (eds.), Eye Movements and Psychological Functions: International Views. Hillsdale, N.J.: Lawrence Erlbaum, 1983a, 223-237.

Andersson, S.I., Eye tracking performance and attention in psychotic patients. In Kolder, H.E.J.W (ed.), Slow Potentials and Microprocessor Applications. The Hague: Dr W.Junk Publishers, 1983b, 467-470.

Andersson, S.I., Eye tracking performance and attention in alcohol abusers and psychotic patients. In Gale, A.G. and Johnson, F (eds.), Theoretical and Applied Aspects of Eye Movement research. Amsterdam: Elsevier Science Publishers B.V. (North-Holland), 1984, 489-496.

Corvera, J, Torres-Courtney, G. and Lopez-Rios, G., The neurootological significance of alterations of pursuit eye movements and the pendular eye tracking test. Annals of Otology, Rhinology and Laryngology, 1973 (82) 855-867.

Drischel, H., The frequency response of horizontal pursuit movements of the human eye and the influence of alcohol. Progress in Brain Research, 1968 (22) 161-174.

Flom, M.C., Brown, B., Adams, A.J. and Jones, R.T., Alcohol and marijuana effects on ocular tracking. American Journal of Optometry & Physiological Optics, 1976 (53) 764-773.

Holzman, P.S., Levy, D.L. and Uhlenhuth, E.H., Proctor, L.R. and Freedman, D.X., Smooth-pursuit eye movements, and diazepam, CPZ and secobarbital. Psychopharmacologia, 1975 (44) 111-115.

Levy, D.L., Holzman, P.S. and Proctor, L.R., Vestibular dysfunction and psychopathology. Schizophrenia Bulletin, 1983 (9) 383-438.

Levy, D.L., Lipton, R.B. and Holzman, P.S., Smooth-pursuit eye movements: Effects of alcohol and chloral hydrate. Journal of Psychiatric Research, 1981 (16) 1-11.

Lipton, R.B., Levy, D.L., Holzman, P.S. and Levin, S., Eye movement dysfunctions in psychiatric patients: a review. Schizophrenia Bulletin, 1983 (9) 13-32.

Ward, J.H., Hierarchical grouping to optimize an objective function. Journal of the American Statistical Association, 1963 (58) 236-244.

Eye Movements and Human Information Processing
R. Groner, G.W. McConkie and C. Menz (eds.)

FREE SEARCH, RESTRICTED SEARCH, AND THE NEED FOR CONTEXT IN RADIOLOGIC IMAGE PERCEPTION

Dennis P. Carmody
Saint Peter's College
Department of Psychology
Jersey City, New Jersey 07306, U. S. A.

Visual search of radiologic chest images is a complex task, one not easily described as systematic or orderly. How does the radiologist choose which areas of the image will receive visual attention, and how large an area of the image is processed accurately with a fixation? Answers to these questions are based on experimental interventions, including restricted search, designed to evaluate the stages of radiographic interpretation which are orientation to the image, scanning, recognition of potential abnormalities, and decision-making. Similarities are discussed between visual search in radiology and other tasks.

INTRODUCTION

Visual search in radiological tasks has been studied to determine if diagnostic accuracy is related to scanning patterns during search (Kundel & Nodine, 1978; Llewellyn-Thomas, 1969; Tuddenham, 1962). A focus of this work has been the chest image, one of the most frequent radiological examinations, and the specific task of detecting the presence and location of tumors or nodules. Clinical studies have shown that 10-30% of solitary tumors are not reported after the chest image is viewed, although the tumors are evident in retrospect (Smith, 1967).

In order to insure adequate visual coverage of chest images radiologists have been advised to follow a preconceived plan rather than a free search technique (Fraser & Pare, 1977; Sutton, 1969). For example, radiology residents are taught to inspect specific anatomic areas, followed by a systematic comparison of the zones of the two lungs from apex to base. Such an orderly search pattern would then be reflected in eye movement behavior, but it is not typical. Radiology instructors and their resident students show comparative scanning of the lungs about 4% of the time when inspecting chest images (Carmody, Kundel, & Toto, 1984). There are some doubts if this orderliness can be taught as attempts to train medical students in the use of systematic scans resulted in poorer decision-making accuracy compared to subjects who used a free search technique (Gale & Worthington, 1983).

A systematic directed strategy of scanning has been advised in textbooks, is taught by instructors and is the method preferred in surveys of radiologists. Why, then, is it not used? To answer this question, several topics are reviewed including descriptions of radiological search, experimental modifications of radiological images, scanning patterns in non-radiological search tasks, and the useful visual field during search. The issues to be addressed are how are areas of radiological images chosen for visual inspection and how large an area of the image is inspected accurately by a fixation.

DESCRIPTIVE STUDIES OF RADIOLOGICAL SEARCH

In many eye movement studies during radiological search, the subjects have included radiologists, radiology residents, medical students, and non-medical research personnel, all of whom will be referred to as readers.

Studies of the fixation patterns of readers show there is some underlying organization, although it is not as systematic as directed or comparative search. The distribution of fixations is influenced by radiological experience (Kundel & LaFollette, 1972) and the object of search (Kundel, 1974). Individual readers repeatedly fixated similar anatomic areas when searching for tumors and different areas when searching for more generalized abnormalities (Kundel & Wright, 1969). These findings suggest that cognitive expectancies direct visual attention, reflected in fixation distributions, to sample image areas which are informative to the task.

Attempts to classify individual scanning patterns have used the distribution of fixations and the sequence of placing successive fixations (Carmody et al, 1984; Kundel & Wright, 1969). Three general classifications emerged: (1) a circumferential scan during which fixations are located at the periphery of the lungs and are separated by long saccades; this scan is repeated frequently with an outer, then inner circular pattern of fixations; (2) a left-right scan during which the reader looks from side to side usually from top down; (3) a complex scan during which fixations are directed at the same features as in the circumferential scan but not in any definite order. When an image contains an abnormality, readers will often fixate the pathology within the first few seconds. If no significant deviations are detected on normal images, readers use circumferential scans about 30% of the time. At times, certain normal features mimic pathology and receive prolonged visual attention which interrupts or terminates the circumferential pattern. Radiology residents use a left-right pattern when inspecting about 30% of the images, and their instructors use this system on only 8% of their inspections, although a majority of instructors (85%) teach this method (Carmody et al, 1984) and a majority of radiologists (62%) believed they used this method (Gale & Worthington, 1983). About one-half of the scanning patterns are classified complex. The distribution of these patterns within the three classifications depends on the task, the duration of the inspection time, and the specific features evidenced on the images.

Errors in radiology have been attributed to variations in perceptual processing, such as an incomplete scan of the image, or variations in the criteria used to decide if an image is normal or abnormal (Kundel, Nodine, & Carmody, 1978). On the basis of eye movement behaviors, three sources of diagnostic error were identified for the task of searching chest images for solitary tumors. A scanning error occurred when the tumor was not fixated by a useful field of view (5.6 deg) and not reported. Approximately 10-30% of false-negative decisions are due to scanning errors, supporting an earlier view that inadequate search contributed to error (Tuddenham, 1963). Recognition errors were a failure to report a tumor that was fixated during search for a duration below a threshold value (480 msec). Failures to report those tumors were thought to be pattern-recognition errors and accounted for 25-45% of the false-negative decisions. When tumors were fixated for longer than a threshold value, and were not reported, a decision-making error occurred, and this defined 45% of the errors. A majority of the false-negative decisions were explained as recognition and decision-making errors, not as search failures.

From the results of investigations of search behavior, errors can occur at four levels in the task (Kundel et al, 1978): (1) orientation to the chest image, which improves in efficiency with radiologic expertise; (2) scanning, when tumors are not fixated with a useful field of view; (3) recognition, when a tumor is scanned but not identified as a perturbation of normal anatomy; (4) decision-making, when ambiguous features are identified and either a tumor is rejected, a false-negative error, or a normal feature is classified as tumor, a false-positive error.

Several experimental interventions have isolated the four levels of the task to evaluate the contribution of each to the overall error rate. These experiments include tachistoscopic presentations, restricted search, and interruption of the circumferential survey pattern.

TACHISTOSCOPIC STUDIES

Under tachistoscopic viewing, radiologists have identified large and gross abnormalities more readily than smaller ones, such as nodules, providing evidence for an initial global response activated early in scanning (Kundel & Nodine, 1975, 1983). During tachistoscopic presentations where readers were directed to specified image locations, exposure time (60-480 msec) was a critical factor for decision accuracy (Carmody, Nodine, & Kundel, 1980a). Identification required at least 360 msec for normal image areas, and 200 msec for tumors, although the visibility of the tumor within the anatomical background directly influenced accuracy (Carmody, Nodine, & Kundel, 1981). Readers improved their tumor identification when they used eye movements to compare suspected areas with other film features, especially for tumors which were less visible against the anatomic details of the image.

There were two differences between the directed tachistoscopic study and the normal viewing situation. First, readers knew the precise location of the tumor and only had to judge presence or absence. In the normal viewing situation, readers are unsure if tumors are present on images and, if present, how many in what locations. Second, a single fixation of limited duration deprived readers of prolonged fixation durations (> 500 msec) and of fixations on surrounding features. In the normal viewing situation, readers will attend to ambiguities with multiple fixations of prolonged duration and will scan the tumor.

The tachistoscopic studies provide evidence for an initial global response which orients the reader to the image and selects areas of the image for detailed study. Other experiments have modified the display of the image to determine if scanning errors could be reduced.

SEGMENTED SEARCH

In an attempt to reduce scanning errors, readers inspected images presented in sections, and their decisions were compared to performance under normal viewing conditions (Carmody, Nodine, & Kundel, 1980b). Segmented viewing showed chest images piecemeal in six sections, and readers could view and review sections for an unlimited time in any order. The study took place over six months with a random arrangement of segmented and free search conditions to reduce any apparent preference for conditions due to learning and fatigue.

Segmented viewing was expected to lead to greater decision accuracy due to a greater coverage of image areas. Not as expected, readers found the same number of tumors in both segmented and free search, and had more false-positive errors in the segmented condition. Segmented search resulted in poorer decision-making performance, except for one observer who reviewed other sections before making decisions about ambiguous features. Could this strategy of comparing segments be similar to the visual comparisons in search when the entire image is displayed?

A review of eye movement records (Kundel et al, 1978) of radiologists searching for solitary tumors found evidence for comparison scans (Carmody et al, 1981). Apparently the information necessary for decisions about suspected tumors was not to be found in the local area that embedded the tumor, but was acquired by fixating features of the normal anatomic structures and using them as a reference.

Eye movements were recorded as readers searched the same images used in the segmented study under modifications of the two viewing conditions. In free viewing readers searched for tumors for 30 seconds, while in segmented viewing readers saw images piecemeal for 5 seconds for each of the 6 sections. Readers pressed a key which marked on the eye movement record the instant a tumor was detected. The tumors were placed into four groups of visibility based on their frequency of detection in the initial study (Carmody et al, 1980b): group A tumors were found 100% (10 tumors); group B, 83% (9); group C, 50% (10); and group D, 2% (8).

Several clear differences were found based on eye behavior. First, in free viewing, the more visible tumors were found more often, sooner, and with fewer fixations than the less visible tumors. Second, in free viewing, the less visible tumors received more comparative scanning than the more visible tumors. Third, decision-making ability, d', decreased as tumor visibility decreased and was better in free viewing than segmented viewing. The comparative scans typical in standard viewing were not evident in segmented viewing.

CONSTRAINED VIEWING AND COMPARISON VIEWING

Another experimental technique combined a tachistoscopic presentation with monitoring eye position (Carmody, 1984). Observers were directed to selected locations on a display by means of five dots which defined a 4° square and its center. The observer fixated each dot and depressed a switch providing a calibration of a 4° window. After a switch depress when viewing the center dot, a chest image was presented which was either normal or contained a 1° tumor. The observer viewed the image area defined by the window with foveal vision and the image outside the window with peripheral vision. Once the fovea crossed a window boundary, the image was replaced by the pre-exposure dot field. Observers had to take part in many practice trials with practice images before testing to insure that the display would not terminate before there was sufficient information to judge the area. This task was similar to the segmented experiment except the area under study was smaller and the entire image was available to peripheral vision. This was the constrained viewing condition.

In a second viewing condition, comparison viewing, observers judged the identical image areas, but were permitted for a maximum of five seconds to leave and return to the window to acquire information. The number of crossings was recorded, and judgments under both viewing conditions were analyzed to determine the effect of comparison scans on local decision-making performance. Subjects saw 200 images, 100 normal and 100 abnormal containing a tumor, for a total of 3800 decisions.

Comparison scans allowed observers to identify 8% more tumors as well as to reduce false positives by 7% and improve true negative decisions by 9.5.%. Signal detection analyses verified significant differences ($p < .01$) in favor of comparison viewing for d' (2.028 vs. 1.683) and the area under the ROC curve (.907 vs. .874).

The tumors in this study were systematically varied on their distinctiveness with the surround by modification of the tumor edge from sharp to dull in five distinct levels (Kundel, Revesz, & Toto, 1979). For sharper edge tumors, there were fewer crossings, and as the edge became duller, thus blending more into the normal anatomy, more crossings were evidenced for all observers.

Clearly, comparison scans were used to improve decision accuracy, to resolve ambiguities, and were relied on when the distinctiveness of the tumor "signal" was degraded in the anatomy "background." Are there similarities in the use of comparison scans between radiological search and other visual tasks?

COMPARISON SCANS IN SEARCH TASKS

Evidence for the role of comparison scans can be found in several visual search tasks. A majority of 6 year old children demonstrated a method of paired comparisons when asked to determine if two schematics of houses were the same or different (Vurpillot, 1968). Vurpillot described an efficient strategy of search for differences as one which systematically compares pairs of features. This strategy appears to evolve from the age of 5 onward and by age 7 the number of comparisons was related to the number of differences between pairs, although children of all ages tend to end search before fixating all possible pairs of features. An increase in the frequency of paired comparisons appeared for older children and for the more accurate subjects in all age groups.

In an embedded figures task, the eye movements of subjects were recorded as they searched through five alternatives to find which one was embedded within a complex target figure (Boersma, Muir, Wilton, & Barham, 1969). The display presented the alternatives and target in one field, allowing subjects the opportunity to shift fixations between figures. Field-independent subjects had a greater number of fixations on target than did field-dependent subjects, and such an increase was due to a shift from alternatives to target. Thus the behavior of shifting visual inspection was related to improved task performance, although it is not clear if the behavior lead to improved decision accuracy, or if both higher accuracy and shifts in attention are due to a common factor attributable to field-independent subjects.

An eye movement study concerned with the development of reading skills had subjects trained to read text with the letters replaced by mathematical symbols (Menz & Groner, 1982). Subjects had to read four lines of text composed of symbols, and the code-table of letters and symbols was always presented on the top of a page in the display. Subjects read 850 slides of material and different types of eye movements were distinguished in the records including decoding jumps which were saccades from the text area to the code-table lines. Decoding jumps showed a decrease from the first slide until approximately 200 slides were read, after which these jumps were rare. Menz and Groner concluded that the process of perceptual learning had advanced to such a degree that is was more efficient for the subject to use a memory search rather than a saccade to the code-table.

The results of these studies suggest that comparisons between a standard and alternatives are used to decide if there are similarities or differences. Such activity appears to be related to improved decision accuracy, and when the standard is novel or new to the subject, comparisons tend to increase (Vurpillot, Boersma). When the standard remains consistent, as in the Menz and Groner study, a period of perceptual learning takes place which is characterized by a high frequency of comparisons at first, with a decline and eventual cessation of comparisons when the features are well known.

COMPARISON SCANS AND THE USEFUL VISUAL FIELD

Several recent investigations have examined the relationship between central and peripheral vision during visual search of displays (Cohen, 1981; Kundel, Nodine, & Toto, 1984; Prinz, 1983). Although the various studies have used different displays, there appear some commonalities of findings. One of these areas that relates to the radiological task is the size of the useful visual field within which attention can be shifted without an eye movement.

Cohen (1981) compared 5- and 8- year old children to college students on a task where subjects judged which alternative was identical to the standard. The four alternatives were located at the corners of a square at 3°, 6°, or 9° distance from the central standard. Search time was divided into two phases: Perceptual phase, from onset of display to first fixation on target; Decision phase, from the first fixation on target to a response. All subjects showed more fixations and time spent in the Perceptual phase than in the Decision phase. The differences between the phases in search time and percent of fixations was most pronounced at 3°, which most probably reflects simultaneous comparisons of foveal and peripheral information without the need for many confirming fixations in the Decision phase. Refixations of the standard and target during the Decision phase became more numerous as the distance of alternatives exceeded 3°. Possibly the refixations for alternatives located more than 3° from the standard are similar to the comparisons used by radiologists.

Prinz (1983) discussed evidence for two mechanisms which influence search for target letters in an array of distractor letters: Automatic Detection (AD) which mediates target detection in eccentric vision; Controlled Search (CS) which mediates target detection in central vision. While the efficiency of AD depends on the permanent distribution of retinal sensitivity, the efficiency of CS depends on a transient distribution of attention over the visual field. These two mechanisms interact such that if the target is detected by AD, search stops, and if undetected by AD, detection depends on the CS. Easy targets, such as the letter D among distractor letters of angular lines, can be detected by AD, while difficult targets, such as Z among angular letter distractors, require CS.

Perhaps the radiologist can use the permanent sensitivity of the peripheral retina to locate high contrast areas and determine the location of the next fixation, in a manner similar to the AD mechanism proposed by Prinz. Targets in the chest image characterized by contrast changes similar to normal anatomy would likely be found only by detailed foveal inspection, in a manner similar to the CS mechanism.

One experimental technique separated systematically central from peripheral vision during search (Kundel et al, 1984). The subject saw chest images in their entirety, but a window was coupled to the dynamic location of the subject's eyes. When the subject moved the eyes, the window would allow a central view of the abnormal image which blended precisely into a peripheral view of a normal image. Thus tumors (0.8^o) could only be seen with central vision. The size of the central window was varied to determine the size of the dynamic useful visual field (UVF). Results showed that a window of 1.75^o lead to poor detection performance, largely due to incomplete central coverage of the image during search. Complete coverage of the image occurred with a window size between 5.25^o and 8.75^o, although there is not a significant improvement in decision performance with central windows larger than 3.5^o. These results suggest that a 3.5^o UVF is sufficient to achieve performance that simulates decision-making under normal conditions.

The question which remains to be answered is what is the relationship of the useful field of view to the use of comparison scans. Previous algorithms used 5° as a minimum distance to identify comparison scans. When a sequence of saccades starts on any suspected area, moves to another image area at least 5° distance, followed by a return to the suspected area, it is defined as a comparison. Was this a reasonable estimate?

To answer that question it would be necessary to determine if the useful visual field exceeded 5°, since a saccade would be unnecessary if the UVF encompassed areas required to make local decisions. Estimates of the size of the UVF can be made from the average or median interfixation distances during circumferential scanning. The rationale is that the viewer is sampling regions of the chest image to determine if detailed inspection is necessary. Estimates from eye movement records for the average interfixation distance are 5.6^o when searching for tumors in chest images (Kundel et al, 1984). This value coincides with a UVF estimate of 5.6^o (2.8^o radius) reported in a separate study of eye movements of radiologists (Kundel et al, 1978).

In the eye movement study where central and peripheral vision received different images, decision-making performance was not improved with a UVF larger than 3.5°. Finally, in the constrained viewing study, subjects did not resolve the presence of a tumor within a 4° square field as accurately as when they could acquire with foveal attention information outside the restricted field.

A recent study was used to examine the size of the zone required around a tumor for accurate decisions to be made. Subjects viewed a single area of a digitized chest image that was visible through a variable aperture. The area surrounding the circular aperture was black, while the chest image was presented at luminence levels equivalent to standard viewing on a viewbox. The circular apertures were concentric with the location of the tumor and ranged from 1.5° diameter to 10.5° diameter (20 to 120 pixels). The series of apertures progressed from smallest to largest with a decision required for each aperture about the presence or absence of a tumor in the image. Images remained available for up to 20 seconds, or less if the subject gave a response. The tumors were created with three distinct levels of edge gradient to determine if this feature influenced the size of the useful visual field. Results suggest that a 5.25° aperture was sufficient to achieve no false positives for normal areas and the maximum average confidence rating for correct decisions about the presence of tumors. Apertures larger than 5.25° did not improve an index of detectability (d'), or the average rating of decisions, or the accuracy of classifying normal and abnormal images.

It appears that the useful visual field during search for lung nodules is between 3.5 - 5.25°. If a confident decision cannot be achieved about a suspected area with the features displayed within that size field, then a comparison scan is initiated which places the fovea at least 5° away, and places the useful visual field in a location that overlaps minimally, if at all, with the UVF on the suspected area.

GENERAL DISCUSSION

Visual search of radiologic chest images is a complex task, one that is not easily described as systematic or orderly. How does the radiologist choose which areas of the image will receive visual attention, and how large an area of the image is processed accurately by the attention associated with a fixation? An explanation of the selection of areas draws from ideas proposed by Hochberg (1970a, b) concerning schematic maps and a search guidance system.

Prior to viewing an image, the radiologist develops a cognitive map to answer questions concerning the health state of a patient. This plan is formed by the reason for the radiographic examination, knowledge of the appearance and location of normal anatomic features, and knowledge of where pathology is evidenced in the image and how pathological features modify the appearance of normal anatomy. A cognitive strategy is developed to guide visual search to these probable locations that, when fixated, will be the most likely areas to provide information to answer the questions about the patient.

A cognitive map serves several purposes similar to Hochberg's schematic maps (1970a). First, the map provides an expectancy of information from different image areas and is modified by features sampled from those areas. Second, it allows recognition of image features regardless of the sequence of eye movements. Third, due to memory abilities, redundancy of sampling is reduced. Fourth, the map has the capacity to recognize features seen peripherally that contain information already recorded, reducing the need for detailed examination of those areas.

Hochberg (1970b) has suggested that sequential fixations are guided during search by two systems: cognitive search guidance (CSG), based on the cognitive map as modified during search; and peripheral search guidance (PSG), based on low acuity information from peripheral vision. The two systems influence a sampling strategy which examines image areas to test expectancies and perceptual hypotheses (Gregory, 1970).

The initial fixations on the image, referred to as a global response (Kundel & Nodine, 1975, 1983), serve to orient and scale the cognitive map to the gross outline of the image. Subsequent fixations are guided cognitively to sample major anatomic areas for pathological findings or deviations from the features of normal anatomy. Cognitive search guidance is characterized by circumferential, repetitive patterns. On the basis of a 5° (diameter) useful visual field, successive fixations spaced 5° apart permit a matching of features to the cognitive map. The ordering of these fixations is not important; each fixation determines if the features of the image are within the expected range of normal features represented in the map. If ambiguities are detected peripherally, detailed examination by foveal inspection is used for resolution.

At times, resolution of ambiguities requires examination of the features surrounding the ambiguity, resulting in many fixations clustered around the suspected area. The radiologist tests hypotheses about whether the ambiguity is pathology or a deviation of normal anatomy. Hypotheses testing requires a comparison of suspected features with criteria developed from two sources: experience represented in the cognitive map, and the features specific to the particular image under study. At times, the criteria based on experience are sufficient for resolution and detailed examination is abbreviated, possibly terminating search. At other times, when the suspected area is less pronounced (e.g., a blurred tumor edge blending into the vascular background), prolonged visual attention, with the aid of comparison scans, is used to develop criteria specific to the range of normal features evidenced on that image.

Comparison scans result when a decision cannot be reached on the basis of information contained in the map. By making a comparison scan, the radiologist updates the map to include the variations of normal anatomy evidenced on that image in either the same or opposite lung field. With these updated criteria, a return saccade to the suspected area leads to a resolution, although not always an accurate one. In one study, radiologists made comparison scans on a majority of tumors falsely identified as normal (Carmody, et al, 1980a).

In summary, the radiologic search task is dependent upon both a cognitive strategy developed before the viewing of an image and adequate visual coverage of image details. An improvement in the detection rates of solitary lung tumors may result from interventions with the strategy as well as with the visual coverage. For example, radiology residents may benefit from a series of images which exemplify the range of variations of normal patterns and how tumors disrupt those patterns. The expected results of such training would be modifications of scan patterns based on well-developed cognitive strategies rather than on mechanical aids which manipulate visual coverage.

This research was supported by Grant CA - 32870 from the National Cancer Institute, USPHS.

REFERENCES

Boersma, F.J., Muir, W., Wilton K., & Barham R. (1969). Eye movements during figures tasks. Perceptual and Motor Skills, 28, 271-274.

Carmody, D.P. (1984).Lung tumour identification: decision-making and comparison scanning. In A.G. Gale & F. Johnson (Eds.), Theoretical and applied aspects of eye movements research (pp. 305 - 312). Amsterdam: North - Holland.

Carmody, D.P., Nodine, C.F., & Kundel, H.L. (1980a). An analysis of perceptual and cognitive factors in radiographic interpretation. Perception, 9, 339-344.

Carmody, D.P., Nodine, C.F., & Kundel, H.L. (1980b). Global and segmented search for lung nodules of different edge gradients. Investigative Radiology, 15, 224-233.

Carmody, D.P., Nodine, C.F., & Kundel, H.L. (1981). Finding lung nodules with and without comparative scanning. Perception and Psychophysics, 29, 594-598.

Carmody, D.P., Kundel, H.L., & Toto, L. (1984). Comparison scans while reading chest images: taught, but not practiced. Investigative Radiology (in press).

Cohen, K.M. (1981). The development of strategies of visual search. In D.F. Fisher, R.A. Monty, & J.W. Senders (Eds.), Eye movements: cognition and visual perception (pp. 271-288). Hillsdale, Erlbaum.

Fraser, R.G., and Pare, J.A.P. (1977). Diagnosis of diseases of the chest (pp. 179-181). Philadelphia: Saunders.

Gale, A.G., & Worthington, B.S. (1983). The utility of scanning strategies in radiology. In R. Groner, C. Menz, D.F. Fisher, & R.A. Monty (Eds), Eye movements and psychological functions: international views (pp. 169-191). Hillsdale: Erlbaum.

Gregory, R.L. (1970). The intelligent eye. New York: McGraw Hill.

Hochberg, J. (1970a). Attention, organization, and consciousness. In D.I. Mostofsky (Ed.), Attention: Contemporary theory and analysis (pp. 94-124). New York: Appleton-Century Crofts.

Hochberg, J. (1970b). Components of literacy: speculations and exploratory research. In H. Levin & J.P. Williams (Eds.), Basic studies on reading (pp. 74-89). New York: Basic Books.

Kundel, H.L. (1974). Visual sampling and estimates of the location of information on chest films. Investigative Radiology, 9, 87-93.

Kundel, H.L., & LaFollette, P.S. (1972). Visual search patterns and experience with radiological images. Radiology, 103, 523-528.

Kundel, H.L., & Nodine, C.F. (1975). Interpreting chest radiographs without visual search. Radiology, 116, 527-532.

Kundel, H.L., and Nodine, C.F. (1978). Studies of eye movements and visual search in radiology. In R.A. Monty, D.F. Fisher, and J.W. Senders (Eds), Eye movements and the higher psychological functions (pp. 317-327). Hillsdale: Erlbaum.

Kundel, H.L., & Nodine, C.F. (1983). A visual concept shapes image perception. Radiology, 146, 363-368.

Kundel, H.L., Nodine, C.F., & Carmody, D. (1978). Visual scanning, pattern recognition and decision-making in pulmonary nodule detection. Investigative Radiology, 13, 175-181.

Kundel, H.L. Nodine, C.F., and Toto, L. (1984). Eye movements and the detection of lung tumors in chest images. In A.G. Gale & F. Johnson (Eds), Theoretical and applied aspects of eye movement research (pp. 297 - 304). Amsterdam: North - Holland.

Kundel, H.L., Revesz, G., & Toto, L. (1979). Contrast gradient and the detection of lung nodules. Investigative Radiology, 14, 18-22.

Kundel, H.L., & Wright, D.J. (1969). The influence of prior knowledge on visual search strategies during the viewing of chest radiographs. Radio-ology, 93, 315-320.

Llewellyn-Thomas, E. (1969). Search behavior. Radiological Clinics of North America, 7, 403-417.

Menz, C. & Groner, R. (1982). The analysis of some componential skills of reading acquisition. In R. Groner & P. Fraisse (Eds), Cognition and eye movements (pp. 169-178). Amsterdam: North - Holland.

Prinz, W. (1983). Asymmetrical control areas in continuous visual search. In R. Groner, C. Menz, D.F. Fisher, & R.A. Monty (Eds), Eye movements and psychological functions: international views (pp. 85-100). Hillsdale: Erlbaum.

Smith, M.J. (1967). Error and variation in diagnostic radiology. Springfield: Thomas.

Squire, L.F. (1975). Fundamentals of roentgenology (pp. 30-45). Cambridge: Harvard.

Sutton, D. (1969). A textbook of radiology (pp. 241-252). Baltimore: Williams and Wilkins.

Tuddenham, W.J. (1962). Visual search, image organization and reader error in roentgen diagnosis. Radiology, 78, 694-704.

Tuddenham, W.J. (1963). Problems of perception in chest roentgenology: facts and fallacies. Radiological Clinics of North America, 1, 277-289.

Vurpillot, E. (1968). The development of scanning strategies and their relation to visual differentiation. Journal of Experimental Child psychology, 6, 632-650.

Eye Movements and Human Information Processing
R. Groner, G.W. McConkie and C. Menz (eds.)

EYE MOVEMENTS IN MAP READING

James R. Antes, Kang-Tsung Chang, & Thomas Lenzen

University of North Dakota
Grand Forks, North Dakota, U.S.A.

& Chad Mullis

U. S. Army Engineer Topographic Laboratory
Fort Belvoir, Virginia, U.S.A.

The attentional processes of subjects as they were engaged in map reading was investigated using eye movement methodology in two experiments. In the first experiment, subjects viewed two thematic maps, one which was prepared according to standard cartographic conventions and another which was poorly balanced. Poor balance interfered with the subjects' ability to fixate informative map components in the early part of the viewing period and resulted in longer fixation durations, especially for more complex maps. In the second experiment, experienced and inexperienced topographic map users examined ten topographic maps in a search for high and low elevations. Experienced subjects performed the task better and had shorter average fixation durations. The results of both experiments are consistent with the view that the informativeness of different map regions influences the distribution of eye fixations and the complexity of the information influences the duration of fixations.

Research on the cognitive processes involved in reading, picture viewing, and other visual activities such as examining radiographs and driving an automobile have benefitted by recording the eye movements of observers as they are engaged in these activities. Indeed, eye movement data have been the basis for models of text processing in reading (e.g., Just & Carpenter, 1980). When applied to picture viewing, eye movement methodology has revealed information about patterns of attention (e.g., Antes, 1974; Yarbus, 1967) and how pictures are remembered (e.g., Loftus, 1972; Parker, 1978).

Another common but complex visual activity, which has received surprisingly little study using eye movement methodology, is map reading. Maps represent a rather unique stimulus in that they contain major components with verbal information and major components with spatial/pictorial information. For example, the title and legend of a map provide a primarily verbal description of the kind of information presented in the map. The body of the map displays information in a spatial format. Thus parts of the map contain verbal information such as is available in text and part contain a spatial representation such as in pictures. In addition, the overall arrangement of the information in a map is such that the viewer has greater choice in the order of processing than is present in reading text.

The purpose of the research reported here was to apply eye movement analysis to the study of the processes involved in map reading. The few studies that have been reported in this area are from the cartographic literature and are primarily exploratory in nature. One finding that parallels results of research on picture viewing is that observers concentrate their eye fixations on the map body and title (Steinke, 1975) and, in general, on regions that are highly informative (Dobson, 1979) when viewing thematic maps. This suggests that the same processes, involving a search for meaning, are directing attention in map reading as in picture viewing and other visual activities.

The present research is part of a program of research involving personnel in cartography as well as psychology and thus the questions investigated have a rather broad and multidisciplinary focus. The first study investigated effects of varying map design on attention in thematic map reading and the second study explored effects of the experience of the observer in reading topographic maps. In the report of both studies special emphasis will be given to findings relevant to the cognitive/attentional processes involved in map reading.

Experiment I: Effects of Map Design

Cartographers follow various conventions or rules in the construction of a map in terms of the placement, organization, and presentation of the information to be represented. For example, Robinson, Sale, and Morrison (1978) have described map design principles involving clarity and legibility, visual contrast, balance, figure-ground relationships, and hierarchic organization. Interestingly there has been little research to indicate whether or not adherence to these principles influences the communication of information to the map viewer. Their use is certainly supported by common sense but empirical verification is needed with the goal of improving map communication. Thus the cartographic interest motivating this study was to make an initial attempt to investigate the effectiveness of these map design principles. Selected for study was the principle of balance which refers to "the positioning of the various visual components in such a way that their relationship appears logical" (Robinson et al., 1978, p. 286). Subjects viewed maps that were well balanced or poorly balanced and their eye movements and subsequent memory for map components were analyzed for the impact of balance on map communication. In addition, the data were examined to study the attentional and cognitive processes involved in the course of map reading.

Method

Four thematic maps were prepared representing information about fictitious places. Each map was prepared in a well-balanced and a poorly-balanced version. For the well-balanced maps the more important, defined in terms of amount and usefulness of the information presented, map components (body, title, subtitle, legend) stood out and the less important components (scale, data source) were placed in recessive positions. Poorly-balanced maps were created by rearranging the map components so that the ordering was disorganized and illogical. For two of the maps the information to be presented was rather simple, having only a single dimension of information and a map body with straight-line borders. For the other two maps, the information was more complex, with two types of information requiring pie chart symbols, and a map body with jagged-line borders. Figure 1 shows one of the complex maps in both its well balanced and poorly balanced versions.

Forty undergraduate student subjects viewed two maps for 20 s each. The visual angle varied slightly for the different maps but was approximately 20 deg horizontally and 15 deg vertically. Each subject viewed a map that was well balanced with simple information and one that was poorly balanced with complex information, or a well balanced-complex map and poorly balanced-simple map. Counterbalancing assured that an equal number of subjects viewed each form of each map the same number of times in both orders of presentation.

Eye movements were monitored by a Gulf and Western Eye View Monitor, Model 1994S, which uses the relative location of the pupil center and corneal reflection of an infrared light to determine eye position. The data, in the form of an X coordinate, Y coordinate, and pupil diameter, were output 60 times per second, and digitized and stored by a PDP 11/34 computer. The data were later reduced to fixations and saccades using a modified version of

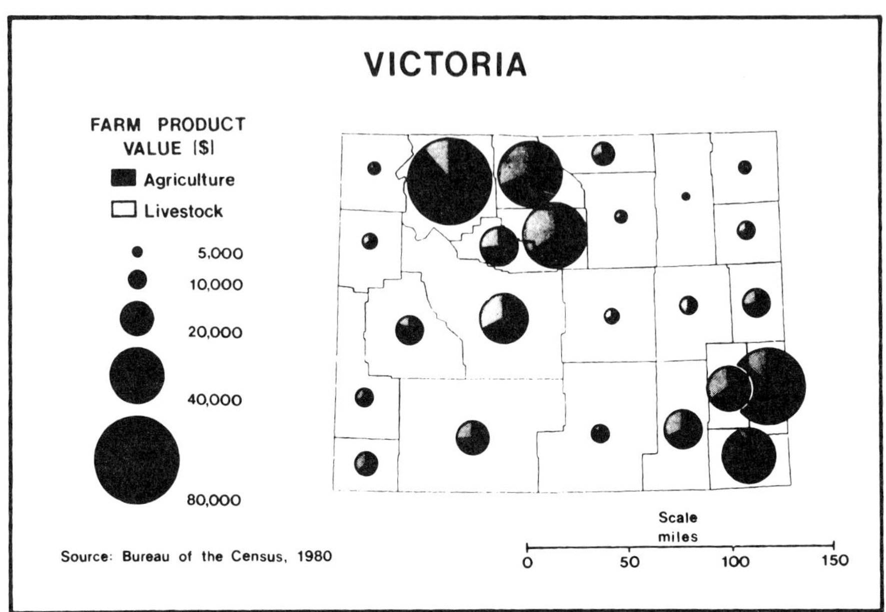

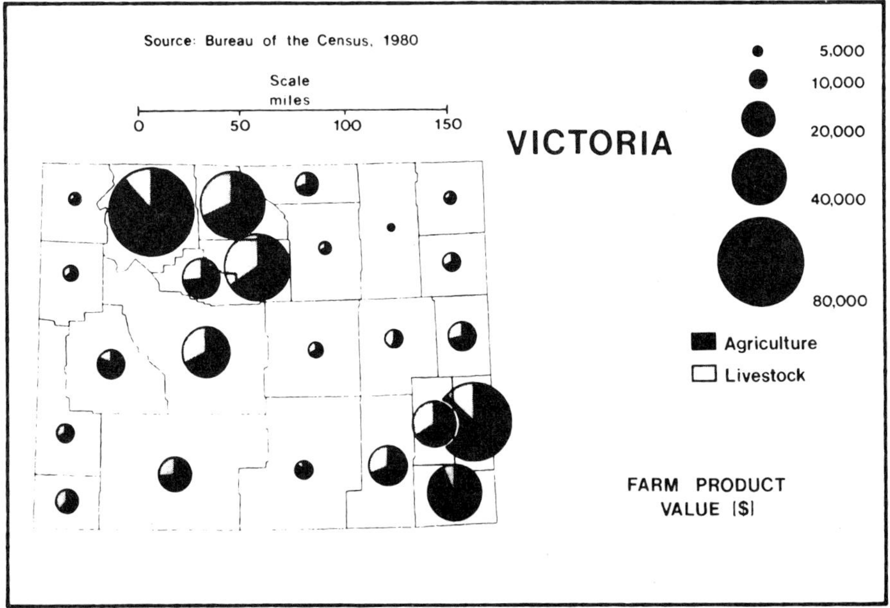

Figure 1. One of the complex maps used in Experiment I in well-balanced (top) and poorly-balanced (bottom) form.

a program described by Kliegl and Olson (1981).

After both maps were viewed subjects were given a separate questionnaire for each map requesting information about the title, subtitle, legend, scale, and body of the maps. They were given as much time as they wanted to complete this questionnaire.

Results

The major eye movement measures that were analyzed were number of fixations, duration of fixations, and interfixation distance.

Table 1 shows the number of fixations (expressed as a percentage) on each map component, broken down by balance and complexity. It is readily

Table 1

Percent of Fixations on each Map Component as a Function of Balance and Complexity

	Map Component						
Map Balance/ Complexity	Body	Title	Subtitle	Legend	Scale	Data Source	Open Space
Good	47.0	4.0	6.4	19.2	6.4	4.4	12.7
Poor	43.9	4.8	5.1	20.9	7.2	5.2	12.8
Simple	45.1	5.0	6.1	18.9	7.5	4.9	12.5
Complex	45.8	3.8	5.4	21.2	6.1	4.7	13.0

apparent that viewers spent most of their time viewing the most important map components, the body and legend. It is also clear that neither map balance nor complexity exerted a major effect on the distribution of fixations. Individual t-tests for each component showed none of the differences to be significant for either balance or complexity.

These data were compiled from the entire 20-s viewing period. It is possible that effects of balance or complexity on attention occurred early in viewing and disappeared later, thus being invisible in this overall analysis. Indeed Antes (1974) and Buswell (1935) have shown that the pattern of attention in picture viewing does change over time. Consequently the location of the first 10 eye fixations on each map was determined and the results are presented in Table 2. The overall pattern of fixations is similar to that seen in Table 1 except that the fixations are somewhat

Table 2

Percent of the First Ten Fixations on each Map Component as a Function of Balance and Complexity

Map Balance/ Complexity	Map Component Body	Title	Subtitle	Legend	Scale	Data Source	Open Space
Good	37.0	8.5	14.8	23.2	2.8	2.2	11.5
Poor	26.8	9.8	7.0	28.8	7.5	6.0	14.2
Simple	33.5	10.8	12.0	20.0	6.5	5.2	12.0
Complex	30.2	7.5	9.8	32.0	3.8	3.0	13.8

more evenly distributed. What is different is the effect of balance and complexity. Individual t-tests showed three differences to be significant for balance and one for complexity. Two relatively important map components, the body and the subtitle, received more fixations when presented in well-balanced form, $t(39) = 2.239$, $p < .05$, and $t(39) = 2.988$, $p < .05$, respectively, and one relatively unimportant component, the scale, received fewer fixations in well-balanced maps, $t(39) = 2.181$, $p < .05$. The legends of simple maps received fewer fixations than the legends of complex maps, $t(39) = 3.315$, $p < .01$.

Further support for differences in the allocation of attention early in viewing comes from an analysis of mean position of the first fixation on a map component. For each trial the number of the first fixation on each component of the map was recorded and averaged across subjects and maps. The data, reported in Table 3, show that the body and subtitle were fixated earlier for well-balanced maps, $t(39) = 2.769$, $p < .01$, and $t(39) = 2.651$, $p < .05$, respectively. Also the title of simple maps was viewed earlier than that of complex maps, $t(39) = 2.348$, $p < .05$.

Table 3

Mean Position of First Fixation on Each Map Component as a Function of Balance and Complexity

Map Balance/ Complexity	Map Component Body	Title	Subtitle	Legend	Scale	Data Source	Open Space
Good	2.3	16.6	11.0	7.6	20.2	21.4	13.4
Poor	5.1	14.0	18.5	5.6	17.6	20.5	11.9
Simple	3.7	11.5	16.0	6.6	17.2	20.5	13.0
Complex	3.7	19.1	13.5	6.5	20.6	21.3	12.3

Table 4 shows the mean duration of fixations on each map component. Subjects fixated significantly longer on the subtitle than any other component. On these maps, the subtitle presents a brief statement of what information was represented on the map (e.g., "farm product value"). The next highest durations were associated with the legend, scale, and data source and these values were approximately equal. Fixations on the map body were shorter than those on any other component, but only significantly shorter than fixations on the subtitle.

Table 4

Mean Duration of Fixations on each Map Component as a Function of Balance and Complexity

	Map Component						
Map Balance/ Complexity	Body	Title	Subtitle	Legend	Scale	Data Source	Open Space
Good	438	468	634	506	460	464	435
Poor	431	485	722	538	557	552	403
Simple	410	492	612	474	484	493	417
Complex	459	459	737	570	541	512	420

Note. Values are given in milliseconds.

Fixations on well-balanced maps were shorter than those on poorly-balanced maps for all map components except the body, although none of the differences reached statistical significance. Fixations on complex maps were longer than those on simple maps for all components except the title. The only component for which this difference was significant was the legend, $t(77) = 2.152$, $p < .05$.

A multiple regression analysis of variance was performed on the fixation duration data across all maps and subjects in order to determine possible joint effects of balance and complexity. The effect of balance was not significant, $F(1,3136) = 0.70$, $p > .05$, but the effects of complexity, $F(1,3136) = 16.20$, $p < .001$, and the balance by complexity interaction, $F(1,3136) = 6.50$, $p < .05$, were. Table 5 presents the means characterizing the interaction. The means were compared with t-tests and there was no significant effect of balance for simple maps but for complex maps the mean duration on poorly balanced maps was significantly longer. Thus the effect of map balance on fixation duration occurred only with complex maps.

Table 5

Mean Fixation Duration as a Function of Balance and Complexity

Complexity	Balance Good	Poor
Simple	450	430
Complex	469	510

Note. Values are given in milliseconds.

Interfixation distance was not analyzed by map component because differences in the location of the components would affect the measure and thus confound the results. However mean interfixation distances were computed over all components and were compared by balance and complexity. The distances were virtually identical (about 4 deg) and t-test comparisons revealed no significant differences.

Interfixation distances were determined for the first 10 eye movements of each trial and again the differences were small and non-significant.

The map memory questionnaires were scored and performance on each question was evaluated by t-tests to see if there were differences due to map balance. The trend was for better performance on questions from well-balanced maps, especially for questions relating to title, subtitle, and legend, but none of the differences reached statistical significance.

Discussion

The manipulation of map balance influenced the distribution of attention, as measured by the number and location of eye fixations, early in viewing, in the first 5 s or so. The relatively important areas of poorly-balanced maps received fewer fixations than the same areas of well-balanced maps and the less important areas received more fixations. Balance thus appears to facilitate the early identification by the viewer of the areas of the map containing important information. The attentional disruption apparently caused by the poorly-balanced maps was overcome to a sufficient extent that by the end of the 20-s viewing period the differences had disappeared.

Fixation duration indicates the difficulty or effort involved in processing the information fixated and thus is a measure of the "intensity" of attention. The effect of degrading the balance of these maps was to increase the fixation duration, requiring more effort in the processing of information. This effect depended, as might be expected, on the complexity of the information in the map. Poor balance was disruptive only if the information was complex.

It was expected that the disruption caused by the balance manipulation would affect the "useful field of view" (Mackworth, 1976) and limit the peripheral range of information use on the part of the viewers. Presumably this should have resulted in differences in interfixation distance, but there were no such differences.

The results generally support the view of attention revealed in picture viewing research. Subjects distribute their attention in such a way as to focus on information-rich areas. This was evident early in viewing as well as later. Maps have a greater orderliness and logical structure than the pictures used in some picture viewing research (e.g., Mackworth & Morandi, 1967) and it is worth noting the differences in the distribution of attention over time. Mackworth and Morandi found the tendency to fixate highly informative areas to be uniform over the 10-s viewing period. In the present study, while informative areas were fixated most often throughout viewing, the effect was less pronounced in the first 10 fixation sample than over the entire 20-s period. Perhaps subjects were becoming oriented to the maps and trying to develop an overall characterization of the nature and location of the information presented. The less structure there is to the stimulus, as in those Mackworth and Morandi used, the longer it would take to develop this characterization and the less the pattern of attention would change in a brief viewing period.

The results also support the finding evidenced in reading, picture viewing, and visual search studies that fixation duration increases with the complexity of the information fixated. Subjects showed a flexibility in processing when viewing maps, which is a kind of metacognitive skill to determine when the information fixated is not fully processed or understood and to allocate more viewing time within the same fixation to fully process the information. It is certainly possible that subjects were also processing information from the previous fixation in addition to information from the current fixation (Antes & Penland, 1981; Russo, 1978), but this study has no data bearing on that question.

In comparing the processing of spatial information in the map (body) with the verbal information, one result seems to stand out. The fixation durations on the map body were considerably shorter than those on the verbal map components, especially the subtitle. However, since the differences in complexity between the spatial and verbal components of the map are unknown (and difficult to measure) the duration differences could potentially be attributed to complexity differences rather than verbal-spatial differences.

In general, the results from Experiment I are consistent with the view of attention in map reading that the amount or importance of information in a map component influences the distribution of attention (selective aspect), as measured by the number of fixations, whereas the complexity of the information influences the amount of attention (intensive aspect), as measured by the duration of fixations.

Experiment II: Effects of Experience

Map reading is a skill, and practice is required in order to extract meaning from a map in an efficient manner. Most people have had some experience with road maps and thematic maps but far fewer have had much exposure to topographic maps, in which the elevation of the land is represented. The range of experience with topographic maps is wide, from those who have rarely seen a topographic map to those who use them daily.

Previous research with other visual tasks has shown the eye movement patterns of experienced and inexperienced viewers to be different. For example, Gould (1969) reported the fixation durations of experienced electronic chip inspectors to be shorter than those of inexperienced persons. Cohen and Studach (1977) found shorter fixation durations and longer interfixation distances for experienced automobile drivers. In a related study, Mackworth and Bruner (1970), in comparing the eye movements of children with those of adults in picture viewing, found the durations to be longer and interfixation distances to be shorter for children. Thus, these findings suggest that less experienced viewers have a more difficult time processing the fixated information (longer fixation durations) and have a more restricted useful field of view (shorter interfixation distances).

In this experiment the study of the effects of experience was extended to map reading by examining the eye movement patterns of experienced and inexperienced topographic map users as they searched a series of topographic maps.

Method

Forty-four students participated as subjects in this experiment, 22 of whom were experienced with topographic maps, and 22 of whom were inexperienced. Experienced subjects had at least two courses in which topographic map reading was an essential component of the course.

The maps were two-mile by two-mile sections from United States Geological Survey topographic maps. There were 10 maps, five in which elevation was indicated by contour lines and five in which there was also shading to promote a three-dimensional appearance. No legends, titles, or other descriptive information (such as "river", "mountain", "butte", etc.) appeared on the maps. The only verbal information was the presence of numbers marking the contour lines and occasional "bench marks" (spot height values). Figure 2 displays two of the maps used in the experiment.

The subjects' task was a search task in which they were instructed to find the points of highest and lowest elevation on the maps and, after viewing each map, to mark those points on a 4 x 4 grid facsimile of the map (absolute height task). Also, following each map, subjects were presented with an outline representing the map and containing three straight lines of different orientation (unique for each map). Subjects were instructed to mark which end of each line overlay a higher elevation on the map (relative height task). Prior to the experiment inexperienced subjects were given a brief description of topographic maps, using a three-dimensional model.

The maps were presented for 20 s each and subtended a visual angle of 27 deg vertically and horizontally. Eye movements were monitored using the same apparatus as described for Experiment I.

Results

Number of fixations, fixation duration, and interfixation distance were analyzed as a function of level of experience. Based upon previous research it was expected that for experienced subjects mean durations would be shorter and mean interfixation distance would be longer. Table 6 summarizes the major results. There was no difference in the number of fixations of the experienced and inexperienced subjects. No particular patterns were evident in examining the overall distribution of fixations. In the debriefing session after the experiment many subjects (both experienced and inexperienced) reported scanning the maps for contour

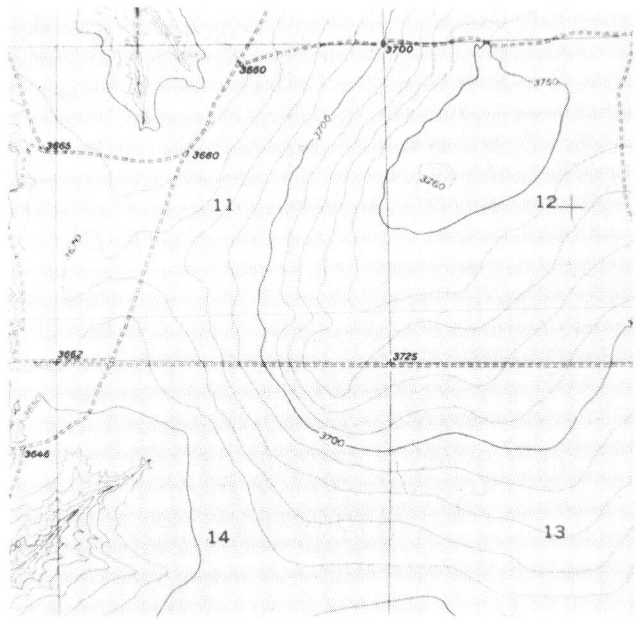

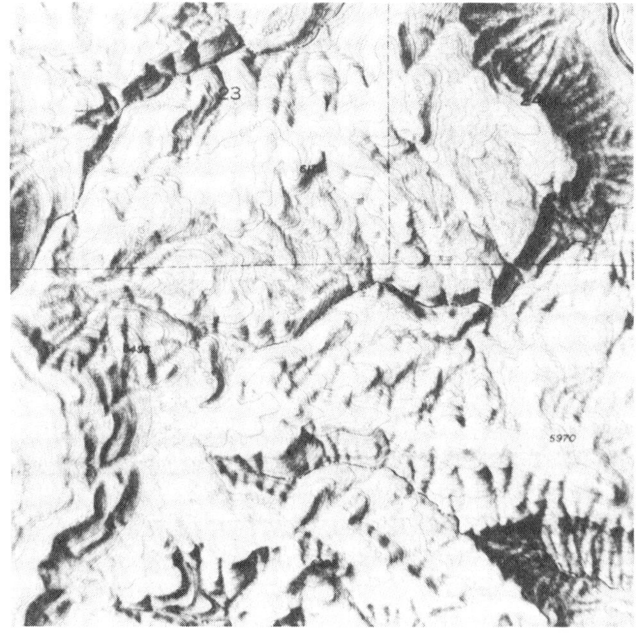

Figure 2. A simple contour map (top) and shaded relief contour map (bottom) used in Experiment II.

Table 6

Mean Number of Fixations, Fixation Duration, Interfixation Distance, and Search Task Performance as a Function of Experience

Measure	Experienced	Inexperienced	t-value
Number of Fixations	43.6	43.2	0.318
Fixation Duration (ms)	345	389	1.788*
Interfixation Distance (deg)	6.2	6.3	0.352
Search Task - total score (%)	58.6	52.2	2.146*
- absolute height (%)	32.2	26.8	1.623
- relative height (%)	76.2	69.1	2.031*

*significant at .05 level, one-tailed, df = 42.

values and bench mark values. Other, more idiosyncratic strategies were reported, such as starting in the middle and working outward in a circular pattern.

There is modest evidence that the experienced subjects distributed more of their fixations to the areas of the maps containing the highest and lowest points. The maps were divided into 16 equal-sized regions, squares roughly 7 deg to a side, and the regions in which the highest and lowest points fell were identified (this grid was the same one that was used in the subjects' determination of the highest and lowest points). The percent of fixations falling within those regions was computed for each map and compared for experienced and inexperienced subjects. Experienced subjects fixated the critical regions 16.5% of the time and inexperienced subjects fixated them 14.2% of the time. The value for experienced subjects was significantly different from what would be expected by chance (12.5%), $t(9) = 2.664$, $p < .05$, but the value for inexperienced subjects was not, $t(9) = 1.749$, $p > .05$. In addition, the difference between the two groups of subjects was not significant, $t(9) = 1.779$, $p > .05$.

Results for fixation duration conformed to expectation. Inexperienced subjects looked 44 ms longer, on the average, during each fixation than experienced subjects.

Interfixation distances for experienced and inexperienced subjects were virtually identical. This failure to find a difference is perhaps best explained by many subjects' reported strategy, described earlier, of fixating the contour values and bench mark values. Such a strategy could limit maximum use of a wider useful field of view. There was evidence, however, that longer saccades were related to better comprehension of the maps, regardless of level of experience. There was a significant correlation between interfixation distance and total search performance, $r(42) = 0.306$, $p < .05$. Subjects who made longer saccades, presumably making use of a wider useful field of view, identified the absolute and relative heights in the maps better.

Performance on the search task indicated that experienced subjects were better than inexperienced subjects in determining elevations, especially for the relative height part of the task.

Discussion

Experience in topographic map reading was related to the manner in which the maps were scanned and the ability to comprehend the maps. The distribution of attention, as measured by the location and number of fixations, was only slightly related to experience. Experienced subjects tended to focus their gaze on the areas of the maps containing the highest and lowest elevations more than inexperienced subjects did. There were no differences in the total number of fixations. The nature of the task almost certainly influenced this measure. Subjects needed to examine the entire map carefully in order to do well, and because of the absolute height portion of the task, subjects needed to look at numbers in order to make comparisons across the surface of the map. Adoption of this kind of strategy would mask any differences in the allocation of fixations that might otherwise be evident.

The differences in fixation duration were most clearly anticipated from the literature. Experienced subjects required less time to process the fixated information and, perhaps, to determine the location of the next fixation. This is consistent with a view of attention as schema-directed processing (Neisser, 1976) in which experience results in a more complete and rapidly constructed schema of the map. Experienced subjects required less time during each fixation because the information was congruent with the anticipations generated by the schema and thus more easily integrated into the evolving schema.

The failure to find differences in interfixation distance, as mentioned earlier, could mean that there were no differences in useful field of view as a function of experience. Since the task seemed to promote a rather systematic examination of the numerical values on the maps, such a conclusion is not yet warranted. The correlation analysis revealed a significant relationship between interfixation distance and performance regardless of experience, which suggests that useful field of view is in fact an indicator of ability to comprehend the maps. In this experiment, though, the compelling nature of the strategy to fixate numerical height values transcended any differences due to experience.

The task performance differences justify the criteria for selecting the subjects. The fact that differences were greater for the relative height portion of the task suggests that the experienced subjects had a better overall conceptualization (schema) of the map (remember that for that portion of the task subjects did not know until <u>after</u> they viewed the map about which areas of the map they would have to make relative elevation judgments).

In general, the results of this experiment support the findings of the first experiment. The allocation of attention was apparently to areas on the maps providing most information for successful performance of the task. Yarbus (1967) and Antes (1973,1974) have shown that what viewers perceive to be informative and consequently what they attend to depends greatly upon task demands. In this task, attention to the numerical height values was required for successful task performance, and subjects indeed reported concentrating on these numbers. In addition there was a tendency to fixate regions containing the highest and lowest elevations.

The duration of fixations in the first experiment depended on complexity. In this experiment duration depended on experience. The first experiment involved a characteristic of the stimulus, the second a characteristic of the subject. Of course, complexity of a stimulus depends upon the ability of the observer to comprehend it. Experienced subjects understood the maps better (their task performance provides good evidence for this) and the information contained in the maps seemed less complex than the same information appeared to inexperienced subjects. Thus complexity was a major influence on fixation duration in both experiments.

Conclusions

This paper began with the observation that very little research has investigated eye movements in map reading. The scant literature that is available comes from the field of cartography and that research seems to support the general view that is evident in picture viewing, reading, and other visual activities that attention is directed by a search for meaning. The findings reported here are entirely consistent with such a view and more specifically suggest that the selective aspect of attention is influenced primarily by the informativeness of the various regions of the stimulus and the intensive aspect of attention is influenced mainly by the complexity of the different regions. In addition, the results suggest that neither informativeness nor complexity can be defined objectively because they depend importantly on characteristics of the subject such as what the task is perceived to be and the expertise the subject brings to the task.

We certainly do not contend that the uniqueness of maps has been fully explored here. There are many kinds of maps and many aspect of map reading and much more research is needed. We believe that the major benefits in map reading research will accrue in addressing applied questions. This research alone has suggested that future research may help improve map design and facilitate map communication. The differences observed as a function of experience could lead to investigations of training topographic map reading. We encourage such research as a fruitful subject of inquiry.

References

Antes, J. R. (1974). Eye fixations as a function of informativeness (Doctoral dissertation, Iowa State University, 1973). Dissertation Abstracts International, 34, 3515B.

Antes, J. R. (1974). The time course of picture viewing. Journal of Experimental Psychology, 103, 62-70.

Antes, J. R. & Penland, J. G. (1981). Picture context effects on eye movement patterns. In D. F. Fisher, R. A. Monty, & J. W. Senders (Eds.), Eye movements: Cognition and visual perception (pp. 157-170). Hillsdale, NJ: Erlbaum.

Buswell, G. T. (1935). How people look at pictures. Chicago: University of Chicago Press.

Cohen, A. S., & Studach, H. (1977). Eye movements while driving cars around curves. Perceptual and Motor Skills, 44, 683-689.

Dobson, M. W. (1979). The influence of map information on fixation location. The American Cartographer, 6, 51-66.

Gould, J. D. (1969). Eye movements during visual search (IBM Technical Report No. RC 2680). Yorktown Heights, NY: IBM Thomas J. Watson Research Center.

Just, M. A., & Carpenter, P. A. (1980). A theory of reading: From eye fixations to comprehension. Psychological Review, 87, 329-354.

Kliegl, R., & Olson, R. K. (1981). Reduction and calibration of eye monitor data. Behavior Research Methods and Instrumentation, 13, 107-111.

Loftus, G. R. (1972). Eye fixations and recognition memory for pictures. Cognitive Psychology, 3, 525-551.

Mackworth, N. H. (1976). Stimulus density limits the useful field of view. In R. A. Monty & J. W. Senders (Eds.), Eye movements and psychological processes (pp. 307-321). Hillsdale, NJ: Erlbaum.

Mackworth, N.H., & Bruner, J. S. (1970). How adults and children search and recognize pictures. Human Development, 13, 149-177.

Mackworth, N. H., & Morandi, A. J. (1967). The gaze selects informative details within pictures. Perception & Psychophysics, 2, 547-552.

Neisser, U. (1976). Cognition and reality. San Francisco: Freeman.

Parker, R. E. (1978). Picture processing during recognition. Journal of Experimental Psychology: Human Perception and Performance, 4, 284-293.

Robinson, A., Sale, R., & Morrison, J. (1978). Elements of cartography (4th ed.). New York: Wiley.

Russo, J. E. (1978). Adaptation of cognitive processes to the eye movement system. In J. W. Senders, D. F. Fisher, & R. A. Monty (Eds.), Eye movements and the higher psychological functions (pp. 89-109). Hillsdale, NJ: Erlbaum.

Steinke, T. R. (1975). The optimal thematic map reading procedure: Some clues provided by eye movement recordings. Proceedings of the International Symposium on Computer-Assisted Cartography (Auto-Carto II), 2, 214-223.

Yarbus, A. L. (1967). Eye movements and vision. New York: Plenum Press.

Eye Movements and Human Information Processing
R. Groner, G.W. McConkie and C. Menz (eds.)

ATTENTION SHIFTS IN PARTIALLY REDUNDANT INFORMATION SITUATIONS

Géry d'Ydewalle, Patrick Muylle and Johan Van Rensbergen
Department of Psychology
University of Leuven/Louvain
B-3000 Leuven
Belgium

Part I gives a general introduction to studies on attention in situations where considerable information is provided simultaneously. The usefulness of analyzing information processing of TV materials is outlined in Part II. It is argued that providing subtitles of a known language from a movie with a partially unknown language provides one track of information more in the situation in addition to the visual image and the spoken sounds. The question arises of how subjects divide their attention among the available information sources. An overview of previous studies (Part III) allows us to specify the main issues of our own investigation as reported in Part IV. Our data are discussed in Part V in terms of the interactive perceptual cycle proposed by Neisser (1976).

PART I - A SHORT SURVEY OF THEORIES ON ATTENTION:

According to Broadbent (1958), a filter mechanism allows only one message at a time to pass from sensory analyses into the attention system. The attention system is required in order to grasp content, context, or meaning. Moreover, switching attention from one sensory input into another takes time. Treisman (1968) and others have modified considerably Broadbent's model to cover findings suggesting that some materials from unattended channels are understood. This line of thought suggests that information in unattended channels is severely attenuated but not excluded for further analyses.

The "divided" attention studies of Broadbent and Treisman emphasized primarily the serial nature of the human information processing system. Neisser (1967) also claims that, while the preattentive stage allows us to process simultaneously separate sensations, "focal" attention is serial: Only one subject can be attended to at any given moment, and each attentive act takes time. This model of the serial nature of attention has been challenged. Schneider and Shiffrin (1977), and Shiffrin and Schneider (1977), for example, have convincingly shown that parallel-processing from multiple external stimuli to meaningful content and context is possible to the extent that automatic-parallel processes for the appropriate multiple inputs are well learned. In the multiple-resource allocation theory (Gopher et al., 1982; Navon & Gopher, 1979; 1980), the human information processing system incorporates a number of mechanisms, each having its own capacity. Those capacities can at any given moment be allocated among several processes. Processing and storage both consume available capacity and activities. They do not necessarily compete for the same resources. This approach gives much more flexibility in the division of attention. Resources can be allocated to all the activities, as long as the total demand on resources does not exceed what is available.

PART II - AUDIOVISUAL PRESENTATION AS A PARTIALLY REDUNDANT INFORMATION SITUATION:

Small countries import a large number of TV programmes from abroad. The imported programmes are generally either dubbed or subtitled in the local language. Although the debate between dubbing and subtitling has been settled by considerations of speed and cost, audience preference has not been studied systematically in the various countries. While almost of all our second-year psychology students (98 percent) preferred subtitling, virtually all foreign films in Belgium are subtitled by the local TV networks. In other countries, such as France, dubbing is more common and it is not impossible that the greater use of one or another technique will change audience preferences. When traveling abroad, it is amusing for Belgians to hear Charles Bronson speaking "fluent" French or German.

If we restrict our discussion now to watching behavior with subtitled movies, it is important to realize that there are at least three different input channels: The visual image, the audio channel, and the text lines. The audio channel contains the spoken language of the actors in addition to special sound effects and background music. The text lines of the subtitle should, ideally, be completely redundant with the information of the audio channel. Most imported programmes are English and French, two languages which are fairly well known by the Dutch-speaking people of Belgium. Accordingly, when focusing the subtitle, a considerable amount of the foreign language is most likely processed by the subjects. Anecdotal evidence indicates that translation errors are often perceived.

We should also not forget that the visual image (not including the subtitle) and the sequence of events in the movie provide abundant information which makes sometimes either understanding the spoken language or reading the subtitle superfluous. Expectations about what will be said play a major effect in comprehending the structure of a story. Moreover, it has been claimed that people unconsciously lipread to a certain extent.

The discussion on attention in Part I raises important issues for research in audiovisual broadcasts. Some people consider the implications from the earlier studies of Broadbent, Treisman, and Neisser as straightforward: At any given time, only one among the audio and visual inputs is fully analyzed. Moreover, it should take time to switch inputs. If one accepts some parallel processing or multiple-resource allocations, more flexibility within the human system is likely to occur. However, research on attention has mainly been focused on simple stimulus presentations with no information redundancy between the input channels. As pointed out above, there is considerable information overlap in film and TV presentations. As most film and TV research does not address attention and processing issues, the main purpose of our studies was to look at the dynamics of attention in this complex information situation.

In order to simplify the research situation, our first study was directed to the viewing time spent on the visual image (excluding the subtitle area) or the subtitle area of the screen (when a subtitle is presented). Considerable research on eye movements in text processing is available (Rayner, 1983). If reading behavior occurs in the subtitle, we also wanted to investigate the positive or negative effects of the same information from the other input channels on reading behavior.

PART III - A REVIEW OF SOME STUDIES ON SUBTITLES:

Surprisingly, little research is available on subtitles. The first studies were mainly concerned with improving television programmes for deaf people and people hard of hearing. An opinion research with normal, deaf and hard of hearing in the Netherlands (NOS Report, 1977) revealed little difference between the three groups in understanding by lipreading what someone is saying during a conversation, with 23 % reporting that they could understand simply by lipreading. This percentage dropped to three when applied to understanding the News. The three groups were quite satisfied with the quality of the subtitles in terms of the presentation duration of the subtitle, their readability and elaboration.

Baker (1981) published guidelines for the subtitling of television programmes for the deaf and hard of hearing. The guidelines are based on the results of analysis of questionnaires and discussions. In this research, eye-movement apparatus seems to have been used on a small scale (as reported in Muylaerts et al., 1983), although the data were not reported.

Systematic age differences have been obtained by Tonla Briquet (1979) in Belgium: Older people report that they have insufficient time to read the subtitles and find the readability not sufficient.

With the help of an eye-movement camera, Schyller (1981) studied how Swedish children scan a subtitled movie and how the eye movements of good and poor readers might differ. In her experiment, there was NO sound track. Good readers scanned the subtitle making fewer fixations than poor readers. Good readers also focused more briefly on the subtitle than did the poor readers.

In many countries, roughly the same rules of thumb are used for timing the subtitles. Two lines together, each with a maximum of 32 characters and spaces, can be used one at a time. If there are two lines x 32 characters and spaces on one subtitle, it is displayed for six seconds. Shorter subtitles are time-scheduled according to this rule (six-second rule). The Dutch-speaking television network of Belgium (BRT), in collaboration with Open University in England, carried out a first pilot study on the six-second rule (Muylaert et al., 1983). Subtitles on a "Dallas" extract were especially constructed in order to investigate variations in eye-movement patterns as a function of the use of one versus two lines, the occurrence of unusual breaks between two lines or between two successive subtitles, and more importantly, as a function of deviations from the six-second rule (shorter and longer presentations). Considerable differences were obtained but detailed analyses on the data were not possible due to technical limitations. For our purposes, it is important to note that the percentage of time spent reading as a function of the projection time of the subtitle is longer with shorter presentations and shorter with longer presentations (the difference is in both cases significant).

PART IV - PRESENTATION TIME OF THE SUBTITLES:

Nobody seems to know how the six-second rule was arrived at. Psychologically, it is at least surprising that presentation time is defined by the number of characters and spaces in the subtitle, especially if reading behavior does occur. The available literature on eye fixation suggests that one reads words in such a situation and that fixation time and its sequence are shaped by the content of the words in the subtitle, and not by an arbitrary string of characters and spaces. Our study was set up in order to describe the eye-movement patterns and attention shifting between the visual image and the subtitle as a function of the six-second rule and some deviations. Three independent variables were included in the study providing an experiment with a 3 x 2 x 3 factorial design. There were all within-subjects variables. The first factor included the use of the six-, four- and eight-second rules. Factor II involved subtitles using either one or two text lines. As the content of the selected movie (ten minutes from a German series "Derrick") could be partitioned in three main parts, the division was also included in analyzing the eye-movement patterns. The equipment, which registered the eye movements in an adjacent room, was based on the pupil-center corneal-reflection method, and provided a registration sampling of 50 Hertz (a sampling every 20 milliseconds). A head-tracking mirror system gave the subject considerable freedom to seat in a relaxed way in front of a regular TV screen (250 cm distance). The data were collected on an on-line PDP-11 computer for further analyses. A videorecording of the eye fixations on the visual scene was also available.

The proportion of missing values correlated with the lack of reliability in calibrating the Y-values ($r = -0.38$) but not so much with the calibration reliability of the X-values ($r = -0.11$). This is rather critical as the division between the visual image and the subtitled area is primarily a function of the Y-values. Accordingly, an ANOVA was applied on the proportion of missing values as a function of our three independent variables. Except one higher-order interaction, no significant F-values were obtained: There is no relationship between our experimental manipulations and the proportion of missing values.

The proportion of time spent in the subtitled area as a function of the projection time of the subtitle decreases linearly as a function of the four- (28 %), six- (23 %) and eight-second (21 %) rules: $F(2, 16) = 3.52$, $p<.05$. This pattern is in agreement with the findings from the BRT study. One also stays longer on a two line of text (28 %) than on a one line (20 %): $F(1, 8) = 5.45$, $p<.05$. There is here one apparent contradiction. With the eight-second rule, more time is available and the subject spends (proportionally) less time in the subtitle. But there is also more time available with two lines, and still the subject typically spends (proportionally) more time on the subtitle with two lines.

In the above analysis, viewing time was compared as a function of projection time of the subtitle. We also investigated viewing time without the transformation in percentage as a function of the four-, six- and eight-second rule. This time, the data show a linear increase as a function of the four-, six-, and eight-second rule: $F(2, 16) = 4.12$, $p<.05$. Also, the eyes fixate more on the subtitle with two lines than with one line: $F(1, 8) = 5.04$, $p<.05$. It seems that with more projection time (according to the time rule and one vs. two lines), the subjects look longer at the subtitle.

Regression analyses were carried out on the viewing time of the subtitle as a function of the number of words and as a function of characters and spaces in the subtitle. The analyses were carried out separately according to the three time-rules and the one vs. two line conditions. Nothing significant emerged from the ANOVAs on the intercepts and slopes of all regression equations.

We obtained an average slope of 124 milliseconds per word. This value is extremely low as eye fixations of adults in text reading are typically much longer (at least above 150 milliseconds). We had some serious doubts about the presence of typical reading behavior in the subtitle. Reading behavior involves as a rule a sequence of eye fixations on words which are preceded and followed by saccadic movements through the text. Further frame-by-frame analysis of the videorecording suggests the following pattern of behavior. Subjects do not read the subtitle. They first look at the visual image, jump quite accurately to the keywords of the subtitle (i.e., the words conveying the most important parts of the conversation) and then go back to the visual image. If the subtitle is still available, they occasionally jump back to the subtitle for more processing of the text. This pattern could explain why there is more time spent on the subtitles with longer presentation time and with two lines. One key issue here concerns what is picked up in peripheral vision. In order to account for the accurate saccadic eye movements from the visual image to the keywords of the subtitle, one has to assume that some processing of the subtitle is possible while looking at the visual image. There may be superficial processing of the subtitles by means of peripheral vision (e.g., by keeping track of the orthographic properties of the words). There is some literature available that the orthographic lay-out of characters in a letter string within a word may help to get quick access to the meaning of the words and the content of the text (Massaro et al., 1980). Understanding parts of the audio channel and implicit expectations of the story structure could also facilitate the efficient processing of simple keywords of the subtitle.

PART V - THE INTERACTIVE PERCEPTUAL CYCLE:

The TV screen was 250 cm from the subject's eyes. At the eye, the screen subtended about 12 deg of visual angle in the horizontal plane and 9 deg in the vertical plane. The area from which information is extracted during a fixation has been considered to be small, possibly equated with the fovea (1 or two degrees). However, it is well known that to some extent people are able to extract a variety of types of information from a much wider area in peripheral vision. The accuracy of the saccadic jump in our experiment suggests that the processing area is much larger than just the fovea and includes substantial amounts of the periphery. Although acuity of the periphery is poorer than that of the fovea, information in the periphery is encoded and could particularly be sufficient in our situation. The expectations one has for the information is likely to be well developed: The information about the events in the movie are at any particular moment provided by the visual image, the audio channel, and the subtitle, and the preceding sequence already contained a number of cues about what will follow.

The encoding of information from the movie revolves around an interactive perceptual cycle (Neisser, 1976; Parker, 1978) in which information in the periphery plays an important role. First, one extracts information from a wide area of the visual field, taking into account information already available in memory and the information from the audio channel which could be understood. This set of information is compared with the expectations one has. The third process guides the selection of areas for direct fixation. Considering the size of the screen and its distance from the subject, the acuity of the periphery is probably adequate for much normal encoding of the subtitle. The full resolving power of the fovea is needed when a word in the subtitle is particularly important to understand what is going on. However, if the subtitle stays for a long time and nothing quite new appears on the visual image, reading behavior will emerge. In fact, many subjects reported that reading behavior was automatically triggered off when the subtitle was given. Our analysis suggests that such reading does not occur at the beginning of the presentation of the subtitle: Only one or two keywords are fixated. The reported experience of reading behavior probably is what happens at the end of longer presentation times.

REFERENCES:

Baker, R. G. (1981). Guidelines for the subtitling of television programmes for the deaf and hard of hearing. Southampton, U.K.: Southampton University.

Broadbent, D. E. (1958). Perception and communication. Oxford: Pergamon press.

Gopher, D., Brickner, M., & Navon, D. (1982). Different difficulty manipulations interact differently with task emphasis: Evidence for multiple resources. Journal of Experimental Psychology: Human Perception and Performance, 8, 146-157.

Massaro, D. W., Taylor, G. A., Venezky, R. L., Jastremski, J. E., & Lukas, P. A. (1980). Letter and word perception. Amsterdam: North Holland.

Muylaert, W., Nootens, J., Poesmans, D., & Pugh, A. K. (1983). Design and utilisation of subtitles on foreign language television programmes. In P. H. Nelde (Ed.), Theorie, Methoden und Modelle der Kontaklinguistik (pp. 201-214). Bonn: Dummler.

Navon, D., & Gopher, D. (1979). On the economy of the human information processing system. Psychological Review, 86, 214-253.

Navon, D., & Gopher, D. (1980). Task difficulty, resources, and dual task performance. In R. S. Nickerson (Ed.), Attention and performance (Vol. 8) (pp. 297-315). Hillsdale, New Jersey: Erlbaum.

Nederlandse Omroep Stichting. (1977). De behoeften van doven en slechthorenden aan ondertiteling van Nederlandstalige televisieprogramma's (Research Rep. No. R77-194). Hilversum, The Netherlands.

Neisser, U. (1967). Cognitive psychology. Englewood Cliffs, New Jersey: Prentice-Hall.

Neisser, U. (1976). Cognition and reality. San Francisco: Freeman.

Parker, R. E. (1978). Picture processing during recognition. Journal of Experimental Psychology: Human Perception and Performance, 4, 284-293.

Rayner, K. (Ed.). (1983). Eye movements in reading: Perceptual and language processes. New York: Academic Press.

Schneider, W., & Shiffrin, R. M. (1977). Controlled and automatic human information processing: I. Detection, search, and attention. Psychological Review, 84, 1-66.

Schyller, I. (1981). Children's eye-movement patterns while watching television - a pilot study. Stockholm: Swedish Broadcasting Corporation.

Shiffrin, R. M., & Schneider, W. (1977). Controlled and automatic human information processing: II. Perceptual learning, automatic attending, and a general theory. Psychological Review, 84, 127-190.

Tonla Briquet, G. (1979). Investigation into the subtitling of film and TV. Unpublished thesis, Hoger Rijksinstituut voor vertalers en tolken, Brussels.

Treisman, A. (1968). Strategies and models of selective attention. Psychological Review, 76, 282-299.

Eye Movements and Human Information Processing
R. Groner, G.W. McConkie and C. Menz (eds.)

EYE SCANNING BEHAVIOR WHEN WORKING ON VIDEO DISPLAY TERMINALS

Helmut T. Zwahlen, Andrea L. Hartmann, Sudhakar L. Rangarajulu and Luis M. Escontrela

Department of Industrial and Systems Engineering

Ohio University, Athens, Ohio 45701, USA

Two exploratory studies were conducted where eye scanning behavior and performance of a total of nine experienced typists working on a video diplay terminal (VDT) was measured, especially as a function of: 1) a data entry and a file maintenance task, 2) the duration of the experiment (three hours each day for three different days or two full working days), and 3) two distinctly different levels of VDT screen viewing time (working with a hard copy or with a split screen). The fairly high visual activities observed reflect the considerable data acquisition and processing demands of the VDT tasks studied. The subjects were capable to perform these tasks successfully using a range of different number of dwells per minute and dwell time combinations, which varied considerably both between and within the subjects.

INTRODUCTION

Surveys of workers who use VDTs indicate that complaints of job-related ocular discomfort and temporary visual difficulties are common (NIOSH, 1981). Although much has been written in the last several years about these problems, there is a lack of research on eye scanning behavior of VDT operators. Such research could help relating objective measures of visual activity in general and screen viewing in particular to subjective complaints of ocular discomfort and to visual difficulties (National Research Council, 1983).

Two consecutive studies (Zwahlen and Escontrela, 1982, and Zwahlen, Hartmann and Rangarajulu, 1984a) investigated eye scanning, pupil diameter, performance, and comfort/ discomfort of VDT operators. In the second study the accommodative state of the eye was also assessed before and after each work session. Both experiments were conducted using longitudinal designs, and the VDT operators were studied while performing meaningful, realistic tasks. Previous papers and reports dealt in particular with the amount of screen viewing involved in different VDT tasks (Zwahlen, 1983), with the effects of very different screen viewing times while working with a hard copy or with a split screen (Zwahlen, Hartmann and Rangarajulu, 1984a), and with the effects of rest breaks in continuous VDT work (Zwahlen, Hartmann and Rangarajulu, 1984b). These two studies also provide a considerable data base on eye scanning behavior of VDT operators, which are presented and discussed in greater depth in this paper.

MATERIAL AND METHOD

Subjects

All nine subjects were females and experienced typists, wearing no glasses or contacts. The three subjects participating in the first study were 20, 24 and 30 years old. The second study investigated six subjects, three of them 18, one (C.S.) 26, one 30 and one (M.T.) 53 years old. All subjects were working under an incentive pay scheme which considered both the key strokes per minute and the errors per file made.

Apparatus

The performance of the subjects (key strokes per minute and errors per file) was continuously monitored by an Apple II computer system which was also driving the Digital VT 100 VDT used in the first study and the IBM 3101 VDT used in the second study. Special lighting and a filter prevented glare. The average distance of the subjects' eyes to the screen was 640 mm in the first study and 786 mm in the second study.

An Applied Science Laboratory 1998 computer controlled eye monitor system (EMS) collected eye scanning and pupil diameter data in a nonobtrusive way. A television camera views the left eye of the subject which is illuminated by a near-infrared illuminator. The resulting picture of the eye is displayed on a TV monitor. A second camera views the scene presented to the subject; on the monitor cross hairs are superimposed on the scene indicating the point of gaze of the subject in real time. By asking the subject to fixate on several preselected calibration points, the eye position can be calibrated and the results can be recorded. The subject's eye rotation (as opposed to eyeball translation resulting from head motion) and consequently the point of fixation is determined by the measurement of the center of the pupil with respect to the center of the corneal reflection. The two features of the eye move together with head motion, but move differentially with eye rotation, hence the difference in their position is indicative of the eye's point of fixation. In this way, the measured eye position is independent of the head position. A third camera and a head tracking mirror allow the system to tolerate limited head motion and to continue the measurement without the necessity of recalibration. Every 1/60 of a second eye movement data as well as the pupil diameter are recorded. The precision of the eye position data is about 1 degree.

Experimental Design and Procedure

The first study investigated each of the three subjects on three different days for three hours each day using a hard copy to screen data presentation mode.

The second study investigated each of the six subjects during two full working days using two different data presentation modes: two half day sessions with a hard copy and two half day sessions with a split screen, where the information which was otherwise displayed on the hard copy was displayed on the right side of the screen area.

The same two tasks were used in both studies: in the data entry task the information had to be keyed in according to an original file, in the file maintenance task the subjects had to find errors on the screen (almost every line had at least one) and correct the whole line according to an original file. The files consisted of names for chemical compounds, stock numbers with 10 characters (e.g. 5VNYJG5CO2), adresses, phone and bin numbers, prices and eight digit location codes. The subjects typed continuously, alternating between 20 files of the data entry task and 20 files of the file maintenance task.

Eye movement and pupil diameter data were usually recorded for each of the two tasks for a ten minute period during each hour in the first study and during each set of twenty files keyed in in the second study.

RESULTS

Figure 1 provides the eye scanning behavior data of the 3 VDT operators in the first study and of the 6 VDT operators in the second study in a hard copy - screen and a screen - screen data presentation; for each condition the average values for the percentage of viewing time, the number of dwells per minute and the dwell times for different VDT areas are shown separately for the data entry and for the file maintenance task. The corresponding performance data (average key strokes per minute and errors per file) are provided in Figure 2.

Figures 3, 4 and 5 show the average number of dwells per minute at the different working areas (screen, document and keyboard) as a function of the corresponding dwell time for each eye movement data recording period for two subjects. C.S. is the subject with the lowest percentage of keyboard viewing, M.T. is the older subject with the narrowest range of eye scanning behavior.

DISCUSSION OF RESULTS

The nature of these studies was more descriptive and exploratory than hypothesis testing, and therefore only a limited number of statistical tests were performed. Statistical comparisons were done between the results of the first study

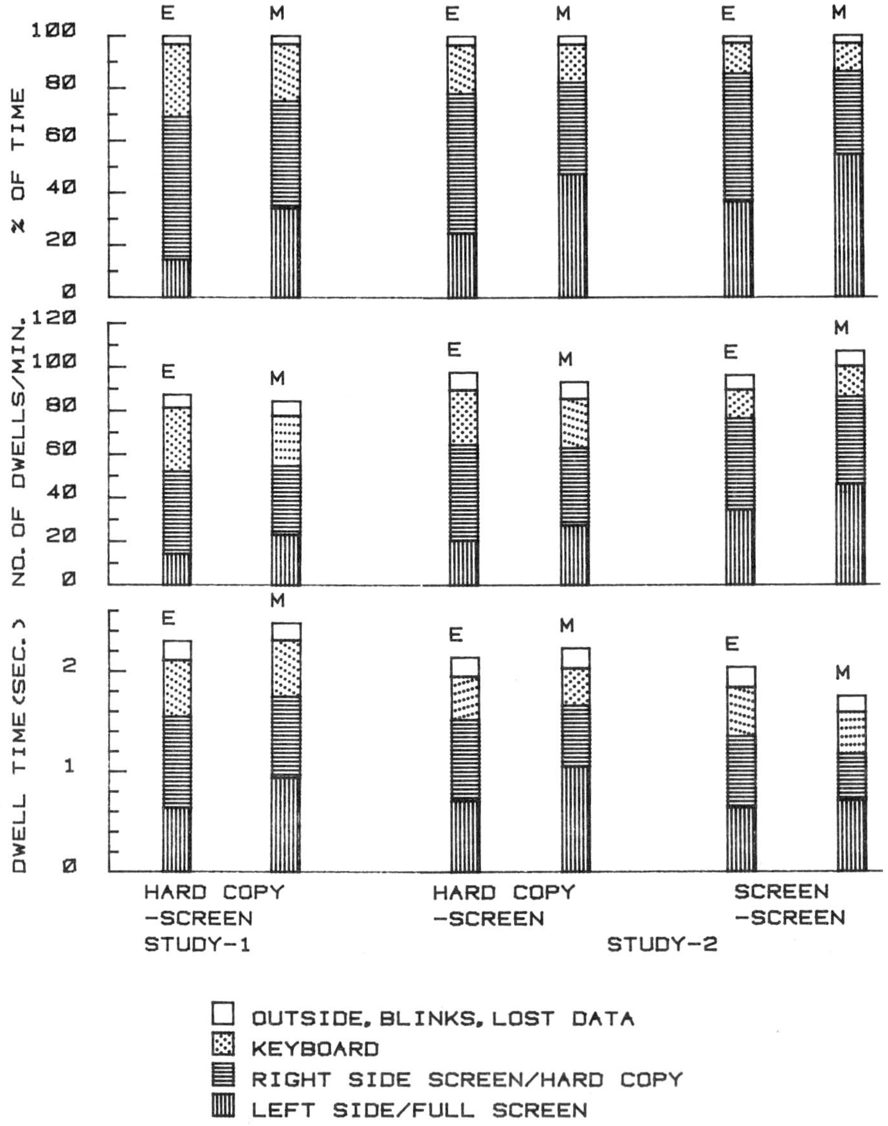

FIG. 1 Eye scanning behavior of 3 VDT operators in the first study in a hard copy - screen data presentation and of 6 VDT operators in the second study in a hard copy - screen and a screen - screen data presentation, for a data entry (E) and a file maintenance (M) task: average values for the percentage of viewing time, for the number of dwells per minute and for the dwell times for different VDT areas.

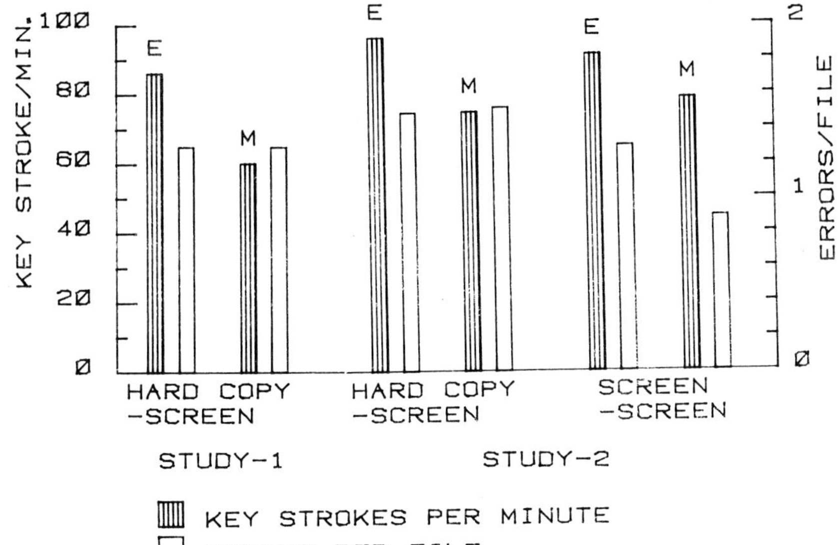

FIG. 2 Performance (average key strokes per minute and errors per file) of 3 VDT operators in the first study in a hard copy - screen data presentation and of 6 VDT operators in the second study in a hard copy - screen and a screen - screen data presentation, for a data entry (E) and a file maintenance (M) task.

and the results obtained for the condition with the same data presentation mode (i.e. hard copy - screen) in the second study using F-tests and t-tests. It should be noted that there are considerable differences between the design of the first study and the design of the hard copy - screen condition in the second study, in particular different work durations, different VDT screens and different keyboards. These differences might have contributed to the differences in eye scanning behavior and/or performance observed between the two studies.

Since in the second study the subjects served as their own controls for the hard copy - screen (HS) and the screen - screen (SS) condition, the differences between the two data presentations were analysed using a pairing of dependent observations t-test. The level of significance was set at 0.05 (two-sided test) for all statistical tests.

Looking at the top section of Figure 1 one can see, that the subjects in the first study (S-1) looked more at the keyboard when compared to the subjects in the second study (S-2) for the hard copy - screen condition (E: S-1 27.6% vs S-2 18.4%, not significant = ns; M: S-1 21.7% vs S-2 14.5%, ns). In the second study it was especially subject C.S. who looked hardly at the keyboard at all (see Figures 3 and 4). However, the percentage of viewing time at the document was almost identical between the two studies for the data entry task (S-1 54.7% vs S-2 53.8%), which indicates that the total amount of time required for the data acquisition from the document was very closely the same for both groups. The file maintenance task required more screen viewing than the data entry task, as the subjects had to correct and detect errors in the files displayed on the screen (S-1: E 14.4% vs M 34.1%; S-2: E 24.6% vs M 47.2%; both highly significant).

In the second study the subjects spent more than twice as much time looking at the screen under the split screen condition, i.e. at the left side of the screen area plus at the original file displayed on the right side of the screen area (E: SS 85.5% vs HC 24.6%; M: SS 86.7% vs HC 47.2%; both highly significant), and they also looked less at the keyboard than they did when working under the hard copy - screen condition (E: SS 11.7% vs HC 18.4%, p .016; M: SS 10.7% vs HC 14.5%, ns).

The average number of dwells per minute are provided in the middle section of Figure 1. The values differ in a similar way between the three conditions (S-1, S-2 HC, S-2 SS) as do the percentages of viewing time. In the first study the subjects used in general a lower number of dwells per minute for the same task (but with a lower performance; see Figure 2) when compared to the subjects in the second study. This difference is statistically significant for the number of dwells per minute at the screen in the file maintenance task (S-1 23.1 vs S-2 27.4, p 0.05).

Furthermore, in the second study the number of dwells per minute at the left side of the screen area were significantly higher for the split screen condition when compared to the number of dwells at the screen for the hard copy - screen condition (E: SS 34.4 vs HC 20.5, p 0.002; M: SS 46.1 vs HC 27.4, p less than 0.001).

There is a natural trade-off between the total number of dwells per minute and the average dwell times a subject can make. The average dwell times are provided in the bottom section of Figure 1. The subjects in the first study had in general slightly shorter dwell times for the screen and considerably longer dwell times for the document and the keyboard when compared to the subjects of the second study, in particular for the file maintenance task (screen: S-1 0.94 sec vs S-2 1.05 sec, ns; document: S-1 0.81 sec vs S-2 0.61 sec, p 0.26; keyboard: S-1 0.56 sec vs S-2 0.37 sec, p 0.002).

The file maintenance task required in all conditions longer

dwell times for the screen area (where errors had to be detected and corrected) when compared to the data entry task (e.g. S-2, HC: M 1.05 sec vs E 0.71 sec, p 0.001).

In the second study the dwell times were consistently shorter for the split screen when compared to the hard copy - screen data presentation; this is statistically significant for the file maintenance task (left side of the screen/ full screen: SS 0.71 sec vs HC 1.05 sec, p 0.009; right side of the screen / hard copy: SS 0.46 sec vs HC 0.61 sec, p 0.007).

As shown in Figure 2, the subjects in the second study typed considerably faster than the subjects in the first study, namely in the data entry task S-2 96.2 vs S-1 86.1 key strokes per minute, and S-2 74.7 vs S-1 60.2 in the file maintenance task. These differences are however statistically not significant at the 0.05 level due to the small group sizes and the large variability between subjects. In the second study the older subject M.T. achieved the lowest performance, i.e. 68.8 key strokes per minute in the data entry task and 51.6 in the file maintenance task..

In the second study the subjects achieved a similar overall performance for both data presentations, as can easily be seen in Figure 2. In the data entry task the key strokes per minute were slightly higher when working with a hard copy (HC 96.2 vs SS 91.6, ns) while the opposite was true in the file maintenance task (HC 74.7 vs SS 78.6, ns). Consistently slightly fewer errors per file were made, when the more compact screen - screen data presentation was used (E: SS 1.3 vs HC 1.5, ns; M: SS 0.9 vs HC 1.5, p 0.04).

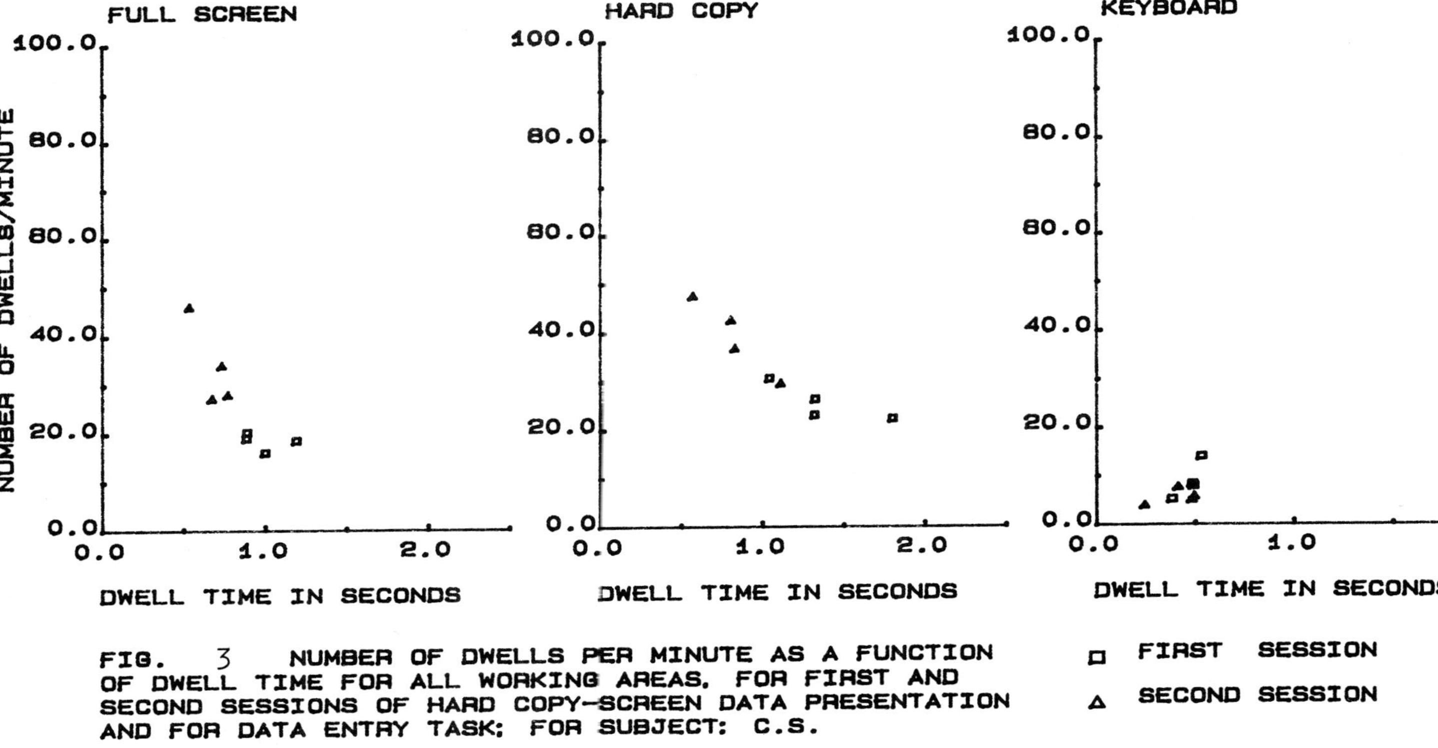

FIG. 3 NUMBER OF DWELLS PER MINUTE AS A FUNCTION OF DWELL TIME FOR ALL WORKING AREAS, FOR FIRST AND SECOND SESSIONS OF HARD COPY–SCREEN DATA PRESENTATION AND FOR DATA ENTRY TASK; FOR SUBJECT: C.S.

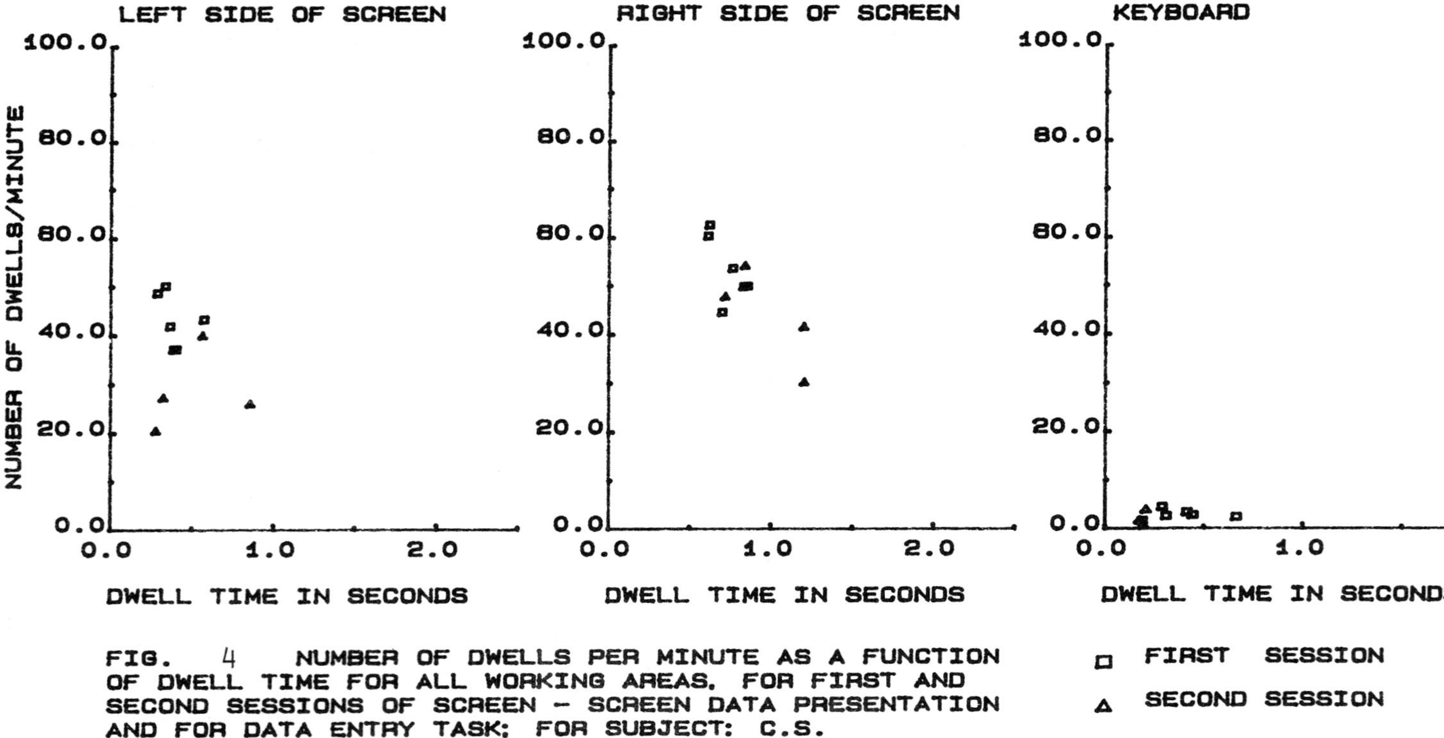

FIG. 4 NUMBER OF DWELLS PER MINUTE AS A FUNCTION OF DWELL TIME FOR ALL WORKING AREAS, FOR FIRST AND SECOND SESSIONS OF SCREEN - SCREEN DATA PRESENTATION AND FOR DATA ENTRY TASK; FOR SUBJECT: C.S.

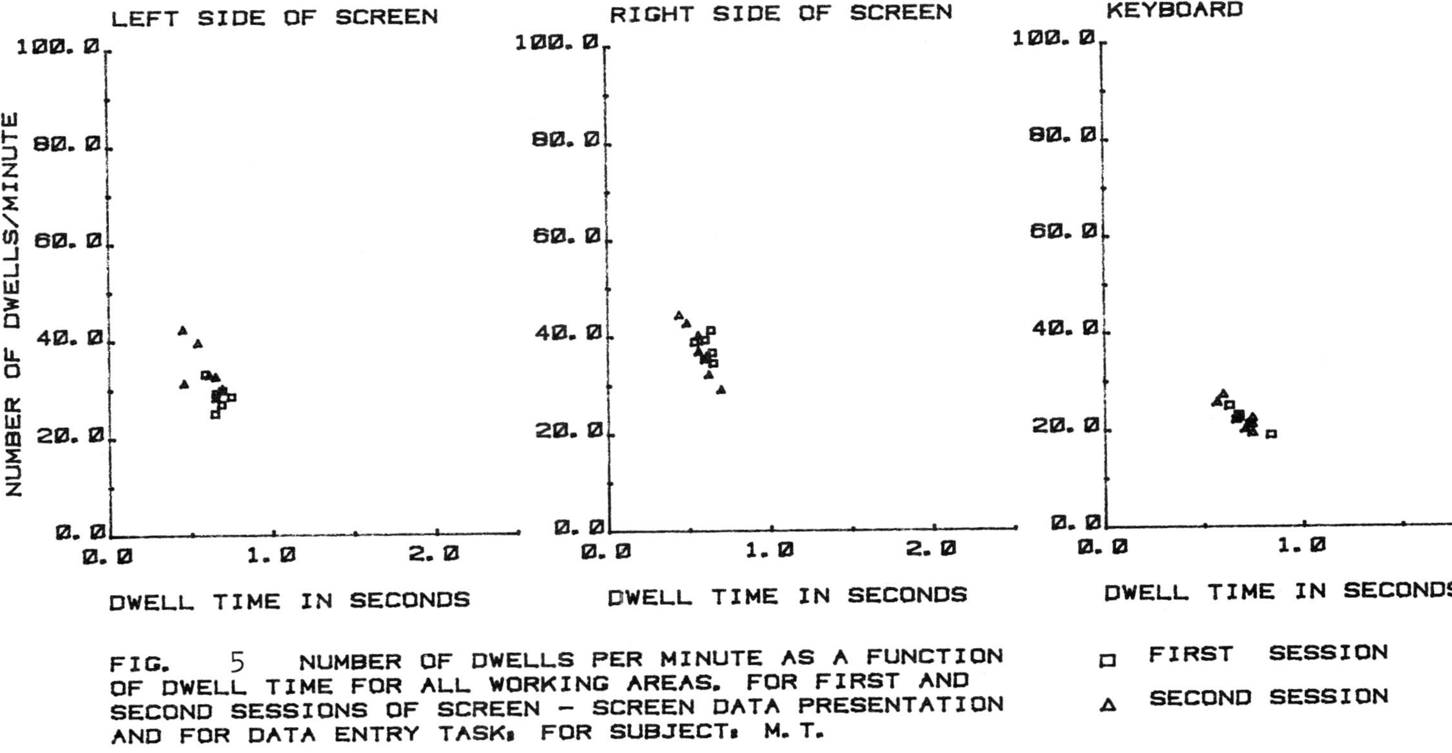

FIG. 5 NUMBER OF DWELLS PER MINUTE AS A FUNCTION OF DWELL TIME FOR ALL WORKING AREAS, FOR FIRST AND SECOND SESSIONS OF SCREEN – SCREEN DATA PRESENTATION AND FOR DATA ENTRY TASK, FOR SUBJECT: M. T.

Looking at the trends of the average eye scanning behavior values as a function of time in the first study (Zwahlen, 1984), it appeared that the subjects preferred to acquire and handle more information per dwell as they became more experienced, i.e. to decrease their numbers of dwells per minute and increase their dwell time. In the second study the opposite trend in eye scanning behavior was observed.
Both trends could be merely due to the high variability of the eye scanning behavior both between and within subjects. Figures 3 and 4 document this for subject C.S. (data entry task, hard copy - screen and the screen - screen data presentation); one can clearly observe three different distributions for the three working areas and that the data acquisition process on the source document and on the screen takes longer than the verification process on the keyboard. On the other hand it is quite obvious that the visual strategies C.S. applies vary considerably over time while she is performing the same task and maintaining a quite stable performance. It appears possible that aging reduces this flexibility; as can be seen in Figure 5, the range of number of dwells per minute and dwell times of the 53 year old subject M.T. was much narrower than the range of subject C.S., in fact considerably narrower than the range of all other eight subjects, who were 18 to 30 years old.

It should be noted that the values in Figures 3, 4 and 5 are averages of the fairly large number of individual dwells made during each of the 10 minute eye movement sampling periods.

The results of both studies show that the subjects are capable to perform the VDT tasks successfully using a fairly wide range of different number of dwells per minute and dwell time combinations. It appears that a subject's visual strategy (dwells per minute and dwell times to different working areas) is only partly determined by the task, the performance, the experience and the data presentation mode, and that the VDT operator has a considerable liberty to select and vary the visual strategy.

CONCLUSIONS

Based on the eye scanning behavior results obtained in these two studies a number of conclusions can be made:

1) The VDT operators looked most of the time at the source document for the data entry task; if the source document is a hard copy, it's visual quality could be as important for the ocular and visual comfort of the operator as the visual quality of the information displayed on the screen.

2) The VDT tasks performed in these studies, which simulate typical clerical VDT tasks in fields such as inventory control, insurance and banking quite well, are characterized by fairly high information acquisition and processing demands, asking for a rather high visual activity.

3) Inspite their experience as typists the subjects made a considerable amount of dwells at the keyboard due to the complex codes they had to key in.

4) Dwell times and dwell time distributions do reflect the amount of information processing involved; the longest dwell

times were required for the document, where the information had to be acquired for the data entry task, and for the screen, where errors had to be detected and corrected for the file maintenance task; short dwell times were sufficient for verifications on the keyboard.

5) The predictive value of a VDT operator's eye scanning behavior for his or her experience and performance is limited due to the capability to maintain a given level of performance with many different visual strategies.

6) It appears that no specific visual strategy (dwells per minute versus dwell times for different VDT areas) is clearly optimal for a given task; many different visual strategies can be used in order to maintain acceptable levels of performance; it is possible that VDT operators might subconciously alleviate the "visual monotony" by varying their visual strategy during the working day.

7) Older subjects might neither be able to acquire the information as fast, nor to handle as much information per dwell as younger subjects, thereby loosing some flexibility in their visual strategies; this could limit their performance and increase their stress in certain VDT tasks. These two studies only involved one older subject; further research is needed to properly address the possible reduced flexibility and the possible limitations of older subjects in VDT work.

8) Considering the lower error rate in the split screen condition when compared to the hard copy - screen condition, the lower dwell times and the higher number of dwells per minute the subjects made while working with the split screen

condition appear to reflect an advantage rather than a disadvantage of this more compact data presentation mode.

9) Looking for more than 80% of the time at the screen when using the split screen as compared to less then 40% when using a hard copy did not result in any other major or consistent changes in eye scanning behavior than the one described in 8) above; the much higher screen viewing time did therefore not result in any disadvantage reflected in a change in the eye scanning behavior, neither for the information processing, nor for the ocular comfort of the VDT operators.

ACKNOWLEDGEMENTS

These studies were partially supported by the National Institute for Occupational Safety and Health. The authors wish to especially acknowledge the contributions of Dr. Olov Ostberg, Visiting Scientist at NIOSH, and Dr. Michael J. Smith, Chief of the Motivational and Stress Research Section, DBBS/NIOSH.

REFERENCES

National Institute for Occupational Safety and Health. Potential Health Hazards of Video Display Terminals. DHHS (NIOSH) Publication No. 81-129, Cincinnati, 1981.

National Research Council. Video Display, Work and Vision. National Academy Press, Washington, D.C., 1983.

Zwahlen, H.T. and Escontrela, L.M. Measurement of VDT operator performance, eye scanning behavior and pupil diameter changes. Ohio University, Dept. of Industr. and Systems Engr. Research Report, prepared for NIOSH, 222 pp., 1982.

Zwahlen, H.T. Measurement of VDT operator performance, eye scanning behavior and pupil diameter changes. In Proceedings of the Human Factors Society 27th Annual Meeting, Norfolk, Virginia, Volume 2, 723-727, 1983.

Zwahlen, H.T. Measurement of visual performance adaptation behavior on video display terminals. In Proceedings of the International Conference on Occupational Ergonomics, Toronto, Canada, Volume 1, 242-246, 1984.

Zwahlen, H.T., Hartmann, A.L., and Rangarajulu, S.L. Video display terminal work with a hard copy - screen and a split screen data presentation. Ohio University, Dept. of Industr. and Systems Engr. Research Report, prepared for NIOSH, 375 pp., 1984a.

Zwahlen, H.T., Hartmann, A.L., and Rangarajulu, S.L. Effects of rest breaks in continuous VDT work on visual and musculoskeletal comfort/ discomfort and on performance. In Salvendy, G., ed.: Human-Computer Interaction, Elsevier Science Publishers B.V., Amsterdam, 315-319, 1984b.

AUTHOR INDEX

D

E

F

G

H

I

J

K

P

Q

R

S

T

U

V

W

Y

Z

SUBJECT INDEX

A

B

J

L

M

N

O

P

R

S

T

COMMITTEES of the XXIIIrd INTERNATIONAL CONGRESS OF PSYCHOLOGY

Honorary Committee

Octavio Rivero Serrano
Rector de la Universidad Nacional Autónoma de México

Guillermo Soberón Acevedo
Secretario de Salubridad y Asistencia

Jésus Reyes Heroles
Secretario de Educación Pública

Antonio Enríquez Savignac
Secretario de Turismo

Héctor Mayagoitia Domínguez
Director General del Consejo Nacional de Ciencia y Tecnología

Jorge Flores Valdés
Subsecretario de Educación Superior e Investigación Científica

Rafael Velasco Fernández
Secretario Ejecutivo de la Asociación de Universidades e Institutos de Enseñanza Superior

Sergio Reyes Luján
Rector de la Universidad Autónoma Metropolitana

Manuel Bravo Jiménez
Rector de la Universidad Pedagógica Nacional

Ernesto Dóminguez Quiroga
Rector de la Universidad Iberoamericana

Juan Manuel Hernández Amenavar
Rector de la Universidad Anáhuac

Sergio Jara del Río
Director de la Escuela Nacional de Estudios Profesionales Iztacala, U.N.A.M.

Rodolfo Herrera Ricaño
Director de la Escuela Nacional de Estudios Profesionales Zaragoza, U.N.A.M.

Organizing Committee

President of the Congress	Rogelio Díaz-Guerrero
President of the Sociedad Mexicana de Psicologia	Mario Cicero
President of the Organizing Committee	Graciela Rodríguez
Secretary General	Isabel Reyes Lagunes
Treasurer	Anne Marie Brugmann García
Executive Secretaries	Sandra Castañeda
	Javier Urbina

Scientific Committee

Juan José Sánchez-Sosa	Víctor Colotla Espinosa
Laura Hernández-Guzmán	Rolando Díaz-Loving
Wayne Holtzman, Jr.	Jorge Peralta Alvarez
Jorge Palacios Venegas	Joseph Ollivier Cuervo

Finance Committee

Darvelio Castaño Asmitia	Lorenzo Ruiz Bouchot

Communications Committee

Fernando Garcia Cortés	Germán Alvarez Díaz de León

Committee on Cultural and Social Events

Olga Loredo	María Eugenia Díaz
Graziella Zierold	

Exhibit Committee

María Elena Alegría	Esther Contreras de Lehr

Public Relations Committee

Xóchitl Gallegos Bañuelos

Advisers the Organizing Committee	Friedhart Klix *(G.D.R.)*
	Wayne H. Holtzman *(U.S.A.)*
	Darvelio Castaño Asmitia *(México)*

Sponsoring Organizations

International Union of Psychological Science (I.U.Psy.S.)
Sociedad Mexicana de Psicología, A.C.
Facultad de Psicología, U.N.A.M.
Escuela Nacional de Estudios Profesionales Iztacala, U.N.A.M.
Escuela Nacional de Estudios Profesionales Zaragoza, U.N.A.M.

Collaborating Psychological Associations

American Psychological Association
German Democratic Republic Psychological Association

INTERNATIONAL UNION OF PSYCHOLOGICAL SCIENCE

Executive Committee 1980-1984

President	F. Klix *(G.D.R.)*
Vice Presidents	M. Rosenzweig *(U.S.A.)*
	T. Tomaszewski *(Poland)*
Treasurer	D. Belanger *(Canada)*
Secretary-General	W. Holtzman *(U.S.A.)*
Deputy Secretary-General	K. Pawlik *(F.R.G.)*

H. Azuma *(Japan)*	B. Lomov *(U.S.S.R.)*
G. de Montmollin *(France)*	D. Sinha *(India)*
R. Díaz-Guerrero *(México)*	A. Summerfield *(Great Britain)*
M.O.A. Durojaiye *(Nigeria)*	R. Taft *(Australia)*
G. d'Ydewalle *(Belgium)*	M. Takala *(Finland)*

Executive Committee 1984-1988

President	W. Holtzman *(U.S.A.)*
Vice-Presidents	R. Díaz-Guerrero (México)
	B. Lomov *(U.S.S.R.)*
Treasurer	D. Belanger *(Canada)*
Secretary-General	K. Pawlik *(F.R.G.)*
Deputy Secretary-General	*to be nominated*

H. Azuma *(Japan)*	F. Klix *(G.D.R.)*
G. de Montmollin *(France)*	M. Rosenzweig *(U.S.A.)*
M.O.A. Durojaiye *(Nigeria)*	D. Sinha *(India)*
G. d'Ydewalle *(Belgium)*	R. Taft *(Australia)*
Q. Jing *(China)*	M. Takala *(Finland)*